Psychiatric Illness

Psychiatric Illness

DIAGNOSIS, MANAGEMENT AND TREATMENT
FOR GENERAL PRACTITIONERS AND STUDENTS

Third Edition

H. Merskey
DM, FRCP(C), FRCPsych

Professor of Psychiatry, University of Western Ontario,
and Director of Education and Research,
London Psychiatric Hospital, London, Ontario

BAILLIÈRE TINDALL · LONDON

A BAILLIÈRE TINDALL book published by
Cassell Ltd,
35 Red Lion Square, London WC1R 4SG

and at Sydney, Auckland, Toronto, Johannesburg

an affiliate of
Macmillan Publishing Co. Inc.
New York

© 1980 Baillière Tindall
a division of Cassell Ltd

First published 1965
Second edition 1974
Third edition   1980

ISBN 0 7020 0790 0

Set by Academic Typesetters, Gerrards Cross.
Printed and bound by Billings and Sons Ltd,
Guildford, London and Worcester

British Library Cataloguing in Publication Data

Merskey, Harold
    Psychiatric illness. - 3rd ed.
    1.   Psychiatry
    I.   Title
    616.8'9   RC454

    ISBN 0-7020-0790-0

To the memory of Erwin Stengel and Lawton Tonge

W. LAWTON TONGE

The partnership which first produced this book was disrupted by the untimely death of Lawton Tonge on 16 September 1976 at the age of 51 years. I feel the loss of my senior colleague and good friend deeply, not only because he had at least an equal share in any of the good features of this book but also for his personal qualities. Lawton was a lively and friendly man with the gentleness of maturity and an outstanding appreciation of the needs of others. Like Erwin Stengel, to whom our first edition owed much in terms of encouragement and advice, Lawton had both an enquiring mind and a natural understanding of human feelings, and these qualities were used to advance the care of patients and knowledge of man. He faced his death with impressive composure and his work in social psychiatry is commemorated in Sheffield by the W. Lawton Tonge Centre for help with stress. It is trite but true to say that he is sadly missed.

Contents

Preface

At the time of the first edition of this book many doctors had qualified with very little training in psychiatry. This lack in medical education was keenly felt by a number of them. It was felt that there was a need not just for a textbook which set out the standard descriptions of illness but for one which enabled them to sort out the muddle of psychological symptoms which many patients seemed to present. In the teaching of medicine there are two main ways in which data can be presented. The first, followed in most textbooks, is to begin with aetiology and pathology where possible, and then to proceed to an account of diseases. The second is to start with symptoms and review their possible causes. The medical student normally undergoes tuition by both these means. He learns about syndromes in the lecture theatre and from his books, and concurrently he meets his patients who tell him about their symptoms. With the help of his teachers he then comes to relate these symptoms to the known facts of pathology and to patterns of illness. In the problems of clinical psychiatry this approach often seems curiously unhelpful. Not only is known organic pathology of less assistance here than in any other branch of medicine but the logic of pathology proves an unreliable guide in unravelling the significance of many psychiatric signs and symptoms. With psychiatric patients the doctor is faced not with a syndrome but with a situation which all too often tends to include himself.

The importance of helping the student or practitioner to cope with these difficulties was made clear by Professor Stengel in his foreword to the first edition. At least 20 per cent of patients in general practice are known to present with psychiatric problems and only a few of them can be referred to the specialist. Every general practitioner must have a working knowledge of psychiatry, and most students are keen to acquire this knowledge. Apart from being important in practice the subject is of central interest in many discussions of human psychology, social relationships and group behaviour. This is not to claim that psychiatry is the key to understanding social problems, but informed discussion of the latter commonly takes account of psychological or psychiatric knowledge, and many in the social sciences look to psychiatry and medicine as an important source both for data and for ideas.

The special purpose of this book was to provide an introduction to the subject through which practitioners and students could resolve some of the problems to which we have referred. There are indeed various excellent standard textbooks, but what seems to be required is one which, besides providing a body of essential technical information, will help the practitioner to investigate different psychiatric problems from the moment they present themselves to him. It sometimes seems as if psychiatric classifications do not fit the patients one meets in practice. An adequate textbook should make clear the principles which underlie this apparent confusion, so that when the doctor is confronted with this situation he can analyse the factors involved with clarity and therapeutic effectiveness. The logic of these enquiries will demand premises very different from those on which the clinical sciences were founded. It will require attention to the basic psychiatric data of feeling and relationship. This is essential if the practitioner is to know, for example, how to proceed when a patient arrives and complains of 'depression' or 'anxiety'—symptoms for which several very different diagnoses may be appropriate—or when parents come to complain that their adolescent son has stopped working.

The aim in this textbook is to remedy that deficiency. In any work there is inevitably some limitation and exclusion; by concentration on problems presented in general practice and outpatient work I have necessarily omitted some topics (such as occupational therapy) and offered only cursory attention to others (such as the indications for leucotomy) which are primarily relevant only to the intramural practice of psychiatry in in-patient units. Other textbooks cover these points thoroughly. What I have attempted to do has been to examine and expound the ways in which the practitioner may manage the psychiatric patient with insight and some hope of success.

Therefore Part I is devoted to the special emotional hazards which await the doctor in face of the demands of an emotionally disturbed patient. In place of the customary systematic exposition of psychiatric disease, Part II proceeds to a discussion of the more common psychological symptoms and the delicate problems of unravelling the differing aetiological strands of which an illness is made up. Clear-cut disease entities are often misleading concepts in this field, and this section of the text is designed to be read as a whole. Special problems such as marital difficulties are dealt with in separate chapters in Part III, while Part IV is devoted to those situations to which the doctor is called in an emergency.

For those who are serving a clinical apprenticeship the book should be of use as a guide to understanding and handling their patients. For those who have had to deal with the many psychological problems of general practice, I hope it will furnish the means for a reappraisal and, if necessary, a reconstruction of their methods of examination and treatment. In both cases I hope it will enable the reader to deal more successfully with some of the problems which may trouble him.

An adequate textbook of psychiatry should give a realistic picture of the way in which doctors and patients relate to each other and of the means by which psychological techniques of treatment, in other words psychotherapy, are used to modify and even cure emotional symptoms. Previous editions were well received, perhaps because in part they seemed to convey how patients are helped by psychological management, yet I still feel considerable hesitation in supposing that we have managed to indicate in a useful way just how this may be done. Moreover, views on the role and use of psychotherapy and other techniques such as behaviour therapy have developed since this book was first drafted. In the present edition I have continued to aim at showing how psychotherapy operates in practical day-to-day consultations. The section on behaviour therapy has also been updated and family therapy and cognitive therapy are discussed for the first time. The sections on drug treatment and on legal matters have been revised to provide information relevant to conditions of practice in Canada and the United States as well as the United Kingdom. Whilst the home of the book is still England alternative North American usages and requirements are also indicated.

As before, there should be sufficient detail to cover the major types of psychological illness adequately for the needs of the general practitioner. In order further to assist the student in reviewing the topics systematically, a supplement (Appendix 2) is provided which sets out in traditional fashion a synopsis of the characteristics of standard psychiatric syndromes. While it remains possible to work these out by use of the Index the tabular arrangement is likely to be convenient for students and practitioners who wish to check common diagnoses. The book is still meant to serve first and foremost as a source of understanding and as a help towards learning the skills of human relationships in medical practice. It will now also, I hope, be of more use to practitioners and students who feel a need for some concrete structure in a superficially intangible subject.

January 1980   H. MERSKEY

Acknowledgements

For reasons of proximity and also because they have special skill and knowledge, Dr M. G. G. Thompson and Dr P. G. R. Patterson have provided the revised version of Chapter 11 on Children and Adolescents, written for the previous edition by Dr R. A. Bugler. Previous editions benefited from helpful comments by Professor E. Wilkes and Dr M. K. Thompson and from the assistance of Dr Wendy Bant in the section on the Treatment of Depression and Hypertension and Dr Gwyneth Sampson on the Premenstrual Syndrome. The benefit continues. Dr Joan Bishop has provided many useful suggestions related to the requirements of North American doctors who may read this book and Dr K. Mesbur provided helpful advice, particularly on the synopsis and on the comments on family therapy. Miss R. deWit advised on drug names.

Part One

Introductory Section

1
The Subject Matter of Psychiatry

Psychiatry is the study and treatment of abnormal behaviour and experience. This is a difficult field to define because opinions differ as to what is abnormal. Moreover, psychiatry is not limited to illness of psychological origin nor to the work of psychiatrists. Many physical illnesses cause psychological change. Other physical illnesses require psychological skill in their management. Many psychological states also must be treated by physicians, surgeons and general practitioners. Anxiety is so common that its treatment is part of the work of every clinician. By contrast certain conditions which are at least partly organic in aetiology tend to be treated by psychiatrists, for example, subnormality, senile dementia, schizophrenia associated with epilepsy. In practice the content of psychiatric work is determined first by the need for extra skill in psychological techniques in diagnosis or treatment. Second, the use of physical measures of treatment, like psychotropic medication, which alter the mental state helps to define the types of illness which are the subject matter of psychiatry. However, there is no fixed line which separates the work of the psychiatrist from that of other doctors in clinical practice and some knowledge of psychiatry is desirable for all clinicians.

A further difficulty is that opinions often differ as to whether a patient should be regarded as morally bad or mentally sick. For practical purposes, however, we can say that the subject matter of psychiatry includes the following:

1. *Organic syndromes* in which the behaviour, experiences or psychological state of the patient are affected by recognizable somatic processes.

Examples of this would be confused states occurring with myxoedema or in senile degeneration of the brain.

2. *Functional psychoses*, that is, illnesses such as schizophrenia or manic-depressive psychosis. In the extreme forms of these illnesses the patient can always be described in lay terms as *insane*. An organic cause for such illnesses is only rarely found, and psychological factors often play a part in the aetiology of these illnesses and are prominent in their clinical syndromes. There is some reason, however, to consider these functional psychoses as likely to be mainly the result of biochemical disturbances. Good results in these disorders are frequently obtained with pharmacological and physical treatments although adequate understanding of the patient's psychological difficulties is essential for the best outcome.

3. *Psychoneuroses and related disturbances.* Psychoneuroses are conditions which sometimes have a formal pattern of psychological symptoms, for example, obsessional neuroses and phobic anxiety states, and in which there is no loss of contact with reality. They are mostly associated, however, with disturbances of personal relationships, whether at the time of the illness or earlier, so that the word *neurotic* naturally becomes extended to include conditions in which such disturbances exist even although a well-defined pattern of compulsion, anxiety or hysteria may not be evident. Examples of this type of problem occur in patients with so-called neurotic depression and in some marital conflicts.

4. *Personality disorders.* These are states in which, again, the patient is not insane in the sense used for schizophrenic illnesses but in which he may indulge repeatedly in forms of behaviour which are harmful to himself or others. In this group it is usual to include the entity of psychopathic (in North America, sociopathic) personality to which the fore-

going particularly applies and which indeed has been described legally in Britain as characterized by abnormally aggressive or seriously irresponsible behaviour. It is also possible to include deviations of sexual behaviour in this group, like fetishism, and other social deviations such as alcoholism. These conditions are characterized by an unexpected failure to learn or change as a result of experience. This failure is not necessarily absolute. Some people with personality disorders can change somewhat either in response to a favourable environment which meets their emotional needs or in response to psychotherapy. In North America the expression 'character disorders' is often preferred for people who appear to have a personality variant which might be amenable to psychotherapy.

5. *Psychosomatic disturbances*, that is, those in which emotional problems or psychological illness influence the course of physical illness. These include some cases of asthma which may be made worse by anxiety, or hypertension made worse by anger or frustration. They may also include illnesses precipitated by emotional stress, for example migraine. It used to be thought that pathological change, for example peptic ulcer, could be induced by continuous emotional tension but this view, whilst not abandoned, is held with more caution today and the tendency is to talk of 'a psychosomatic approach' to illness, rather than of psychological causation. Psychosomatic conditions still imply a pathophysiological disturbance. They do not include such states as hysterical paralysis in which the bodily disturbance is a psychological, rather than a physiological, consequence of the emotional state. These are best described as psychological rather than psychosomatic.

6. *Reactions to physical illness*. Conversely, physical illness may be an important cause of emotional reactions. These are often accurately but cumbersomely called somatopsychic reactions, although that term also includes a suggestion of somatic compliance in which a particular organ is held to be vulnerable to psychological effects. The psychological illness promoting physical illness or resulting from it is often regarded in North America as part of the work of the 'liaison psychiatrist', a term occasionally used in Britain. The

traditional appointments of physicians in psychological medicine to some British teaching hospitals used to provide for the same function and in some places still do.

7. *Subnormality of intelligence*, whether or not the result of detectable organic cause. In North America subnormality is called mental retardation.

The common factor in nearly all these conditions is some disturbance of the individual either in his relationship to the external physical world or to his fellows or in his experiences or behaviour. The presence of such disturbances does not necessarily mean that the case must be regarded as a psychiatric one. Disturbances in at least one of these categories will be found in every patient who has noticed something wrong with himself—even if it is a lump which he brings to the surgeon. But whenever the behaviour of the patient differs greatly from that of other people or his experiences appear psychologically abnormal it is usual for the psychiatrist to be consulted. And in general practice where the condition is not such as to warrant referral to a specialist it is likely that in these cases the doctor will regard himself as dealing with a psychiatric problem.

With this subject matter it appears that the doctor's problem is twofold. First, whilst it is not possible to set hard and fast boundaries to the subject matter, the doctor has to learn to recognize those syndromes and aetiological agents which can usefully be defined. For this purpose, as elsewhere in medicine, he needs to know for what information he should be looking and how to obtain it. Second, in approaching these groups of patients, and especially the neurotic ones, he needs to be able to deal with problems of personal relationships which are peculiarly delicate and for which his standard medical training does not always prepare him. This is particularly important in general practice where it is generally held that at least 20 per cent of consultations are for neurotic or psychosomatic complaints. Chapter 2 is, therefore, mostly devoted to the special difficulties which doctors may have in handling their own relationships with psychiatric patients, particularly the neurotic ones.

2

The Doctor's Problems

Irritation with the patient

Most people who deal with psychiatric patients find many of them extremely difficult. Such patients engender varied feelings like pity, sympathy, amusement, concern, contempt and anger in those whom they encounter. This happens even in the surgery or consulting room. Why it happens is a matter of great interest. As already mentioned psychological illness, especially neurosis, is seen very often in general practice. Since nearly all these patients are convinced that they are ill, and, since many of them present with somatic complaints, the problem is one which the family doctor is forced to try and solve in some way. In analysing this situation we shall discuss, first, the patient who has a bodily complaint (frequently hypochondriacal) and, second, the patient with a frankly psychological symptom or symptoms.

The patient with a bodily complaint

When a patient calls on his doctor for help he generally implies that his own efforts are not enough. He asks his physician to make decisions for him, and he offers to depend upon this medical guidance. When the doctor regards the patient as not responsible for his complaint, or not able to manage it sufficiently well himself, he accepts this dependence with satisfaction even though he may be quite unable to influence the disease significantly for the better. Whether the illness is a recoverable pneumonia or an intractable chronic neurological complaint the doctor is gratified at the trust shown and willingly accepts the responsibility that is put upon him. The doctor believes, correctly, that this is what he has been trained to do.

The doctor becomes dissatisfied, however, when he examines a sane patient with bodily complaints, cannot find a cause for them and does not believe that there is an organic cause. Often he has suspected that this will be the outcome of his examination long before he has finished taking the history. He then commonly says to the patient: 'There is nothing wrong with you.' This is an odd statement since the patient has already found something wrong. Paradoxically, the patient may be grateful for the observation. He is pleased because the interchange of speech, facial expressions and gestures between doctor and patient invariably mean more than the words alone make explicit. The patient has usually implied: 'I have some unusual bodily feelings. I shall be content if you will tell me that they are not important,' and the doctor with very imprecise words has told him that he is not physically diseased. The doctor may also have shown that he is friendly to the patient or sympathizes with him. Often this suffices to allay the anxiety which the patient has felt, and often, too, it leads to the relief of symptoms. Even where a medicine is prescribed it needs little insight to recognize that it is the personal interchange which has 'cured' the individual. Both doctor and patient may also recognize that the patient has been worried because of some change in his personal life. They are aware that the consultation gives the patient an opportunity to turn to some person he may trust and receive support and reassurance even though the actual source of the worry has not been mentioned. Provided that this is an occasional happening and provided that the trusting patient accepts the doctor's conclusions the latter remains content. The patient's demands have been limited and the doctor has been able to satisfy them. The doctor has also been able to function in the role, which he is happy to accept, of a beneficent authority.

A large number of these patients, however, refuse to accept

the statement 'There is nothing wrong with you'. Even if it is put more tactfully there are some who will challenge the doctor's words. They say correctly: 'There must be something wrong, Doctor. I feel so awful.' Others less bold think this but keep their thoughts to themselves. There can be few doctors faced with this situation who have not felt exasperated and the causes of this exasperation must be considered.

We dismiss as unimportant the fact that the doctor's professional opinion has been challenged by someone who may be ignorant of medicine. The patient is concerned with his own case and medical opinion agrees that the most unreasonable person in suffering is entitled to ask for a second opinion if he is sufficiently troubled by his complaint. Most doctors are mature enough to accept this. What they do not accept is that it is justifiable for the patient to persist in his great concern with his symptoms after a more or less thorough physical examination has been completed. This is one cause of their exasperation.

The doctor in these circumstances also has an uneasy suspicion that the patient will not take 'No' for an answer and insists on prolonging an interview which the doctor feels has already served whatever useful purpose it might have had. The doctor comes to the conclusion that the patient wishes to determine how the physician shall act without regard to the latter's own view. He feels the patient is imposing on him even if he is merely asking for extra time and attention. We are only willing to spend spare time with people with whom we are in a friendly or affectionate relationship. It may be that the patient is asking for such a relationship. If so, the doctor does not want to respond in the way the patient wishes and the doctor feels the demand to be unreasonable.

For these several reasons the doctor feels that the patient is making unfair demands. This situation is made worse because it seems to the doctor that the patient is making an attempt at false pretences. The hypochondriacal patient who persists with his complaints does not give up his claim to have an organic illness. Such a claim carries with it the requirement of appropriate treatment, or at least sympathy, and the doctor particularly resents the suggestion that he should sympathize with someone who, while apparently bent on deceiving him, has the impudence to be indignant when his deceitfulness is laid bare. A time when the doctor feels this especially keenly is of course at night when his own proper rest has been disturbed. It is, therefore, particularly interesting and striking that Clyne[15] has found the majority of his night calls to be motivated by anxiety.

Lastly, the doctor is liable to become anxious when faced with these patients. There is sometimes a risk with them that he will be persuaded to recommend unsuitable treatments which may be dangerous or potentially toxic. In so doing he exposes himself to criticism of his professional skill from himself or others at having been tricked by a neurotic. The source of this threat becomes an object for his hostility, and this is the more grievous because it is his unfortunate patient who has asked him for help and towards whom his first feelings were intended to be sympathetic.

If there are any who think that we have painted too gloomy a picture they should listen again while they and their colleagues discuss neurotic patients. We do not exclude from this either ourselves or most other psychiatrists. There can be very few practitioners who are not troubled by these difficulties to some extent. But those who admit the problem are clearly in a much better position to deal with it.

The patient with a psychological complaint

Similar problems to the foregoing also arise with the neurotic patient who explicitly appeals for the treatment of a psychological difficulty. The patient of this type does not offend the doctor by seeming to wear a deceitful mask of organic disease. The doctor is therefore less ready in this case to indulge in moral indignation against his patient for shamming but, because he may consider that the patient should 'pull himself together' and 'help himself', he is still liable to feel that an illegitimate request for help has been made by someone who is not sick. Because he doubts his own ability to deal with this situation and yet has a feeling that it should be within his competence to do so, the doctor becomes uncomfortable. He is asked to take responsibility to cure yet he feels neither properly trained nor equipped. In addition he may suspect that he is being asked to share some personal difficulties of the patient and that this is an unreasonable demand. This makes the doctor either reluctant to sympathize or even indignant, and the indignation is reinforced by the fact that it is his patient, for whom he should feel sympathy, who has put the doctor into this awkward position. As with the hypochondriacal patient, so with the agitated, hysterical or demanding patient, the doctor is subjected to emotions which impair his professional skill. Yet there is no question of deceit—only the problem of coming to terms with the doctor's own response to psychological illness.

The psychotic patient

Similar problems arise with the grossly irrational or insane patient. Fear of such patients is common but experience helps here to give the doctor confidence that he can deal with the situation. It is one, however, in which lay people expect the medically trained to be particularly skilful and where they tend to think that they can see the proof or otherwise of that skill. It has been said that a doctor who fails in such a situation will lose much prestige. We are not unaware of this in handling such patients. Often we see it as a test which puts us on our mettle instead of as a clinical situation needing calm appraisal. In consequence it is not surprising that doctors often share the fear of psychotic patients and the defensive jocularity towards them which is widespread amongst all classes of the population.

Adopting a suitable attitude

Having presented the problem we would say that to us it seems clear that the psychiatric patient and his physician are at cross-purposes. In consequence, the doctor often fails to respond appropriately. It may be that there is no complete solution for the patient's difficulties. But it is at least essential for the doctor to find a way of handling such people which is practical and helpful to them because decisions on their welfare which are taken in a mood of suppressed or repressed hostility are not likely to be good ones; whereas

those decisions which are made with detachment, consideration and care are nearly always worth while. It is for this
reason that the excellent standard advice given to the trainee
in psychiatry is to treat his patients with a neutral sympathetic attitude. Not only does this provide the most effective
means of helping the patient in his difficulties, it also safeguards the physician from making a variety of emotionally
determined mistakes. For example, it helps him to avoid
taking sides when the patient is in conflict with other people.
It is not the doctor's function to be a judge even when both
parties to an argument are present. It is much less his role to
take sides and become involved when, in the nature of the
circumstances, he can know only part of the facts. The doctor's best aim is to be useful to his patient as a guide, helping
the patient to manage his emotional problems. The patient
may have a natural wish to enlist the doctor's support in a
particular role. In principle and in practice such a step has
to be avoided.

Nevertheless, there are certain ways in which we do consider it helpful for the therapist to intervene actively, rather
than continue to be simply a passive listener. However, the
recommendation to take a neutral sympathetic approach is
a precondition which must be satisfied before intervention
can be successful and not dangerous.

More active intervention should not be taken lightly. An
example may illustrate the limits of suitable intervention. If
a patient wishes to change his job the psychiatrist may well
arrange psychological testing of his abilities and make an
appraisal of the man's potential. He will then tell him what
is suitable, perhaps encouraging him quite strongly in seeking
alternative employment. At this point the doctor is using
persuasion. This is a reasonable step but one that must be
consciously recognized and not pushed against the resistance
of a patient. The time when the individual himself is vacil-
lating and wants support is the best moment for such active
intervention.

A more difficult problem arises when the choice is to do
with one of the great events of life: marriage, having a child
or divorce. Specific advice to undertake one of these steps
for the sake of relieving psychological illness is notoriously

unwise. To encourage someone to plan his or her life in a way which yields normal satisfaction is helpful and is sometimes essential. To push him in such a direction is nearly always a mistake. If the patient is already in a situation which is clearly harmful it is justifiable firmly, even warmly, to encourage change. An instance of successful intervention of this type occurred with a girl suffering from epileptic fits. Attractive and of above-average intelligence she had become the mistress of a man who would not marry her. She described him, however, as marvellous. Since the start of the affaire, her fits increased in frequency, because of her state of unhappiness and tension. Firm advice to change her boyfriend was eventually heeded and in a happy relationship with a new man who did indeed marry her, the frequency of her fits was substantially reduced.

The conditions for intervention are rarely, if ever, discussed in psychiatric papers or books. We would suggest that the minimum conditions are as follows: first, it should serve an acceptable personal aim of the individual; second, it should involve no conflict with the proper interests and concern of others; and, last, it must be reasonably attainable rather than a visionary counsel of perfection.

Thus we think that the case of the girl just described met all these criteria for she needed a different relationship, the existing relationship could not continue indefinitely, and, finally, she was more than sufficiently attractive as a person to be able to find a satisfactory partner. By contrast, recommending divorce could rarely be expected to have as much justification.

The disturbance of personal relationships

A disturbance of personal relationships is a cardinal feature of nearly all psychiatric illness. Consideration of this fact will help explain why the physician is liable to encounter this special hazard of emotionally determined mistakes. It has been acknowledged already that certain patterns of disturbed behaviour do occur. It is of value to know about these in order to be able to tackle the therapeutic problems of prescribing the appropriate treatments and resolving the pathological

relationships whenever possible. But the need to define the
disturbed personal relationships is nearly always present, and
this fact provides us with an important further clarification
of the reason why most people find psychiatric patients difficult and why the doctor finds personal difficulties in dealing
with such patients, especially the neurotic ones. With these
patients the doctor has to fulfil a different role from the currently accepted one of curing disease entities, despite the
patient's implied suggestion that this is what is required. His
task is to recognize the sources of different emotions and their
modes of expression and to help modify the effect of these
emotions. Moreover, he has to do this with people whose
emotional relationships are usually faulty in more than one
respect and who, in turning to him for help, may well involve
him actively and personally in their difficulties. Frequently
the relatives of these patients are disturbed as well, they may
indeed be the cause of the patient's trouble, and they, too,
may take the attitude that the doctor has a personal obligation which greatly exceeds his professional one. It is not
surprising, therefore, that in many cases the doctor will
become unhappy at the situation. If our analysis is correct
this will happen whenever the patient makes what are felt
to be undue demands upon the doctor, unless the doctor can
adopt a different point of view. We would again emphasize
that this different point of view must be an attitude of neutral
sympathy. Although intervention is sometimes needed, it is
clear that the moment when the doctor's sympathies are
aroused is the one when he must be most scrupulous in his
detachment.

The emotional reaction to physical illness

If we can define the emotional situation of the patient and
the doctor in relation to his illness we may understand the
patient much better and his management should benefit.
At the least, some of the common criticisms of hospitals and
the medical profession should then become less justified or
less common. Now it has been pointed out that in neurotic
illness there is a disturbance of relationships in which the

patient may seek to involve the doctor. In physical illness the position is somewhat similar even if not quite identical. The patient with a physical illness, whether more or less neurotic than the average, comes to depend upon his doctor in a special way. The patient comes to him for physical help with his own person—something he may not have sought since childhood from anyone except perhaps from his wife. He is indeed most likely to form towards the doctor the sort of attitude he once had to his parents, especially his father. Occasionally as a variant on the foregoing he forms towards the doctor the attitudes to medical figures which his parents exhibited; these may be worshipful or antagonistic. If the attitude is antagonistic this is soon noticed as a rule. If the attitude is worshipful the doctor may accept it complacently. If the parents responded with excessive concern to physical illness the patient may show the same pattern of behaviour and expect concern from the doctor. If the parents had to be coerced to take notice, the patient may seek to coerce the doctor. And intelligence in the patient is not a bar to the formation of such irrational attitudes. Amongst these attitudes the first obvious reaction, common to all mankind, which we expect from our patients is anxiety, even terror. Most doctors cope with this well enough whenever there is an organic basis for it, for example, angor animi appearing with severe angina or cardiac infarction, or in the woman who develops a breast tumour. Practical and sympathetic handling of such situations is part of the stock in trade of almost every general practitioner, physician and surgeon. Many also learn that anxiety may show itself as resentment, even hostility, a demanding or critical attitude or a stubborn refusal to cooperate and accept appropriate measures such as radical surgery. Experience here teaches the practitioner that most patients can be got to accept necessary treatment provided that they are handled considerately and are given time for additional consultations either with relatives or with other doctors. These are aspects of physical illness in which the general clinician will probably have much more experience than the psychiatrist, and we, therefore, do not comment further on their management. There is, however, another situation in which psychiatric knowledge may give additional understanding. This is the case where the patient actually welcomes illness.

There is little doubt that many neurotic patients and even some psychotics cheer up when they learn they have a proved physical complaint—even, say, a tedious and uncomfortable one like haemorrhoids. One reason is that many of these patients always feel they ought to receive the attention and sympathy which are given to the organically sick. They are also wearily aware that their psychological complaints are not considered 'genuine'; or else they are aware that they have some need to be considered as physically ill and intuitively recognize that it is 'safer' to have an actual physical illness than a psychogenic one. In the latter case, apart from running the risk of further rejection by their associates and by their doctors, they are also exposed to the danger of further enquiries being made into the reason for their psychological illness. If it is accepted that many such psychological illnesses represent the solution to a conflict it is clear that to probe their origins would be painful. The patient is better defended against this possibility if he is given a convenient physical complaint which will meet his need to be ill. Moreover, rightly or wrongly, it is usually less damaging to his self-respect if he has an objective organic disorder. There are, therefore, quite sufficient reasons for the paradox that the patient would rather have 'something wrong' than 'nothing wrong'. Yet more reasons may be adduced to show that there is often an irrational welcoming attitude to physical illness.

The view that some individuals have a positive masochistic need to suffer is commonly accepted in ordinary life as well as in clinical psychiatric practice. For such people there must be an obvious satisfaction in physical illness and operations—especially if they are painful. If we accept, as seems most likely, that the intense masochist represents merely one extreme of human variation, it is reasonable to suppose that there will be many more people who derive a moderate unconscious satisfaction from physical disability or illness, even to the extent of entrapping the unwary surgeon into unnecessary operations.

There are also advantages in physical illness which, if not carried to extremes, may be considered as relatively non-neurotic. Increased sympathy from relatives and friends and relief from pressures at work are common and indisputable gains which sometimes follow from physical illness. Midway between such inadvertent benefits and the extreme neurotic gains mentioned, come such other advantageous happenings as enforced leisure to think and read or a change of role to a dependent position which is more or less welcomed by the invalid.

In dealing with physical illness, therefore, the doctor will encounter both anxious and hostile patients on the one hand and those who are irrationally pleased or satisfied with the situation on the other. Having learned to be patient, tolerant and detached with the first group, he will also need to learn to be friendly and yet also detached with the second group. For whilst it is not necessarily important to spoil the irrational pleasure which some patients may take in being physically ill, it is essential to recognize when this happens that there is always some risk of self-pampering or else of hypochondriacal perpetuation of the original physically based dependence upon the medical world. And if one of the larger aims of medicine is to support people in physical sickness or psychological ill health so that they are free to lead a full and independent life it is essential not to maintain people as patients merely because they have an organic disability from whose cultivation they obtain pleasure.

Difficulties of definition

Compared with the foregoing, the technical difficulties which the doctor faces in psychiatry are less, but one matter which deserves special mention is the problem of terminology. Terms are often used in psychiatry which have a different meaning in ordinary speech. This is probably unavoidable since, even if such terms were not taken from the vernacular into psychiatry, the reverse process would be certain to occur. *Hysteria* and *schizophrenia* are terms which present such difficulties. To the doctor hysteria technically means a conversion process whereby an unpleasant conflict is resolved with the production of a physical (or psychological) symptom and repression of the conflict into the unconscious mind. It may also mean to the doctor the behaviour of a certain type of extraverted or dependent personality. To the layman it means uncontrolled or demonstrative or jittery behaviour often occurring in a state of alarm or despair. The doctor also sometimes uses it with these latter meanings. It is perfectly legitimate to use the same term in a number of different ways provided it is recognized that this is being done. Failure to recognize the necessary distinction leads to confusion. In the case of schizophrenia this has happened with a term which had quite precise meaning when it originated. It meant then, and technically still means, a syndrome with certain characteristics and a particular prognosis, in which there is a progressive splitting or disintegration of emotions and thought. Many nonpsychiatrists now take it to mean no more than a dissociated personality indulging in two contradictory types of behaviour, for example, Dr Jekyll. This is also quite a precise idea but very different from the intended one. Likewise many difficulties with the body-mind dichotomy are based upon confusion of meanings. Fortunately in the practice of psychiatry this need not trouble the doctor so long as he remains alert for the exact meanings of the terms used.

In appreciating these exact meanings two terms which are much used require special care. These terms are *neurosis* and *psychosis.* Contact with reality is maintained in the neuroses and in many ways they represent an excessive development of normal feelings. This contrasts with psychosis in which contact with reality is lost and in which the patient is described in common sense terms as mad and is so regarded by ordinary people as well as for legal purposes. A patient who is afraid to cross a bridge because he invariably experiences attacks of panic in such a situation is neurotic if he recognizes that there is no objective reason for his fears. He will generally say: 'It's silly but I can't help it.' We would call him in fact a case of phobic anxiety. A patient, however, who is afraid to go out or cross particular bridges because he believes that foreign spies armed with death rays or poisonous bullets are lying in wait for him is obviously psychotic and, if questioned, will maintain that there is objective evidence for his fears. Even though it may be difficult to distinguish between neuroses and psychoses, and how far they depart from 'normality', these examples indicate that there may be a useful distinction to be made.

Confusion in the use of these terms arises, usually, because they are being used in two different ways. On the one hand they refer to groups of illnesses and on the other hand to degrees of rationality. Schizophrenic and manic-depressive illnesses as well as gross brain disease usually lead to a serious loss of contact with reality. Because of this we class the whole group of illnesses as psychoses. But in mild forms of these illnesses sufficient contact with reality may be maintained for it to be difficult for us to say that the patient is irrational. The converse phenomenon may occur with reactive depression. This is more often grouped with the neuroses but may give rise to a situation where we regard the patient's wish to take his life as psychotic so that on occasion such patients are compulsorily detained in hospital. To avoid misunderstanding it is important to keep clear the twofold technical meaning of each term.

3

Examining the Patient

The practitioner should be able to investigate his psychiatric patients according to the manner in which they present themselves. For example, if he is asked to see a young man who has ceased to work, this may be because of the start of an insidious schizophrenic illness or because the youth, being educationally subnormal, has always had a precarious tenure of his job and has at last been sacked because of failure to adapt to minor changes in the work required of him. To distinguish between these and other possibilities the practitioner must know the relevant questions to ask, just as he would be most particular in a case of jaundice to enquire about the colour of the stools and less concerned to ask questions about diplopia and parasthesiae which would be appropriate to a suspected case of disseminated sclerosis. It is our aim to provide guidance in these situations from Chapter 4 onwards. At the same time, whilst most clinical situations are investigated by special emphasis on particular points, these special enquiries are always related to an appreciation of the state of the different bodily systems. To match this for psychiatric patients the practitioner should be able to take a good general history and indeed if anything may be said to be the secret of success in psychiatry it is the ability to take such a good history.

Taking the history

In medicine generally, and in psychiatry in particular, it is often held that it is difficult to collect precise information by clinical means. This may happen, of course, because a lesion, for example, a tuberculous infiltration in the lung, fails to produce detectable clinical signs. It may also happen because the disturbance in which we are interested is intermittent, as for instance the fast pulse rate of paroxysmal tachycardia. This is especially true for those changes of mood which are reflected in the tone of voice, the movement of facial muscles, the inclination of the head, the stance taken and so forth. Yet, just as the careful observer can note changes in the pulse when they do appear, so he can also make a record of an interview which is reliable and meaningful. Sometimes he will simply note that the patient appears anxious or cheerful or suspicious. If he does not trouble to consider why he thinks this, or if it is difficult to specify his reasons he may, somewhat guiltily, say he based his opinion on intuition. This 'intuition' is probably the summing-up of a number of un-expressed inferences. The art of psychiatry is to make these inferences, often explicitly, from the material of speech and behaviour which the patient presents and to couple them with an interpretation of his history, but first of all to elicit this material and the history with skill and finesse. We would stress that with but a little care and sensitivity this art can be acquired by nearly every practising doctor. Once acquired the art serves not only for diagnosis but also, frequently, as a means of therapy. Even in these days of multiple ancillary techniques it remains the basis of good medicine and psychiatry and, when properly used, is the supreme justification of the clinician. In practice, in psychiatry, the process begins with the entry of the patient into the consulting room or surgery and with the taking of the history from the patient. Where the patient is not sufficiently cooperative to give a history there is much that can still be done and even where he does give a lengthy history himself it is often advisable to supplement it with information from other sources. This latter point will be discussed subsequently. For the moment we would just mention that much of this information may well be available to the general practitioner. This is the case even with seemingly negative observations. For instance, it is very valuable to know that the patient may have been on the practitioner's list for a number of years without ever having sought his doctor's help.

Of course, as we have remarked already, it is always easier to take a good history if the practitioner has some idea of the items for which it is important to search than if he is puzzled by the complexity and uncertainty of the material which initially comes to his notice. Because we know that a lump in the scrotum is quite likely to be a hernia we are accustomed to see if we can get above it and what is the effect upon it of coughing. Similarly, the knowledge that depression is frequently precipitated by bereavement or the loss of a loved object will lead us, once we have this knowledge, to make appropriate enquiries. There is a certain body of technical information of this sort in psychiatry which the practitioner will find invaluable in making his enquiries. Initially he may have to learn some of this in a routine way, and he will need to ask his questions systematically even though some of them are not likely to be relevant. Ultimately his proficiency in taking a routine history and his increased background knowledge will enable him to deal expeditiously with the seeming complexity of the subject and its apparently conflicting implications, as well as with the problem of clarifying his impressions of the patient and recording them.

Proficient history taking is not of course the sole skill which the practitioner must acquire. He must recognize that the patient has to be seen not just as a source of information but rather as someone with whom he is dealing in a personal relationship. We have emphasized this already with respect to the difficulties which the patient causes for the doctor. It is just as important to remember that if the doctor makes his relationship with the patient devoid of feeling and simply aims at collecting facts, the patient, too, will suffer. A balance between the need to help the patient be at ease and the anxiety to acquire relevant data must and can be found.

It is notorious that the practitioner with a full waiting room feels oppressed or irritated when faced with a patient having a psychological complaint. This is often explained by the practitioner's inability to find the time to deal with the case. There are other reasons, however, why the practitioner may feel such disturbing emotions, and we have already discussed some of them. We assume here that if the limited amount of time available when the patient first calls does appear to be a practical difficulty the practitioner will make arrangements to see the patient soon at greater length. The claim is probably justified that one interview of moderate duration (say three-quarters of an hour) takes less time than a series of calls for prescriptions by an unsatisfied patient whose problem has never been adequately investigated. Such an interview also stands more chance of contenting the doctor.

It is best to begin the interview with a standard enquiry as to the patient's complaint. Having made this enquiry the doctor should remain (and look) interested and wait for what the patient has to say. As in medicine generally it is often invaluable to record the patient's actual words as far as possible. There are few patients who will then talk for more than two minutes if the practitioner keeps quiet and does not interrupt with further questions. Some psychiatrists, especially in North America, then encourage the patient to talk about the detail of his current problems, describing when he first felt ill, what causes seem to be important to him in producing his altered feelings, and so on through the whole history of the present complaint. Others with more concern for systematic collection of the data will not encourage the patient to expand the initial complaint immediately but will quite quickly start to review the life history in order to further enquiries on specific points. Whatever the order favoured in the approach to the life history, these enquiries should be directed to three major ends. They should amplify knowledge of the symptoms, explore the family and medical history and the nature of any difficulties in the life of the individual and, perhaps most important of all, secure for the practitioner a picture of the temperament and characteristics of the individual. If the doctor has already established a sympathetic atmosphere by listening quietly to what the patient first had to say the patient will then usually reveal the necessary information on these latter themes. And the doctor, in obtaining his information, will be proceeding in a systematic way which both he and the patient will feel to be different in kind from a mere exchange of good will of a type that might happen in any social conversation.

Whilst the average general practitioner will not want to make his record a detailed or lengthy one he will probably still wish to have asked the relevant questions. These are best grouped under headings which give an indication of the life pattern of the individual, and they may be found in the formal scheme for case-recording which follows at the end of this chapter. Although larger and more comprehensive schemes exist, this one should provide most of the essential information required.

We have stressed that the questions in a psychiatric examination are intended to help elucidate the case in the way that similar questions and observations may do for physical illness. In connection with these item headings some comment is therefore desirable on the main points of enquiry.

We ask about place of birth or, if we know it already, we nevertheless still remark upon it, saying 'You were born at ...' because this prepares the patient to give a full history. Frequently if one says 'I should like to ask you about your past life' patients offer to cooperate and assume that this means talking about their adult experiences only. Asking the place of birth permits a wide enquiry to be made with ease. It may give surprising information as with a white man working as a factory storekeeper who answered Jamaica, and who it turned out was the son of a prosperous planter. In turn we wish to know details of this sort about parental occupation in order to note whether the patient has advanced or fallen from his original status in life; this may give clues to his intelligence and social stability. The temperaments of the parents may have conditioned similar, or opposite, traits in the children. If they died in the childhood of the patient it is very important to know whether this affected him or whether he had satisfactory parent surrogates. The number of siblings leads to further questions. If the patient is depressed and has quarrelled with many siblings he is obviously different from another sort of individual who is anxious and fearful but on excellent terms with numerous brothers and sisters. Again, one boy in a family of girls may have played a very special role, and our enquiries can serve to establish whether or not this was the case. Thus, from the past history, it is often possible to gain information of great importance in assessing the current problem. This is true for all those other topics listed, such as delinquency, education, employment record and past illnesses.

The relevance of sexual and marital relationships will be discussed in subsequent chapters. The relevance of recent stress, particularly bereavements and altered personal relationships, likewise needs no extra emphasis here. It is important to recognize, however, that whilst work difficulties can be blamed for precipitating illness, usually by means of 'overstrain', it is more common for psychiatric illness to be brought on by bad relationships with other people, whether at work or at home, than by mere pressure of work.

The sequence given here is quite a common one, and we find it is one which permits tactful and often successful enquiries to be made on intimate matters. Furthermore, it tends to follow a chronological order which makes it easier to remember but allows the interviewer to return to early and more delicate topics in the patient's life when a related subject has been broached (for example, premarital intercourse when discussing marriage). Often enough, given a suitable lead, the patient will amplify his answers, for example, if he is frankly complaining of anxiety or depression he will respond readily to the questions about childhood fears or lifelong tendencies to worry.

At other times it will obviously not be appropriate to ask certain questions. If the patient will not or cannot give a history this is noted, and the examination is confined to the mental and physical states; the other information is obtained so far as possible from a relative or close acquaintance. Generally, with a little practice, a history may be taken on these lines as efficiently as a physical examination in which the practitioner is well-versed; and the medical setting usually makes it possible even with uncooperative or hostile patients to move on with ease from enquiries about illnesses to enquiries about feelings and behaviour.

If the patient remains persistently garrulous or evasive this itself is of clinical significance and should be treated as such. It helps to save the doctor from exasperation with such patients if he can treat the feelings which irritate him as clinical material instead of feeling them as thorns in his own side. Early on in their clinical career medical students learn a stereotype of a 'good patient' which most doctors keep throughout their professional lives. This (almost mythical) 'good patient' answers questions in a certain way, gives his symptoms and not his views and does not harass the beneficent practitioner with extra complaints or persistent requests for explanations. This type of patient may well be as abnormal as the type who is experienced as objectionable, but his abnormality takes a different form. He is often satisfied to be passive and dependent, to suffer in silence and to be quiet about suppressed anxieties which in fact can be the cause of his symptoms. Besides, therefore, recognizing that the 'good patient' may be sick in ways of which he does not complain, it should also be realized that the 'bad' patient by his behaviour and talk can always provide the doctor with significant data.

It was said above that where the patient fails to give a history the examination will proceed to the assessment of the mental state. In such cases it becomes relevant to establish if the patient is correctly orientated and whether he is in proper touch with his surroundings; the presence of speech defects and/or poor orientation will be used to help gauge whether or not there is an organic confusional state. The presence or absence of hallucinations, delusions, ideas of guilt and self-blame and so forth will help to establish what sort of psychiatric process may be occurring.

At other times the assessment of the mental state will be founded mainly on the history; this is the situation which the general practitioner most often encounters.

Patients with an explicit history of phobias may already have betrayed their anxiety; others may have revealed past hysterical or obsessional symptoms. If not they should be asked specifically about such experiences as a lump in the throat, difficulty in swallowing or speaking, paralyses, fears of various types and a tendency to check and recheck taps, locks, doors, etc. By these techniques, which can be fairly reliable and are in no way mysterious, the practitioner will often be able to make a realistic assessment of the patient's pattern of illness.

The pattern which emerges

As with the physical examination for organic complaints, so with the psychiatric examination the point of the procedure is to define patterns of illness or disturbance which will guide the subsequent management of the case. Such definition, without necessarily excluding the presence of physical disease, will usually establish whether or not there is a psychiatric condition which accounts for the patient's state. If it fails to show such a psychiatric condition one may of course still be present, but the chances of this being so are probably less than when physical examination fails to show an organic cause of illness. And in respect of the latter we must stress that a negative physical examination is one of the least sound reasons for regarding any complaint as functional. If a psychiatric condition is to be diagnosed this should almost always be done for positive reasons and quite frequently, if this is done, needless physical investigations, including laparotomy, may be avoided.

In these psychiatric histories the most important comparison is probably that between the present state and the previous personality. Patients with depression provide a good illustration of this antithesis. The sort of man who has always been conscientious and hardworking and cheerful, whose performance at his job in fact is regarded as excellent, may now have come to regard himself as a useless failure for whom the best thing to do is to end his life. He is likely to be suffering from a type of depression with a good prognosis. In another man with the same present feelings who has always been gloomy and a worrier there is a greater likelihood that his present complaint, although also constitutionally determined, is more closely related to recent stress. In both instances considerable amelioration if not complete recovery to the premorbid state may be anticipated with appropriate treatment. But in the second instance the presence of current stresses will require more attention, and the best final outcome for which one may hope is that he will return to his previous, basically pessimistic state. In this respect it may be noted that while the unthinking often expect psychiatric treatment to change a personality dramatically this can rarely be done, and it is as logical to expect this as to expect the treatment of the oedema of chronic nephritis to renovate the structure of the kidney.

Another type of pattern which often emerges is of the man or woman who has always been anxious and perhaps had one or two unimportant phobias (for example, of the dark or heights) and who now develops a disabling symptom such as fear of travelling in cars, buses, trains and public vehicles of all types.

In the young adult such a development may prove to be related to anxieties about a forthcoming marriage or to difficulties in a badly established one. The problem and pattern are then formally those of neurosis. In yet another case, where in fact the person has always been anxious, shy and somewhat suspicious, the problem may seem at first to be a similar one of neurosis, but when the patient becomes increasingly detached and withdrawn with dulling of affect (emotion) and perhaps hallucinatory experiences or delusional ideas the pattern is then clearly different and is one type of insidious schizophrenic illness. All these are patterns which can be established quite clearly from a routine case history of the type we recommend.

In doing this the practitioner will recognize that there is often a particular reason for the questions: 'What did your father die from?'; 'Did you live with your parents?', just as there may be for such enquiries as: 'Do you get short of breath going up stairs?'. Ultimately these enquiries in psychiatry should answer three questions for the doctor—questions which have been summarized by Halliday[28] as:

1. What sort of person is it who has fallen ill?
2. Why did he fall ill at this particular time?
3. Why did he fall ill with these particular symptoms?

With the answers to these questions the practitioner is in a position to treat or to refrain from mistreating psychological complaints. These answers will almost certainly point to the diagnosis and give an indication of the sorts of measures which can be helpful.

In analysing a case history, some find it helpful to draw up a life chart in which the events of the patient's life and the history of the patient's illness are noted in parallel columns with the date. If psychological features are important the onset of the illness, its remissions and exacerbations can all be seen to relate to events in the patient's life. If this is not so, one may conclude either that the illness is organically determined or that the patient is withholding important facts. This type of analysis also allows one to determine which of a number of stresses are related to the illness. The following extract from the life chart of a patient shows clearly that her symptoms began almost immediately after she gave up her job and began to work as a partner in her husband's business. It suggests that the conflict of roles (wife versus colleague) may have played an important part in the production of her symptoms.

Date	Life Events	History of Illness
1964	Onset of menopause Patient working	
1969 Dec.	Patient relinquishes job	
1970 Jan.	Began working in husband's business	
1970 Feb.		Onset of depression
1970 July	Hysterectomy for fibroids	
1972 July		Psychiatric consultation

Both the patient and her husband were reluctant at first to admit that working together was the cause of her trouble because they knew it would be difficult to change the arrangements. The patient had associated her illness with the operation, but could not explain how it could have caused symptoms which predated it by five months. Her husband attributed her illness to the menopause, but could not account for the six-year time lag. Only a careful scrutiny of the history convinced the psychiatrist, the patient and her husband of the true precipitating cause of her illness.

Item headings

Present complaint (from patient). Short or long form according to circumstances or preferences.

Past illnesses.

Family history and background. Father's (or mother's) occupation. Parents' age/age at death; their illnesses and cause of death; their temperament, for example, whether easygoing, prone to worry or to debt, strict, cold, affectionate, habitual drinkers, and the like. Relationships between parents and patient's feelings towards them. (These points are easy to ask about and often very helpful.) Details of any other marriage by either parent. Siblings; number; position of patient in family. Relation to siblings and parents.

Childhood and premorbid personality. Whether happy or otherwise. Whether patient was 'nervous' then, for example, shy or self-conscious, frightened of dark, prone to nail-biting or temper tantrums, or whether considered 'delicate'. Whether jumpy or frightened of heights then or since, or uneasy in trains/buses/crowds/small rooms/open spaces, and the like. Whether prone to worry unduly; obsessional traits (checking); touchiness, sociability; moral standards; whether quiet and retiring or cheerful and zestful. Mood swings.

Education. Type of school and postschool training. Standard reached. Age on leaving school. Examinations. Attitude to schooling.

Delinquency. Truanting from school. Trouble with police/ in army.

Employment. Jobs held. Reasons for changing. Longest

job. Attitude to work, superiors, subordinates. Military service, if any.

Medical history.
(a) *Physical illnesses* ⎫
(b) *Psychological illnesses* ⎬ Dates and treatments.
(c) *Use of drugs on prescription*
(d) *Use of drugs, for example, cannabis, amphetamines, barbiturates and narcotics*

Menstrual history.

Marital and sexual history. Age and occupation of spouse. Date of marriage. Number of children, pregnancies, relationships with spouse including sexual adjustment. Other sexual relationships including engagements, other marriages, masturbation, extramarital intercourse and homosexuality.

Present illness (if not already obtained). An account from when the patient last felt well. Bodily symptoms and psychological ones; sleep, appetite, weight, whether better in morning or evening.

Recent stress. Bereavements, health of relatives, broken engagement, employment worries, financial worries, marital difficulties, and the like.

Present mental state (especially when patient is unable to give a coherent account of himself). Abnormalities of dress and demeanour. Disorders of speech—dysarthria, dysphasia, thought disorder. Orientation for time and place; is he in touch with his surroundings? Disturbance of memory for past or recent events. Presence or absence of hallucinations of hearing, sight or smell. Presence or absence of delusions, for example, persecutory, guilt or self-contempt, grandeur.

Physical examination.

Results of investigations.

History from relatives. Information which supplements or provides a check on the patient's history should be sought from the relatives whenever possible. The history is rarely complete without it. Interviewing members of the family with the patient may later be an important part of the treatment.

Clearly some of these questions, for example, about employment in the case of children, will not always apply; also, the general practitioner will know the answers to many of these questions and will only need to ask a selection of them.

Part Two

General Problems
in Consultation

4

Common Symptoms

Of the large number of patients who present themselves at their doctor's surgery with a psychiatric disturbance, there are few who do not complain of anxiety or depression. Yet, in spite of this plethora of clinical material, there seems at first sight to be little agreement and much confusion regarding diagnosis, classification and treatment of these syndromes. Many also have hypochondriacal or hysterical complaints, and it is not uncommon to hear of diagnoses such as anxiety neurosis with hysterical and depressive features. Even with a single diagnosis the situation may seem as perplexing, and no one can blame a general practitioner for being in despair if, after he has referred a middle-aged lady with typical symptoms of anxiety to a psychiatric clinic, where she is successfully treated by electroconvulsive therapy (ECT) (in North America, electroshock treatment, EST), he then hears or reads the same psychiatrist teaching that ECT has no place in the treatment of anxiety states. What is proposed in this chapter is not a new classification of the syndromes of anxiety and depression (with which our colleagues would be bound to disagree) but some guiding principles which will help the general practitioner and student to think more clearly about this problem.

It will perhaps help here if we begin with a survey of the symptoms under discussion.

Anxiety

Anxiety is a widespread feeling of apprehension or uneasiness which fills the patient's mind. It can be experienced in a variety of ways. It may occur acutely, as in the panic attack, in which the patient feels acutely frightened, and often complains of symptoms of adrenaline release: palpitations, sweating, breathlessness, and the like. These attacks may occur spontaneously or for a reason which appears to be insufficient. It is an essential characteristic of morbid anxiety that it occurs in situations where no fear is apprehended by others, and yet in other circumstances, when there is real cause for anxiety, the patient may rise to the occasion and behave normally. This characteristic of anxiety will be discussed more fully later on when the psychological causes of anxiety are explored. In panic attacks the patient is usually at a loss to explain the content of the panic; he feels frightened and does not know why. In between attacks he may feel well.

The same unaccountable discomfort is also experienced by the sufferer from chronic anxiety—a pervading mood of spontaneous apprehension. Sometimes, especially in chronic anxiety, there is little primary disturbance of mood but heightened awareness of the physical symptoms of anxiety, such as tachycardia, which are often mistaken by the patient for organic disease.

Phobias

More frequently, anxiety is experienced not as a free floating apprehension but bound down to certain situations or events in which an irrational fear is experienced. In effect the patient behaves as if he believed: 'I will not be anxious provided that I can avoid . . .'.

It is important to distinguish between two clinical situations because these require different treatment. In the first place there are the phobias which occur alone. These are the monosymptomatic phobias and are usually concerned with a well-defined object of fear such as cats, thunder, water, and the like. These symptoms often respond well to behaviour therapy. Then, there is the very common phobia of streets, which may imprison the patient in a type of house arrest. We have seen patients who have not dared to leave the house for twenty or thirty years. This disorder, often called *agoraphobia*, almost always occurs in the setting of a more complex psychiatric disturbance. It tends to occur more often in housewives. Depression is the most common underlying disturbance, and it is sometimes associated with an unhappy marriage. It is occasionally the result of a severe personality disorder of the schizoid type. Successful treatment of the underlying disorder will often relieve the symptom, but sometimes behaviour therapy is necessary to clear a residual habit of staying indoors. In one follow-up study of house-bound housewives, only 55 per cent made a complete recovery.

Dizziness

Dizziness is one of the most common complaints of psychiatric patients. It must be distinguished from vertigo in which the patient feels that either he or his environment is rotating, and from postural hypotension, which is commonly caused by either medication or vasomotor instability in the patient. It is most often described as a feeling of unsteadiness, as if the patient were about to fall. Actual falls are, however, rare. It is usually regarded as an hysterical symptom, vividly portraying the subject's anxious insecurity.

Depersonalization

Many people have a transitory feeling of unreality. This is especially likely to occur with fatigue or intoxication. It is not particularly unpleasant and is often regarded as a fleeting curiosity of experience. It also occurs as a symptom of many psychiatric illnesses when it can be dense and prolonged and cause distress to the patient.

The state of depersonalization is hard to describe accurately. Although the subject is fully in touch with his environment and behaves perfectly normally, he feels cut off from what is taking place around him. He is a detached observer of himself and others, as if he were watching a play in which he is taking part. Usually it is the individual who feels that he is not 'really' there; on occasions it is his surroundings which appear to be remote.

The nature of this disturbance has provoked much controversy. Most authorities regard it as a preformed mechanism present in about 40 per cent of the population. It would seem to occur more frequently in depression, but it has been recorded in many different types of disorder, including brain disease and epilepsy. Lysergic acid and, probably, cannabis can also provoke it.

Compulsions

Some compulsive phenomena are concerned with actions, such as persistent hand-washing or checking gas taps; at other times the patient feels compelled to entertain thoughts of an obscene or disturbing nature. These are called obsessions. If the patient experiences a compulsion to brood on disturbing thoughts or indeed anything which he cannot voluntarily dismiss from his mind this is often termed *rumination*. It is characteristic of these symptoms that the patient realizes that the compulsive urge is irrational and struggles against it. Nevertheless, he often experiences great anxiety until he submits to it.

Worry

Worry is perhaps the most common complaint of patients and their relatives and, psychopathologically, is a more complex phenomenon than they realize. It consists mainly in an emotional over-reaction. The anxiety which is constantly present attaches itself to any difficulty or deviation from routine which presents itself. So the housewife is filled with fear when her husband is late or her child hurts himself. The clerical worker becomes anxious and angry when new documents have to be used in the office. Anxiety, however, is not the only background to this symptom. More commonly, a mood of depression with lack of self-confidence may present each molehill as a mountain. In an extreme form, agitation appears, with hand-wringing, complete inability to cope with daily tasks and restlessness. For other patients worry is a compelling preoccupation with anxiety-laden problems, a type of rumination.

Hypochondriasis

Probably all of us have had irrational fears concerning our health at some time or other. In the absence of psychiatric illness these fears either subside spontaneously if the symptom is unimportant, or resolve when medical advice is sought. In hypochondriasis such an easy solution does not happen. Frequently, it is a symptom of anxiety which attaches itself to minor physical symptoms. This is facilitated if physical symptoms of anxiety are present. It is easier to worry about one's health (which is the doctor's responsibility) than about one's feelings (which are one's own responsibility). Sometimes it is no more than 'an uneasy awareness of bodily function' (Mayer-Gross et al.[46]). Some fears of illness bear a closer relation to the psychological problems which activate them, for example, fear of venereal disease. Sometimes they represent a translation into physical terms of a depressed mood, for example, a fear of death from cancer. Fear of insanity may be an expression of the fear of increasing tension or of letting go unacceptable feelings such as anger or rage. A distinction must be made between a fear of illness, in which the patient will (temporarily) accept reassurance, and a false belief that he is suffering from illness. This is a delusion and does not respond to medical reassurance.

However, the most outstanding problems of hypochondriasis appear in patients who will accept reassurance for a brief while but soon return with renewal of the same symptoms or with different ones. The keynote of these cases appears to be their constant need to demand medical help for bodily complaints despite assurances that this is not required.

Dissociative symptoms

The description *hysterical dissociative symptoms* is currently applied when the feelings involved in a mental conflict are thought to be converted into symptoms which serve to resolve the patient's problems. For example, a soldier who is afraid to go into battle, guilty at the thought of running away, and frightened at the risk of court martial may suffer a paralysis of the legs which enables him to escape from the dilemma by means of illness. However, what we have just said is an explanation of the symptoms rather than a description. Chronologically the delineation of symptoms which served this sort of purpose preceded their explanation.

In the late nineteenth century, Charcot demonstrated that certain symptoms corresponded to the patient's idea of an illness rather than to a lesion affecting specific nerve pathways. A paralysis of an arm would involve the whole arm rather than the muscles supplied by given nerve roots or nerves. In addition it was possible to show that function was preserved in muscles which the patient believed to be paralysed. If asked to raise a supposedly useless forearm the patient may contract the flexors while resisting movement with his extensor muscles, thus agonists and antagonists would cancel each other out. In practice the delineation of hysterical symptoms tends to start from a neurological examination which demonstrates these patterns. The common symptoms of this type are paralyses of limbs, ataxias and aphonias. Other symptoms lack this certainty of diagnosis, but there is nevertheless an important discrepancy between objective findings and a complaint of subjective loss. Such symptoms include some visual impairments, some complaints of deafness and anaesthesia, certain types of attacks of loss of consciousness and some instances of amnesia. It needs to be emphasized that for a firm initial diagnosis of a symptom as hysterical the anomaly demonstrated must be positive in the sense that it must be shown that the patient can do things which he believes he cannot. It is not enough for the doctor to suppose that lack of an adequate physical explanation establishes the occurrence of any psychological symptom, much less an hysterical one.

When it is established that the symptom is hysterical it then often appears that the symptom solves a conflict. It happens that any kind of symptom can be exploited to solve a problem even though it is not always, or even often, possible to demonstrate its hysterical character on physical examination. Dizziness, pain and fatigue are good examples of symptoms which may or may not be hysterical. In practice these less reliable symptoms are associated with those which can be proved. Where any of the symptoms in question affects the body it is known as a *conversion symptom*. Both conversion symptoms and non-somatic symptoms like amnesia are regarded as being due to dissociation in the sense that there is a split between aspects of consciousness or between consciousness and feeling.

The psychological explanation given so far is extremely important. It is particularly relevant in times of war. There are, however, indications that in times of peace and in more settled conditions a substantial minority of patients with hysterical symptoms have a physical disorder involving the central nervous system and particularly the higher levels of the brain. Although such patients are not confused, demented or delirious their cerebral function seems to be abnormal in predisposing them to have neurotic symptoms which in form are dissociative. The full explanation of this is an unsolved problem, but no concept of hysteria will be complete that fails to take into account the high frequency of cerebral organic disease in civilian patients with dissociative symptoms. When dissociative symptoms occur they must be distinguished from malingering, which is a deliberate attempt to simulate illness to deceive others; the 'patient', however, is not fooled. In hysteria, the patient succeeds first in deceiving himself, and the cause of his illness is not, therefore, under his voluntary control. It may be remarked here that malingerers rarely attempt to return to work, and that their 'disabilities' do not interfere with their pleasures.

Some physical symptoms in psychological illness have no meaning as a symbolic expression of a psychological conflict but arise through a direct physiological mechanism. The tachycardia of an anxiety state or the muscular pains which are caused by increased tone in the muscles, demonstrable by electromyography, are examples of this. Such pains are often relieved by physiotherapy. No doubt this is partly due to improved muscle relaxation as well as suggestion and other psychological factors.

Depression

Perhaps the most important single question in the psychiatric examination is the enquiry into the patient's spirits. Few depressed patients will miss this opportunity of describing their low state of mind. Unintelligent patients of poor education may not at first grasp the meaning of the question until it is rephrased as 'Do you feel like crying? Do you feel miserable?'.

Those who have not suffered the mental pain of depression frequently dismiss it too lightly, unmindful of the fact that it is probably the most unpleasant experience to which the human organism can be subjected. A patient who had suffered from both depression and a compound fracture of the humerus was in no doubt that he preferred the latter as less distressing. It has been said that the most important reason why depressives kill themselves is because their sufferings are so unbearable.

Depression does not come in one way only. For some patients it is primarily a guilt experience, and they are bowed down under the torment of self-accusations which flow ceaselessly through their mind. One patient reproached himself endlessly and bitterly because he had kept seven shillings which he had found in a park—the occasion may be as trivial as that. Self-contempt suffuses the whole of their conscious experience. Such patients may at first sight appear to be suffering from delusions of persecution until it is realized that they are only looking for what they think they deserve: 'I should be in prison, not such a lovely hospital'. Such ideas are naturally classed as delusions (of unworthiness and self-reproach) and are not open to reason.

For other patients, depression occurs in the setting of anxiety. In the more severe examples, agitation and hand-wringing are apparent, but in others there is only a morbid lack of confidence and a conviction that there will be no satisfactory outcome to any of their endeavours. Hopelessness is often felt by such patients: 'I will never get better'.

Many depressions bring about a significant decrease in the patient's interests and output of energy. There is a generalized slowing of response (retardation), which is noted in movement, speech and thinking. Such patients complain of difficulties in concentration. In extreme forms, retardation can lead to a striking lack of spontaneous movement, and even occasionally stupor. In retarded patients, their complaint of being unable to cope is often confirmed by those with whom they work. It is important at this stage to prevent such patients from going to work, not only to secure the treatment they need but to prevent serious consequences at their place of work.

In yet other patients, depression is experienced as loss of love; they feel unwanted, desolate and lost. This feeling is often accompanied by an excess of self-pity, against which the patient struggles in vain. Many patients complain that the most disagreeable aspect of depression is the self-absorption in their own troubles and the incapacity to take an interest in others. Even the most favoured pursuits lie unattended. Irritability, malicious thoughts and angry outbursts make serious difficulties for the relatives of depressed patients. Few depressed patients avoid turning this anger against themselves, and for this, as well as other reasons, suicide is always a potential hazard.

Pain

It may seem surprising to list pain as a common psychiatric symptom. On *a priori* grounds, it is generally assumed that pain is a symptom of physical disease. Yet over 50 per cent of patients seen by us in consultation have a complaint of pain and the same finding has been noted by other psychiatrists.[49] In addition many patients with pain from tissue damage respond completely or largely to suggestion or placebos, and pain can be abolished by hypnosis. The assumption that pain signifies physical disease is, therefore, less valid than it seems, and Beecher[5], an anaesthetist, has shown that most potent so-called analgesics exert their effect partly in the same way as do placebos—by allaying anxiety. Beecher has also shown quite convincingly in studies of soldiers that the attitude of the patient to his wound is of critical importance. Even where there is indisputable local damage the circumstances of the individual may make an enormous difference to his response to this damage and to his appreciation of it. As Montaigne[58] observed: 'We feel one cut from the surgeon's scalpel more than ten blows of the épée in the heat of battle.' We would, therefore, emphasize the importance of pain as a sign of psychiatric illness as well as of physical illness; in the many psychiatric patients who have this complaint, it can usually be seen to be a direct consequence of their mental state.

Pain in psychiatric illness is sometimes bizarre. However, this is not so with the majority. Many pains of psychological origin are presented as a simple complaint unadorned with helpful exaggerations. 'Just a pain' or 'an aching pain' are the commonest descriptions. Frequently the pain is persistent but gains some relief from simple traditional measures, for example, aspirin, heat. Frequently, too, it is acknowledged to be made worse by worry. Most often it is a headache and although of course headache can be caused by serious organic disease it is often a functional disorder. However, it can be hard to distinguish pain of psychological origin from other sorts of pain due primarily to organic lesions by means of the symptomatology alone.

The pains which occur in psychological illness have two main causes. First, they may be of purely symbolic significance. They represent an idea or problem which bothers the patient. At its simplest this is seen when a patient comes to the surgery, mentions a pain, and then proceeds to talk about apparently unrelated troubles. Here the complaint of pain is the patient's passport to his general practitioner whom he trusts. At other times the pain may have a more specific symbolic significance as where it represents the memory of a beloved relative who died from a painful illness of the same part, and gives vent to a fear that the patient may have a similar trouble. A pain in the left side of the chest may indicate that the patient's father had angina rather than that he has it himself. In this sense pain is most often a hysterical conversion symptom or an expression of anxiety.

Second, pain may be psychosomatic in nature, that is, arising from bodily (physiological) disturbances which in turn are due to emotional factors. The anxiety which causes painful muscle tension has been mentioned. It has been shown that muscular relaxation goes *pari passu* with the relief of this pain. Once such pain is felt, of course, it may itself become a source of worry and a focus for irrational fears. This type of pain is particularly common as headache and is often described as a feeling of pressure, or a vice or a band round the head, or a steady dull ache anywhere in the body. It is associated primarily with anxiety and to some extent with depression. It responds particularly well to mild sedation and to psychological methods of treatment, including simple explanation and reassurance. There are also indications that pain may occasionally occur as a result of depression without the mechanism necessarily being one of conversion or tension. In these cases the depression is not obvious and the pain is sometimes called a 'depressive equivalent'. What this means is not clear. It is best simply to recognize that pain and depression may be linked without the mechanism always being ascertainable. But it appears that pain may occur as an hallucination in some patients with endogenous depressive illnesses.[49]

One aspect of physical illness which is somewhat neglected is the effect which chronic disability or suffering has on the personality of the afflicted individual. It is commonsense to suppose that a chronic physical disability, and especially one that is accompanied by discomfort or pain, may make patients more anxious, depressed or complaining. Surprisingly this is often ignored and the changes in personality which accompany chronic illness, for example, ulcerative colitis, rheumatoid arthritis, the pain of nerve lesions, are often regarded as causes of the complaint rather than effects. In our view this is often done without sufficient warrant. Indeed, there is evidence that such patients may see themselves as having been brought low by their illness; they acknowledge that they are distraught, yet emphasize as do others with physical disabilities, that they used to be fit and effective people. This seems wholly reasonable.

These are some of the more common morbid experiences which the patient will anxiously bring to the doctor. This list is not exhaustive nor are the sections mutually exclusive. Each sick personality makes its own unique selection from the repertoire of psychopathological responses which are latent in the individual's constitution. The processes which lead to the appearance of these symptoms may now be considered.

There are in general four ways in which people fall ill with anxiety and depression. First, there are the emotionally immature and vulnerable personalities, in whom anxiety and depression are frequent responses to life stress. This is the condition of psychoneurosis and is discussed in Chapter 5. The fundamental disorder is at a psychological level rather than physiological. Second, current environmental stresses have to be considered. The physical environment of the human being has to satisfy certain requirements if health is to be maintained; the same is also true for the social and psychological milieu. The more common stressful situations are discussed under this heading in Chapter 6. Third, there are endogenous (physiological) disturbances which can produce similar syndromes, especially depression, and although psychological considerations are by no means irrelevant to the understanding of these disorders it seems likely that the basic disturbance is pathophysiological. These are discussed in Chapter 7. Finally, the effect of organic disease on mental health requires notice (Chapter 8).

Like other psychiatric concepts, these four pathological processes are not mutually exclusive. Successful management and treatment consists in the correct evaluation of these factors, which may all be present in varying degrees in an individual case, rather than in assigning the disturbance to one of a number of separate diagnoses. This is discussed in Chapter 9.

5
Neurosis

If a careful history is taken, it will be found that some patients
fall ill apparently as a response to certain events in their lives.
While some of these events would generally be accepted as
stressful, for example, a bereavement, in many cases they
would appear to be relatively trivial. One of our patients
complained of severe anxiety and phobias after an illness of
his mother, although the latter made a good recovery. Another
patient developed depression when a grandson for whom she
cared started to attend school and she missed his presence
during the day.

THE NEUROTIC PREDICAMENT

By neurosis, therefore, we mean a psychiatric illness which is
primarily a disturbance of adaptation. This implies, first, that
the personality before the start of the illness was to some extent emotionally immature, sensitive, vulnerable. Second,
minor psychiatric disturbances will probably have occurred
before in times of stress. This is common in childhood in
those who later do not suffer neurotic breakdowns, and universal in those who do. This is a point of some significance
with neurotic symptoms occurring for the first time in middle
life; it is very unlikely that the vulnerable neurotic personality has survived unstressed until this time, and, therefore,
other pathological processes must be sought for, such as a

space-occupying lesion. Sometimes, of course, previous break-downs are concealed from the physician for fear that the latter should correctly diagnose neurosis! Third, the onset of the illness must be demonstrably related to an emotional disturbance. The patient frequently does not realize that such a connection exists; therein lies the value of a careful history of the patient's life. This will often indicate interesting 'co-incidences', albeit in psychiatry it is unwise to dismiss correlations as coincidences. The factors which appear to be associated with the onset of frank neurotic symptoms are almost invariably disturbances in emotional relationships, usually at home but sometimes at work. If at this stage this is pointed out to the patient, he often decries their significance; he has good reason to do so. The material stresses of life, such as poverty, have much less effect on neurotic patients although they may play an important part in the psychosomatic stress disorders which afflict more mature individuals. Anniversaries are important. One patient deliberately made his wife pregnant against her will, and fell ill exactly twelve months later to the day; although unaware of it at the time, during psychotherapy he came to realize the significance of the date of onset of his symptoms.

Lastly, the clinical symptomatology must be consistent with the diagnosis of neurosis. Morbid ideas are open to discussion and (temporarily) respond to reassurance. Depression, even if marked, is rarely accompanied by retardation. Although lack of concentration is a frequent complaint, it is due to anxious preoccupations. If the patient can be detached from these he can perform intellectual tasks with his normal efficiency. Spells of depression are more often precipitated by events, and become deeper as the day wears on when the patient is fatigued. Although complaints of sleeplessness are common, early waking is rare. Some loss of weight is to be expected in the acute stages of neurosis, but this is rarely well marked, or sustained.

It must be stressed at this point that the diagnosis of neurosis does not rest only, or even mainly, on the clinical symptoms, but on the demonstration of a life pattern of breakdown associated with emotional stress. Atypical symptoms may indicate the effect of other and different psychopathological processes concurrent with the neurotic disturbance. There are also illnesses which present neurotic symptoms at the outset and develop depressive or organic symptoms later on. The practitioner must be able to review his diagnosis if the illness does not respond to treatment as expected.

It follows from this account of neurosis, that to alleviate the symptoms of anxiety by a tranquillizer or a change of environment is almost as rational as prescribing an expectorant mixture for a coughing patient without further investigation. The tranquillizer, like the mixture, is of use but should not be the only measure employed. The next period of stress can be predicted to produce a fresh outbreak of anxiety. The essence of the disturbance must lie within the personality and its characteristically fragile relationships. It is this network of disturbed relationships which unsettles so many physicians when consulted by neurotic patients. It is certainly a curious disturbance which is activated by the emotional experiences which healthy people can accept easily or joyfully, and yet is left untouched by non-personal catastrophes. If the doctor is to cope successfully with such patients, it is necessary, as has been said earlier, for him to have some insight into the nature of the neurotic predicament.

The first point to be made in discussing the psychology of the neurotic personality is that the symptoms arise out of a conflict of feelings or wishes inside the mind, and that the patient is not directly aware of this conflict. A simple example may make this more clear. An intelligent, unmarried girl in her late teens consults her doctor in great distress because she is pregnant. She then recounts that she has regularly been having intercourse with her boy friend over many months without either of them taking any contraceptive precautions. She is so troubled about her pregnancy that she has thought of suicide if an abortion is not arranged. In such an example there can be no doubt that the patient is genuinely horrified at the thought of her pregnancy, yet her actions tell a different tale: that she deliberately invited the social problem which has now overtaken her. The only conclusion that can be drawn is that the wish to be pregnant is as strong as the fear of pregnancy, and that the patient was unaware of this conflict in her mind; she therefore failed to guard adequately against her unconscious wish to be pregnant.

The case quoted illustrates very well the ambiguity of much human behaviour. When we see patients acting in such ways we speak of them as being 'ambivalent'—turning in two directions. This is a key word since ambivalence is manifest throughout the range of human behaviour from procreation and marriage to fighting and war. Nor is it an accident that we sometimes hear talk of 'the battle between the sexes' or of situations where men and women seem obliged both to cherish and to attack each other. This basic dichotomy of feeling has been obvious to writers throughout the centuries. The mainsprings of such conduct have been described, in physical metaphor, as forces of love and hate. They have been regarded, notably by Freud, as primary sources of energy, that is to say as inborn drives or instincts. There is some dispute on the technical issue of whether aggressive drives are primary or merely established in response to frustration, but of their strength and power there can be no doubt. The erotic (libidinal) force also should be interpreted more broadly than just in terms of sexual-genital interests although clearly the latter play a great part. The term may properly be extended to refer to all friendly forms of social contact and to much of our interest in the material world. Bowlby[10] has produced important evidence that attachment behaviour is a fundamental biological phenomenon. This is best seen in the links formed between parent organism and the newborn or infant. It has survival value and when attachments are ruptured other consequences follow including states of inertia and apathy or depression. Some anxiety responses and personality disorders may also be attributed to failures in proper attachment (bonding).

It can be seen that Freud's primary division of mental forces into two is too simple but more complicated schemes have not found lasting favour and sufficiently complex theories are available to explain the transformations and changes of direction which these forces may undergo. Such explanations depend largely on a further concept, that of the unconscious, in which is hidden the origin and much of the strength of the libidinal and aggressive forces. We may realize the necessity of such a concept if we consider how little people are able to explain their own behaviour when it is of the conflicting type so far considered, although they may well think, correctly, that they understand the behaviour of others.

The word *unconscious* invites misunderstanding for many people. It seems to create a myth of a submerged cavern in the mind in which frightening and obnoxious fantasies rule, like the dragons of a fairy story, and into which the psycho-analyst descends as an intrepid potholer. The true meaning is much simpler than this, although more profound. An unconscious wish is only one of which the subject is unaware, but which nevertheless exerts an effect on behaviour or experience. The question then arises as to how this 'unawareness' comes about. It can hardly occur deliberately; it is very hard to forget distressing thoughts. This type of forgetting, as automatic and protective as a reflex, is termed *repression*. The essence of repression is the denial of importance, which may extend to frank amnesia. One patient became depressed when her brother emigrated. She was devoted to him and had brought him up after their mother's death. She was, therefore, angry and bitter when he deserted the family to go overseas. At first she denied that the loss of her brother played any part in her depression. She could not admit to herself that she felt his behaviour to be a rejection of her love. When the point was pressed she broke down in tears and admitted that this was so. Unreflectingly, she had assumed that her brother would show to the family a devotion equal to hers. She was wrong and her assumptions made a fool of her. Repression, like other mental mechanisms, has the purpose of protecting us from painful insights about ourselves and others. This insight was too painful to be faced until it was inescapably brought to her notice.

Although this process of repression occurs at all periods of life, it seems likely that the serious consequences (for neurosis) arise from repressions in childhood. It is unavoidable for children to experience impulses and feelings which are utterly unacceptable to the environment of adults. While it is hoped that the child can be trained to discipline these impulses, a situation easily arises when an intractable conflict ensues: to indulge in these impulses and feelings appears to the child to invite rejection at the hands of the adults on whom he is dependent, which is an unthinkable alternative; on the other hand, the child may well find that he cannot deny the existence and strength of his feelings. Faced with this impasse, the child retreats so far from the problem that he is no longer aware of it.

The difficulties thus encountered naturally vary according to the society; in our own society greatest stress is laid on disciplining the drives of aggression and sex. Until recently many people believed (and some still do) that children do not experience sexual feelings in spite of the fact that children's play affords many illustrations of their preoccupation with sex and reproduction. This attitude shows clearly the effects of repression. Naturally, all the instincts (including sex) are present in the child although in an immature form.

The harmful effect of repression is seen when it prevents the developing individual from coming to grips with important problems. In the same way as the intellectual functions of the child fail to develop properly if they do not receive adequate stimulation, so the emotional life of the child fails to develop properly if all sexual and aggressive feelings are experienced as taboo. Kept apart from the maturing stimulation of everyday experience, persisting unchanged into adult life, their emotional demands will not have progressed further than the child's need for mother love. Sexual feeling will still be 'naughty' or 'dirty'. Aggressive drives too will not have matured, so the individual will be incapable of the controlled self-assertion which a position of responsibility demands, and yet will still be liable to petty outbursts of rage which are essentially temper tantrums.*

Immaturity and emotional maladjustment are also attributed to the failures of parents, or those who occupy their role, to provide an adequate model for the growing child. The absence of a father or a father-figure can lead to homosexuality in a male, or a relative deficiency of masculine characteristics. Harsh or unloving parents not only leave the child with feelings of rejection and all their consequences, but also deprive him of the opportunity to learn essential attitudes,

---

*See Chapter 11 for a further discussion of these childhood difficulties.

patterns of feeling and behaviour which he will need for mature adjustment in adult life.

A person in this condition is peculiarly ill-equipped to cope with the emotional load of a mature sexual life, the responsibility of parenthood or the burden of leadership in his job. Hence the stresses which provoke neurotic breakdown are not the worries experienced by mature men and women but the everyday occasions; engagement, marriage, buying a house, parenthood, promotion at work. These are intolerable emotional burdens to the neurotic patient. One patient, after her recovery, traced the start of her breakdown to caring for her young baby. 'When my baby cried at night,' she said, 'I felt it was I who really needed a mother's care, and I was resentful of the baby's demands.'

Worries which are appreciated by emotionally mature men and women frequently leave neurotic patients unmoved. During World War II air raids produced an increase in perforations of peptic ulcers, but did not materially increase outpatient referrals for neurotic patients.

The loss of a parent is a tragic event to all of us, but it is an insupportable catastrophe to a neurotic patient who is still childishly dependent on his parents. Even moving away from home may be sufficient to precipitate symptoms.

It might be thought at this point that a completely free upbringing would eliminate neurotic personality development, but this is not so. First, it is impossible to bring up a child free of prohibitions, for example, toilet training and, second, discipline provides a framework which is essential to the child's security. Without that security, the child's anxieties would become unmanageable.* In our view the best prophylaxis is to ensure that the child can freely discuss his problems with his parents. It is impossible to avoid problems arising; it is essential that there should be a way of helping the child to cope with them.

It must not be thought, however, that the responsibility for neurosis lies only with parents. Many neurotic patients have perfectly healthy siblings, reared in the same atmosphere. It

---

* William Golding's novel, *Lord of the Flies*, is a convincing account of this situation.

may be that innate differences in temperament render communication between parent and child well-nigh impossible. Genetic factors too play a part; some nervous systems are more unstable than others, as has been shown in twin studies. More stress is being laid on psychological than genetic factors, not because the latter are less important, but because a grasp of the psychological factors is essential in the treatment and management of neurosis.

THE MECHANISM OF SYMPTOM PRODUCTION

The manner in which symptoms arise in neurotic states is perhaps clearer now. When the neurotic personality takes on an increased emotional load, as in marriage, the repressed sexual feelings are aroused, and considerable tension and anxiety arise inside the personality in the attempt to maintain the state of unawareness of these feelings. Tension and anxiety also arise as the individual tries to cope with the demands of the situation from his inadequate emotional resources. This anxiety and tension is experienced directly as an anxiety state or transformed into phobias or hypochondriacal fears. The following discussion, which deals with more complicated processes of symptom formation, is not really essential for the simple treatment and management of neurosis, but it should be of special interest to readers concerned with the psychological mechanisms involved in the handling of their patients.

Hysterical dissociative symptoms

Hysterical dissociative symptoms differ from the palpitations and breathlessness which are the physiological expressions of an anxiety state, in that they possess meaning and purpose for the patient. Correctly interpreted, the conversion symptom expresses the conflict in the patient's mind and goes some way, either in fact or symbol, to providing a solution. The following is an example of a simple type of conversion symptom.

A man in his early twenties had always suffered from a stammer which caused him no great disability. He was a miner by occupation, but disliked working underground. He could not afford a surface job because of the lower wages, and yet was dissuaded from seeking employment elsewhere because his house was tied to the job. Following a roof fall he and six others were entombed for eighteen hours in a small gallery twenty yards long and four feet high. For the first twelve hours there were no signs of their rescuers. On being brought to the surface it was noted that he had an aphonia for several hours, and this was succeeded by a severe exacerbation of his stammer which made it impossible for him to continue working underground. It was clear that he was in mental conflict between his overwhelming fear of the pit and the impossibility of finding alternative employment. Moreover, as with most miners, the hardy tradition of the pit prevented him from admitting to himself the true depth of his fear. Faced with this impasse, like a child he was unable to recognize the problem (repression). The automatic defence mechanisms of his mind made use of his stammer to produce disablement and this led to his referral to the clinic. His symptom then served as a signal to those who understood that he could no longer withstand the stress of the coal face, and ultimately led to his rehabilitation in new employment.

It is worth remarking at this point that the origin of his aphonia probably had a different mechanism from its continuation. Overwhelming fear is well recognized as producing temporary paralysis. This effect has been regarded by some authors as hysterical, and it may well serve a biological purpose. The symptom in those circumstances does not necessarily resolve a conflict and could equally be regarded as one which is the result of excessive physiological discharge. Stammer too may well be a physiological dysfunction promoted by anxiety. However, the continued exacerbation of his stammer can be attributed both to anxiety and to the function the stammer served in providing an escape from his problems.

A more complex and important example is provided by a woman patient who complained of backache. During psychotherapy it was noted that she had difficulty with her sexual feelings, but the connection between this and her symptom was not clear until she dreamed that she was being attacked by a 'sexual maniac'. She fought bravely for her honour until the man placed his hand on her back, on the exact site of the pain, whereupon she was paralysed and could resist no further. She then woke up. This dream suggests the way in which the backache provided an outlet for her conflicting feelings: her desire for sexual pleasure and the guilt engendered by this desire. The backache not only represents the satisfaction of her need for punishment for her guilty sexual feelings but provides a symbol of her inability to struggle any longer against accepting satisfaction for these desires. Moreover, by obtaining satisfaction by means of rape, she could not be held responsible for giving in.

In this case the backache and the dream not only express the problem but offer a compromise solution of the conflict of feelings in her mind in terms of symbols. This was one of those relatively uncommon cases where the hysterical character of the symptom was established by means of the patient's own discovery of her unconscious motives. Unlike the first example, in this case the conflict is entirely *endopsychic*. It will be recalled that in the discussion of the immature personality attention was drawn to the external conflict between the child's instinctual feelings and parental prohibitions. This example shows clearly how later in development the prohibitions of parents are taken over by the child and built into his personality where they provide the beginnings of conscience. Normally they develop under the influence of experience into the function of providing enlightened moral judgement. If, however, because of repression they are secluded from conscious experience, they fail to mature and remain a system of rules and prohibitions which are utterly inappropriate for adult life, in conflict with feelings which would otherwise be free to provide a full emotional life for the adult.

Finally, this case also illustrates how the primary gain of a neurotic illness is to maintain the state of unawareness, and so protect the patient from the disturbance of recognizing unacceptable feelings. The conflict is never even acknowledged, and this goes some way to explain the definite impression that most neurotic patients are reluctant to get better. This is in part true; what is more true is that neurotic patients are unwilling to face the truth about themselves which full recovery entails. This type of gain, of which the patient is often not aware, must not be confused with the advantages which often accrue from any illness, organic or psychological, and which may impair the patient's will to recover. This is sometimes known as secondary gain.

The mechanism of conversion hysteria is open to all of us if under sufficient stress. However, it can be expected to occur more frequently in hysterical personalities. Most often conversion symptoms are found in people who attract descriptive terms like 'immature' or 'dependent'. However, there are also other personality traits which are usually linked with the word *hysterical*. Perhaps the essence of this type of personality is the need to project an image of oneself. In clinical practice this is frequently coupled with a dependent, appealing attitude or with histrionic behaviour. Necessarily, the first person to be deceived by this manoeuvre is the hysteric himself. Self-deception, therefore, comes more easily to these people than to others. Their capacity for personal relationships is impaired by their need constantly to have in mind the effect they are having on other people. Consequently their displays of feelings (which come easily) often give the impression of not being entirely genuine. It never fails to surprise that after a stormy interview with much shedding of tears – and having to borrow the doctor's handkerchief—the hysteric will rise, repair her make-up, and sail brightly out of the consulting room as if nothing had happened. Certainly it is true that much less has happened underneath than might be thought from the surface display of emotion.

It has to be said that the notion of hysterical personality is widely and sometimes inaccurately used. Chodoff and Lyons [14] pointed out that no less than seven groups of features have been called hysterical. These range from self-centredness, vanity, exhibitionism, attention-seeking, mendacity and unbridled and labile affects of emotional shallowness, lasciviousness, frigidity, and suggestibility. It is clear that there is room for refining the concept of hysterical personality. Moreover, hysterical symptoms have only a limited association with hysterical personality. Between 20 and 40 per cent of patients with conversion symptoms have a personality which is of the immature or histrionic type. Yet there probably is a meaningful association between immature, dependent, histrionic and manipulative traits on the one hand and hysterical symptoms on the other.

At its best, people with this personality type fulfil a useful function in society, for example as salesmen, where their capacity to project an image of themselves and the concern which they represent is much appreciated by those responsible for selling and advertising the products. With a more immature personality things are very different. The childish emotions of the immature are given free expression, and life with such people is exceedingly stormy. With the frigidity of the psychosexually immature goes the need to be loved and admired, leading only to unsatisfying flirtations and frustrating sexual experiences. Some women of this type have a tendency to be assaulted and raped on more than just one occasion. The childish need to gain attention may lead, especially in older women, to a stubborn and sometimes bizarre hypochondriasis.

Although the basic structure of this type of personality is probably determined genetically, much can be done to help these people by promoting emotional maturity with the help of judicious psychotherapy. Once the tensions and anxieties inside the personality are relieved, the characteristically hysterical behaviour becomes less obtrusive.

Obsessional and compulsive disorders

In obsessional and compulsive disorders it is noticeable that the content of the compulsive thought or action is often a direct or symbolic expression of the feelings that have been repressed. A patient who had much difficulty with her aggressive feelings was horrified to experience an impulse to hit the bald head of the man who sat in front of her in church. Sometimes the compulsive thought takes the form of a fear that the forbidden act may be carried out. The same patient was in anguish for fear that she might harm her children. Sometimes it is feared that the harm has been carried out unwittingly. One patient, when driving a car, was sorely tempted to turn back to verify that the bump in the road was not in fact a person whom he had run over without realizing.

Patients of this type develop checking rituals to make sure that accidental harm will never arise from their actions, for example, checking gas taps, searching for pins. Another patient refused to go out of doors for fear that a sleeping tablet hidden in her coat might drop out and be picked up by a child. The basic psychopathological mechanism appears to be a splitting of feeling and impulse: the impulse to hurt is dissociated from the feeling of anger and is allowed to enter consciousness on its own. This represents a partial discharge of the repressed feeling associated with it, yet because it appears in the patient's mind without the appropriate feeling the patient does not understand its significance; the state of unawareness is maintained. Moreover, these patients are usually horrified at the compulsive thought, and the anguish thus caused assuages the hidden sense of guilt which accompanies the anger. The feelings of such patients are more primitive and more disorganized than those of hysterics: the uncontrollable black rage of the toddler compared with the more socially oriented anger of the five-year-old. Corresponding to the violence of their feelings, the discipline of their parents is also experienced as savage and demanding, and provides the foundation for guilt feelings of brutal intensity. In the emotional life of these patients, sexual and excretory functions are scarcely distinguished, and the disgust associated with the latter cannot be dissociated from the former. Sex remains a sordid experience for many of them. Therefore, such people are often crippled with guilt when sexual or aggressive feelings are aroused in them. To some extent the mechanism of repression succeeds in shielding these distressing complexes of feeling from conscious awareness, but when this breaks down the characteristic obsessional manoeuvre occurs of splitting feeling from impulse, and symptoms result.

Although this psychopathological mechanism may occur in any personality, it is most often found in obsessional personalities. In an attempt to control the turbulent emotions which they possess, they react by developing a rigidity of conduct with which they seek completely to control their environment. Tidy and methodical in their habits, with plans prepared for any eventuality, they also find it necessary to impose their prohibitions on the lives of those associated with them as otherwise they might be confronted with disturbing feelings or situations. Like people living on the edge of a precipice, they build a high wall of rigid rules around their lives for fear of falling into the abyss. Yet they find it hard to escape their fate; their repressed feelings of love and hate insinuate themselves into their experience of life. Often they perceive the world as a hostile and sordid place in which there is no security, and in the depths of their own minds the unacceptable impulses reappear as obsessional thoughts. Many, however, make a reasonable adjustment. The reaction-formations in their character against angry affects change them into quiet and reserved people with a horror of violence. Lacking flexibility and sometimes assertion they often fail to reach the highest positions in life, but flourish in occupations where an orderly method is required, in banks, in offices, in accounting. Less stable variants of this personality are more difficult to live with. Alongside rigid and often irrational prohibitions, there go unpredictable outbursts of rage and a compulsive sexual drive which are not sufficiently checked by the obsessional character traits.

At the risk of repetition, it must be pointed out again that an important cause for a flare up of neurotic symptoms is a concealed minor depressive illness. This appears to be true relatively more frequently for obsessional illnesses than for other neurotic disorders, probably because the obsessional personality is especially prone to depression.

Mechanism of the depressive reaction

The mechanism of the depressive reaction is well illustrated by the case of a woman in her late thirties. Complaining of depression, she described how her childhood had been made miserable by her father's drunkenness. Brought up in a remote Welsh village in a society with rigid Calvinistic morals, she was frequently humiliated through having to bring him home when he had been overcome by the effect of drink. She was painfully aware of the censorious attitude of the community and was bitterly ashamed of the poverty into which her father's habits had plunged the family. In spite of this, she was very fond of her father, who was a gay and lovable companion at other times. They both enjoyed music, she playing the organ with more than average competence, while her father, before his evil habits completely overcame him, was well known locally for his fine voice.

He died painfully. A carcinoma of the oesophagus made necessary a gastrostomy, and the patient nursed him devotedly through his last illness. Some time after his death the patient became depressed.

During psychotherapy the patient became increasingly preoccupied with a conflict of feelings towards her father. She found that she was full of both love and hate towards him. She became very guilty about the hate, wondering if his tragic death was not in some way retribution for his evil ways. It was as if the hate and humiliation which he had brought about in her had magically found expression in his agonizing illness. She then dreamed that she was seated at the chapel organ in the village of her childhood, but the music before her was not organ music but singing music (tonic sol-fa). She commented spontaneously: 'How shall I play my father's part?' She was soon to find out. From that time she developed a replica of her father's illness, with pain and difficulty in swallowing. The psychiatrist treating her waited anxiously as her depression deepened, seemingly as impotent to help her as she had been in nursing her father. When the anniversary of her father's death was reached, the symptoms began to clear quickly, and she was soon fit to leave hospital.

Depressive reactions are prone to occur in the setting of ambivalent relationships where love and hate are equally strong. With the loss of the loved person (by death or separation) the mourner reproaches himself for the bad and hateful feelings. He feels as if they have magically taken effect and brought about the disappearance of the loved person. Guilt and depression are unavoidable. This case, however, illustrates another and more serious mechanism. It has been noted earlier that the attitudes of the parent are taken into the child's personality. This process is accelerated by loss of the parent. If the relation with the lost person was fundamentally healthy no harm arises. Indeed, the very opposite is the case. To incorporate the image of a loving parent at the heart of the personality is to ensure a sense of security which cannot be undermined by any external stress or emotional trauma. This is probably a crucial process in the building-up of a mature personality. If, however, the relationship with the lost person is dangerously ambivalent, the image which is incorporated is bad as well as good, is hated as well as loved. Hence the depressed person feels as if he hates himself; more accurately, he hates the lost person who has now truly become part of himself. Destructive impulses towards the lost person are transformed into an urge to kill oneself, and the danger of suicide is not small. In the case under discussion, the dream predicted how the patient would have to take over the bad part of her father as well as the good, how she would have to play an unaccustomed part, and accept his pain as well as his love.

Disturbances of behaviour

Behaviour disturbances are very rarely lacking in neurotic disorders. The difficulties which those with neurosis have with their feelings, and hence with their personal relationships, have been a constant theme of this chapter. While this causes suffering to the patient through the production of symptoms, it also inevitably causes upsets to those who live and work with them. This comes about in a number of ways.

In the first place, those with neurosis are abnormal in their demands on those who are with them. Since they are emotionally immature anyone with whom they are in contact runs the risk of being transformed into a parent surrogate. Normal adults meet usually on a basis of friendship or contract; the person with neurosis demands attention or help. While many have sufficient insight to try to control these demands (at least outside the family) a few, more disturbed and socially imperceptive, know no restraint. Continually telephoning friends, seeking reassurance and sympathy from all whom they meet, they quickly build up antagonism in family, friends and neighbours by a ceaseless importunity which could be acceptable only in a sick child calling his mother. Many neurotic patients, because of their great need for affection, are sensitive to the slightest change in the emotional atmosphere; indeed they often suspect a cooling of relationships without cause.

Second, inner troubles distort perception of the environment. By a mechanism of projection the patient protects himself from a disturbing complex of emotions by locating it outside himself. This is very common in the neurotic patient's dealings with the medical profession. Doctors are irrationally pictured as all-powerful, threatening, dangerous, untrustworthy, tireless, perfect, omniscient. In the ambivalent relationship with his parent, the patient is often aware of only one feeling; the contrary is repressed. It is the repressed feeling which is often projected. At other times the projected feelings are fully ambivalent—antagonistic and dependent at the same time. Patients who argue as to the merits of a doctor are being more informative about their relationships with the dominant parent than about the quality or skill of the physician in question.

Third, in neurosis, the individual may be under such great pressure of instinctual feelings that he acts them out, without being able fully to account for his behaviour. Some patients are antagonistic and hostile, picking quarrels with all and sundry. Other patients become involved in sexual adventures. This type of behaviour, which may lead to great social difficulties, temporarily relieves the tension of internal conflict while still maintaining the state of unawareness concerning their inner problems. The following case history concerns a girl who sought relief from her problems with her mother by acting out her feelings.

Her history was that for two years she had led a life of extreme promiscuity. Whenever she was near a man she felt sexually aroused, and she found herself encouraging his advances whether or not he was personally acceptable to her. Yet she found these relationships profoundly unsatisfying both sexually and emotionally. Frequently she found herself conducting several affairs concurrently.

In the course of psychotherapy, a number of points emerged. Her mother was a hard woman, liable to violent physical assaults on her children and incapable of giving them affection. She was also morbidly suspicious of sexual misbehaviour in her children and at times accused them of sexual misconduct, especially of a homosexual nature, without apparent cause or reason.

The patient's need for love and affection was frustrated not only by her mother's unloving nature but also by the latter's insistence that the sensual experience of affection was immoral. This was a further barrier, the patient felt, to feeling love for her mother. This so-called moral training, therefore, forbade the patient even to recognize in herself her physical yearning for her mother. The erotic desires are not, however, so easily suppressed, and the forbidden and unrecognized feelings found an outlet later on in her experience with men. Of course, these attachments proved unsatisfactory and transient; it seemed likely that it was not a male lover she was looking for but her mother: a homosexual feeling masquerading as heterosexual, so that the forbidden nature of these impulses remained unrecognized. The guilt she felt about her liaisons served also to placate her mother's morality.

The climax of this patient's treatment came when she asked the question: 'Is it wrong to love?'—and with this the taboos erected in her by her mother began to crumble. She began to see her mother's 'morality' for what it really was, and the way was open to develop more realistic and truly responsible attitudes to love and sex. Soon she was capable of stable and mature attachments to a man, untainted by the need to secure a mother's love from him, and later became engaged.

This patient's promiscuity, therefore, like all neurotic symptoms, was a compromise arising out of several conflicting impulses: the need to find an outlet for her desires for her mother, the need to remain unaware of the nature of these impulses, and the need to feel guilty. She was, of course, unaware of this conflict; her early training had successfully stifled any tendency to examine the state of her feelings for her mother. When she first came for treatment she was aware only of feelings of resentment for her mother. She hotly denied that she had any tender attachment to her at all and scornfully repudiated the suggestion that this had anything to do with her promiscuity. The truth, of course, was otherwise, but at that time the force of her mother's morality was such that intolerable anguish would have been caused if she had caught a glimpse of the true state of her feelings. To avoid that intolerable anguish by maintaining a state of unawareness about inner feelings is always the primary purpose of neurotic illness.

In an earlier chapter the emotional difficulties of the doctor with the neurotic patient were pointed out. The inner nature of these difficulties may now be clearer. In the neurotic patient the symptoms indicate not a disease but an emotional disturbance. The nature of this disturbance is such that peremptory demands are made on the doctor to save the patient from his difficulties and to love him. The doctor is always perceived by the patient through the distorting haze of unsolved emotional problems with his parents. He appears more often as frightening or as an object of love than as a professional adviser. More rarely, but embarrassingly, the doctor may be the recipient of powerful instinctual feelings which the patient is acting out.

The doctor has as well his own professional difficulties. The emotional conflicts which produce the symptoms are shielded from his enquiries by powerful defence mechanisms of which the patient is entirely unaware and which he will only relinquish after much patient psychotherapy. It is indeed a formidable task in therapeutics. Yet it is one of the most pressing. Most neurotic patients know that they are different from other people, but they are not clear as to the nature of this difference. They frequently have no insight as to how unreasonable their behaviour appears to others, and they are hurt and offended by the antagonism of others which, without realizing it, they have created themselves by their own actions and demands. As well as these troubles they have to endure the suffering and disabilities which arise from the symptoms. From all this they wish to be rescued; by themselves they are helpless.

In summary, it can be said that neurotic illness is due to tension and anxiety which arise out of conflicts in the mind. These conflicts are concerned with the fate of the instinctual desires and the feelings which accompany them. Opposed to these instinctual forces are the taboos and moral axioms ingrained in the personality by the weight of the individual's upbringing. If this conflict is too massive, the individual unconsciously protects himself by maintaining a state of unawareness towards this conflict. Repression, projection, acting out, dissociation of feeling and impulse are all devices which try to maintain this state of unawareness at the cost of symptom formations.

The conflict arises in the first place because the instinctual drives of love (which is experienced bodily as sexual feeling) and aggression (experienced as anger and hate) are directed towards the parents. Insofar as the child feels that these impulses are unacceptable, then conflict arises. Some conflict is unavoidable, but provided that the tension engendered is below the limit of tolerance, the individual remains well. In the neurotic patient this equilibrium is sufficiently precarious to be upset by the sexual and aggressive demands of adult life, and he falls ill. This probably rarely happens when significant people have provided adequate love and training during the individual's childhood, or adequate patterns of behaviour which may serve as a model for feelings and relationships.

The views put forward in this discussion are offered as a working hypothesis for the understanding and control of neurotic phenomena; they do not do justice to the complexity of these conditions, and indeed at times simplification has approached the point of distortion. Classical writers on this subject have at different times laid stress on other points as well as those covered in this chapter, and their works should be consulted *in extenso* if a full understanding of these perplexing problems is to be reached.

6

Social Factors

The discussions of the patterns of psychiatric illness and psychopathology have so far concerned the patient on his own. Yet patients live in families and other groups, and it is impossible to understand and control psychiatric disturbance without considering the family setting in which it occurs.

Who is the real patient?

The family is the basic group in our society, and, therefore, when one of its members seeks advice about an emotional disturbance it can be taken as an axiom that the whole group is more or less disturbed. The first task in the psychiatric formulation is to locate the disturbance, and it may not be in the patient who first seeks treatment. The person with least tolerance is usually the one who first shows signs of distress. The family tensions may be arising from an emotional disturbance elsewhere in the family circle, and so on occasions it may be true to say that the patient is showing the symptoms of someone else's neurosis.

This is shown most clearly in the psychological disorders of children (see Chapter 11). Being immature and vulnerable personalities they are especially sensitive indicators to the emotional tensions set up by their parents. This was well shown by one of our patients who had a grossly hysterical personality. She was frigid in her emotional and sexual relationship with her husband, which no doubt was a factor which facilitated an extramarital liaison on his part. She was incapable of warm affection towards her children, one of whom she rejected outright; from time to time she threatened to kill him. The first 'symptom' of this woman's character disorder was the encopresis of her rejected son. When admitted to hospital he had perfect control of his sphincters but relapsed immediately he returned home to his mother's threats.

A valuable clue to what is going on in the family is often given by the person who accompanies (or fails to accompany) the patient. Mothers who complain of the behaviour disorder of their children will often say: 'I can do nothing with him', thus revealing a conflict between mother and child, and the mother may not be aware that it is her neurotic demands which have precipitated the conflict.

Even more revealing are the relatives who stay away from the consultation. When one woman sought advice for her unhappy marriage her husband stayed outside in the car throughout the interview. As it was his behaviour which was largely the cause of his wife's difficulties, his desire to stay away from the psychiatrist's questions can easily be understood.

If the behaviour of relatives often provides valuable clues to the emotional pressures inside the family, the same can sometimes be said of occupational groups. One patient failed to respond as expected to treatment until a director of his firm sought an interview. Then it was revealed that the manager of the office in which the patient worked was overbearing and tyrannical and loved to humiliate his subordinates. This patient was the second psychiatric casualty in that office, and three others had already left. A small epidemic of psychiatric illness in a place of work always suggests a focus of infection of emotional disturbance. One of us treated in quick succession the wife and colleague of a very disturbed man who acted the part of tyrant both at home and at work. The patients were being treated for the effects of this man's disorder. Industrial medical officers can play an important part in preventing and dealing with these situations, which are often undiscovered by the patient's own medical advisers.

In the first example, the office manager was persuaded to leave, and this brought about a quick recovery in the anxiety states of his subordinates.

The effects of psychiatric illness

Before going further we should perhaps state explicitly what is implied above: the effect on others of the patient's disturbed behaviour will often demonstrate the important motivations which underlie that behaviour. These motivations are 'unconscious' in the sense that the patient is unaware of them and will often deny them even when taxed, but the facts speak for themselves to any unbiased observer. In one case, the patient's behaviour produced great suffering and anxiety to her family. When removed from her family her symptoms were greatly ameliorated, only to relapse when she was sent home on leave. She had a well-marked obsessional neurosis so that she spent all her time washing and prepared no meals for her family. Her children were often fed by neighbours. She had very strict rituals regarding letters which led her to destroy or conceal important mail from her husband. Her family were not allowed into the kitchen except for brief intervals. In the course of psychotherapy it became clear that the patient was full of hate towards her husband and yearned for the time when she was a single woman unencumbered with a house and a family. This confirmed the surmise that could be drawn from her behaviour: her illness had such devastating effects on the family, but produced so little disturbance when she was isolated in hospital.

Similar conclusions can be drawn from similar covertly aggressive behaviour; the poor housewife who consistently overspends her allowance, the husband who appears to prefer his work to his home, and the like. Any behaviour which produces genuine distress in others is likely to be aggressively motivated, although the patient may deceive himself by denying it. This is one reason why those with neurosis can be so unpopular; the effects of their hidden aggression are so painful to others. In other instances, psychotic and psychopathic behaviour can be the main cause of much emotional disturbance in the family. The behaviour of a psychotic patient can be more damaging to the mental health of the children than the inheritance of the genotypes of mental illness. The development of community care services in which more patients are treated at home increases the responsibilities of general practitioners to make sure that an intolerable burden of psychiatric nursing does not fall upon the family. The unpredictable outbursts of a schizophrenic mother, the self-absorbed depressive, unoccupiable, irritable and gloomy, the old lady with senile dementia who stumbles around the house, incontinent at night and who is periodically missing are only examples of the way in which mental illness can destroy the equilibrium of a household and bring about further breakdowns in mental health in other members of the family.

Physical illness in the parents is also the cause of emotional disturbance in children, which may be expected to affect their attitudes in adult life. A daughter may be prematurely cast in the role of a substitute mother. A son fails to complete his education and all may fear similar suffering to come if this disease is believed to be hereditary.

Psychopathic (sociopathic) character traits (as described in Chapter 16) can be equally damaging especially as they may well be overlooked. There are occasions in many families in which one of its members drinks too much, gets into debt or is in trouble with the police. When these difficulties occur in non-psychopathic families, the ordinary measures of society, for example, the probation service, are quite sufficient to restore the family to its former adjustment to society. There is a small proportion of families who do not seem to benefit, and these are of special interest to the psychiatrist. One reason is the presence of psychopathic subjects in the family who are unable to learn how to adjust to society. In other cases the families are conforming and adjusting to a minority culture whose way of life is so different as to be regarded as antisocial by the majority. Some delinquent and 'problem' families come into this group.

The significance of antisocial behaviour is considered more fully in Chapter 16, but some of the implications of psychopathy for family life need to be mentioned at this point. When the psychopathic subject is the husband the family soon learn the demoralizing effects of an uncertain income, unforeseen debts, alcoholism, outbursts of rage and perhaps prison sentences. Repeated admissions to mental hospitals are not uncommon, and for long periods of time the family is left on its own. It is surprising how often the wives and families of such men remain in their support, when they could appear to have so much to gain by obtaining a separation. Such a view, however, neglects not only the affection which some of these men inspire in their wives but also the very real difficulties which confront a working-class woman who attempts to leave her husband and fend for herself and her children.

MISFORTUNE AND SOCIAL STRESS

There is a tendency, among psychiatrists and others, to assume that misfortune does not occur. As our knowledge of neurotic psychology deepens we come to believe that human beings create their own particular social environment, and if later they find it distasteful, they have no one but themselves to blame. Most psychiatrists receive the impression from time to time that psychological treatment largely consists in helping the patient to scramble out of the pit which he dug for himself. No doubt there is a lot of truth in this, but we must not be deceived into ignoring the fact that the current social and psychological milieu of our patients may in itself provide stresses which would make anyone anxious, nor must we be blinded to the fact that chance can deal some very grievous blows. The maxim that 'Character is Destiny' is, of course, comforting—provided one can be sure of one's own character, and it is often difficult to accept the fact that life is full of uncertain chances and unpleasant surprises, both for ourselves and our patients. To think otherwise courts the risk of losing one's compassion for those to whom misfortune occurs.

In the section on neurosis we point out that the stresses which precipitate neurotic illness are often to be found in events which stable people do not regard as stressful. In this section we are concerned with those personal disasters which test the adjustment of the stable and which are catastrophic for the vulnerable. Such stresses are more frequent than we may easily recognize and their effects go further than is often supposed. Widows within a year of bereavement have six times the expected death rate.[64] Redundancy or unemployment saps the morale of men who have been stable all their lives. The victims of concentration camps have an exceptionally high rate of chronic schizophrenia.[20] Former prisoners of war held by the Japanese under harsh conditions appear liable to prolonged emotional instability which appears when, superficially, there has been a return to normal life and health. The implication is that where such misfortunes have played a part in the production of psychiatric illness, no amount of treatment either psychological or medical can be expected to restore the *status quo*. However, attempts to ameliorate the social environment may be an essential part of therapy if medical and psychological treatment are to be effective.

Following the analogy of physical medicine, one thinks of stresses as a trauma of inflicted injury. A more apt comparison would be the deficiency diseases, where physical health breaks down because of the absence, for example, of essential vitamins. We believe it to be more helpful to regard misfortune as engendering states of deprivation which hinder psychological well-being.

The ego (or self) is vulnerable from three directions; intimate personal relationships, social success and the esteem of peers, and scope to develop and create a characteristically personal existence. Misfortune may deprive the subject of satisfaction in one or more of these spheres.

Loss of love is the most important example of disaster in personal relationships, and its gravity depends upon the age at which it occurs, the young and the old being especially vulnerable.

Bowlby and others have written on the psychological consequences of the loss of maternal love[9] before the age of 5 or 6 (see Chapter 11). Naturally, not all separations produce irreparable psychological damage, but it is a hazard which is to be avoided or mitigated when possible. Separation from father does not appear to have such grave consequences, but there is some evidence to suggest that in vulnerable male children it may be linked with difficulties later in life in assuming the masculine role. Loss of the father in childhood occurs more frequently than the average in the histories of both homosexuals and unemployed neurotic patients.

The loss of a loved person in adult life by bereavement or permanent separation always leads to serious psychological consequences. It is important to know the normal process of bereavement; lack of psychological response may be as pathological as an excessive response.

Murray Parkes[63] and others have given us a clearer insight into the process of mourning. The initial reaction is one of shock or numbness. The afflicted person can scarcely believe what has happened; he is dazed and frequently requires assistance in making the necessary arrangements. This is quickly followed by a long period of anguish. The bereaved person is often restless, talking of selling up and moving away. This phase of the reaction has a resemblance to the searching behaviour shown by animals who have lost a mate or an off-spring. It is important at this point to reassure the bereaved and to dissuade them from making important decisions about their life which they might regret afterwards. During this time they often suffer acute pangs of yearning: 'Why did this have to happen?', a question requiring not a philosophical or theological reply but a kind understanding that such a loss is hard to accept. At this time, quasi-hallucinatory experiences are common, sounds are misperceived as well-remembered footfalls, a patch of shade in the garden becomes the shadow of the husband digging.

In a few months this period of acute distress gradually gives way to a more settled depression, as the bereaved person begins to count the cost of the loss. This is the period of loneliness, when widows realize how much of their social life depended on their husbands, when widowers realize just how much their wives contributed to the home. Serious practical problems of money or care of children have to be solved. In time, the individual readjusts and organizes his life into a new and acceptable pattern.

This sequence of events can take up to twelve or eighteen months when a marriage partner is lost. There seems to be no point in trying to shorten this period. Those who cut short their grief work and get themselves reorganized in a few weeks are liable to fall ill with a reactive depression a few months later. Contrary to what might be expected, young people have mourning reactions which are more severe than the old. Unexpected or violent death produces more disturbance than a long-awaited bereavement. Yet the survivor in the latter case misses the demands made by the dying person and the relief from nursing duties leaves life pointless.

Mild guilt reactions are common and natural. We could all have done more for those we love. Severe guilt and depressive reactions are more likely when the survivor has a strained relationship with the dead person, as in the case quoted on page 60. Young people often behave badly, committing legal or sexual misdemeanours, getting drunk or becoming unsettled at work. As well as psychiatric illness, physical illness is also more common; the increased mortality of widows has already been referred to. Occasionally the period of mourning may become morbidly prolonged, with constant visits to the cemetery, the dead person's room preserved unchanged. For various reasons, some are unable to complete their mourning.

With increasing age, the capacity to love fresh people diminishes and the pathogenic effect of bereavement is correspondingly increased, especially in childless women. It is a tragic spectacle to see such a woman on her own except perhaps for distant relations whom she has hitherto ignored. Having devoted herself to her husband she has not troubled to cultivate friendships outside the marriage and now finds herself unable or unwilling to care for strangers. It is not a depressive delusion which makes existence barren and hopeless to such women; it is a future which many younger women fear. We have written here mostly of the death of a spouse since this is the commonest cause of bereavement. Obviously the death of a child must be very painful to parents and although such bereavement occurs more rarely it seems from time to time to be a persistent cause of depression. It is not uncommon for the parents to be unable to share their grief with each other and with their children. The family atmosphere becomes tense with unexpressed feeling. This may lead to behaviour disturbances in the children and marital problems between the parents. In men, grief over a lost son can be a cause of impotence. John Emery[21] has written about the consequences for the family from the most poignant of bereavements—cot deaths.

'The mother is utterly confused.... Her confidence in her motherhood has its roots cut. Hers was a normal baby—everyone said so.... What went wrong? Guilt is inevitable.'

We do not blame the parents now as we used to do for smothering their child, but it is still almost impossible for them not to blame themselves.

Responsibility for caring for the bereaved is shared by the general practitioner with his colleagues in community care: health visitors, social workers, clergy. General practitioners do not always have the time which the bereaved need, but we believe that they have a special responsibility to make sure that the family is visited by someone who does care and does have the time.

To come down in the world is always a bitter blow. One patient for long held the post of manager of a high-class shop. Due to no fault of his own the shop was closed and he was dismissed. Being in his late fifties he was unable to secure fresh employment. He fell ill with a hypochondriasis which did not respond very satisfactorily to treatment.

The factors concerned in this type of problem are status and income. To some men the sympathy of friends becomes intolerable, while to others the damage to their self-esteem is the serious injury. The drop in income which accompanies such misfortunes makes public the loss of status (having to sell the car), as well as producing difficulties in budgeting. It is not easy to live on half (or less) of the income which one has come to rely on over the years. This, however, is the situation of many men who are disabled with chronic illness and may well be a hindrance in treatment.

If any reader is tempted to comment that such setbacks are part of life and must be taken with a good spirit, it may be salutary to reflect upon one's own feelings if for any reason one was debarred from the practice of medicine (for example through blindness). Yet the security of any profession is not inviolate, and most occupations are considerably less secure than that.

The relationship between poverty and mental ill health is

still far from clear. It is certainly true that loss of fortune or earning capacity is a severe stress, and this is borne out by the statistics of suicide. It is also true that the prevalence of schizophrenia and of neurotic disorders seems to be increased in the less affluent sections of the community. Research in this difficult field reveals a complex situation. Mental illness itself (especially schizophrenia) can cause a downward drift in social class, and even when a true increased incidence of psychiatric illness can be demonstrated in underprivileged groups, it would appear that social and cultural factors are of more significance than poverty.[75] We do not wish to suggest that the financial relief of poverty is not worthwhile, but the grounds for action are humanitarian rather than as part of a mental health programme.

The third state of deprivation may be less obvious but is no less far-reaching. Often the patient is aware only of a vague dissatisfaction or a sense of frustration. A pertinent question in considering these problems is to ask what satisfactions are being offered to the patient by his current life. It is true that patients who find themselves in this situation have very often brought it about unwittingly either on account of the neurotic traits in their personality or through thoughtlessness. An interesting definition of mental health might be the ability to foresee and avoid the social milieu in which the subject's personality is at a disadvantage. Notwithstanding these points, a situation of chronic frustration constitutes a very real social problem which merits its own treatment apart from the neurotic and other factors which have brought it about.

There are three ways in which this state of affairs commonly arises: in the work situation, in marriage and in the plight of the single persons who have devoted a major part of their lives to the care of aged parents.

Neuroses arising from chronic dissatisfaction at work are not as common as might be expected. There are occasional examples of men who find themselves in the wrong occupation. A patient who complained of anxiety was successfully occupying the post of factory manager with a comfortable salary. He had always been a talented amateur singer but had not pursued a stage career because of his family responsibilities.

In his early forties the financial responsibilities for his family were drawing to a close, and the crisis came when he was offered an audition by a television company. Once he decided to take the risk of accepting their contract he immediately lost the anxiety symptoms which had been accumulating over the years although he was facing the hazards of a most insecure livelihood in place of his factory job.

Failure to be offered promotion and doing their work for incompetent seniors are also potent factors in the production of this type of frustration. Two patients (a journalist and a bank manager) were cured by promotion. We felt that the striking improvement was due not only to a rise in status and salary but to the extended opportunities of putting their professional ideas into practice and making use of long frustrated initiative. It also shows that the presence of neurotic symptoms does not necessarily show that the patient is unfit for higher responsibilities; he may be needing them. One of the more trying occupational situations is to be second in command, with divided loyalties to the working group and the boss. A very irritating variant is to be in charge of a family business where the senior member of the family has nominally retired but continues to interfere.

Another type of work neurosis could be called 'work addiction'. The nature of work varies more than is realized. In many jobs the worker does not control the amount he has to do. The doctor's task is finished when his surgery is empty, the clerk has to leave the office when it shuts. There are other jobs in which the worker sets his own targets. This applies to salesmen, who are only 'as good as their last sale', to housewives who finish when they judge that their house is clean enough, and to executives. In these work situations it is essential that the worker be able to set realistic limits to his output. Obsessional personalities who are prone to make excessive demands on themselves are unable to do this. One patient, a managing director, sought advice because of a tension state from overwork. A tranquillizer was prescribed and on his next visit he said he felt fine, 'I've done twice as much work!' He relapsed later and only made a complete recovery after he had retired. It is important to help the patients to limit their output of work, sometimes by a change of occupation.

Chronic frustration is often seen in the married woman whose children are growing up. In spite of the romantic myths embedded in our culture, it is hard to believe that marriage and the care of children are sufficient aims to satisfy the total life of a woman. In the fifth decade of her life she may find herself with too little to do, endeavouring to extract from a tired husband and irritated children the emotional satisfactions which they find in part in their occupations outside the home. Much is written in the popular press about the social evils of women who go out to work, and it is true that few women can do this and also care satisfactorily for young children. But where the demands of the family are diminishing it is surely better to have a stable and contented mother even if she has important commitments outside the home, than a tense, irritable and frustrated woman whose sole mental stimulus is the routine of housework. Part-time jobs are helpful for the married women who have sought treatment for psychiatric disorders.

The care of the aged by the younger generation is a pious duty which is found in most religions and civilizations. Although the social good sense of this is too obvious to need discussion, it is as well to draw attention to the price paid by some vulnerable individuals in the course of carrying out this duty. The following case history is illustrative.

A man in his early forties sought advice for anxiety symptoms. Although he gave a history of symptoms for only a few years previously, the patterns of his earlier years showed only too clearly the influence of neurotic motivations, although he was unaware of this at the time.

His father had suffered a setback in the early 1930s due to the economic depression and was demoted to being a poorly paid clerk. Despite this drastically lowered income, they strove to maintain a façade of bourgeois respectability, although they scarcely had the financial means to sustain it. His mother was an hysterical personality who had the unfortunate tendency to fall ill if her wishes were not fulfilled. For many years the patient believed that these attacks might endanger his mother's life, and this led on his part to an attitude that at all costs he must prevent harm to others. If he failed in this perfectionistic task he was beset by a disabling feeling of guilt.

When the patient was in adolescence his father fell ill with a psychotic illness and was a patient for five years in a mental hospital where he died. The patient reacted by vowing never to marry but to support his widowed mother for the rest of her life. True to his pattern the patient held himself to blame for his father's illness and death, and by denying himself the emotional and instinctual gratification of marriage he managed to assuage his feelings of guilt. Moreover, believing mental illness to be hereditary, he could not contemplate inflicting himself—whom he regarded as a potential psychotic—on to a wife, nor could he bear the thought that such tendencies might be inherited by his children. This resolution was made easy by the fact that because of his neurotic conflicts he was almost entirely unaware of his sexual needs and was ignorant of all but the simplest physiological facts concerning reproduction. His mother naturally found this development in her son agreeable and did nothing to discourage it.

His overt illness was precipitated by falling in love. This relationship foundered very quickly, but it was sufficient to upset the precarious balance between his instincts and his guilt.

With the help of psychotherapy he obtained much insight into his problems but little relief. Although this unsatisfactory result was due in part to technical difficulties in the psychotherapy, a real and daunting obstacle was uncovered. He arrived at the stage when he could contemplate a sexual relationship with a woman and overcame his reservations to marriage. He then found that unmarried women of his own age group were uninviting regarding matrimony (naturally, as the others had married twenty years previously), while he found it hard to make contact with girls twenty years younger than himself. Moreover, as he pointed out, if he did meet an attractive woman of his own age group, it would be foolish to ask her to share a house with his mother who was still alive, and his salary would not support both a wife and his mother unless they lived in the same house.

This sort of difficulty is not uncommon in both sexes. Having refrained from marriage in early adult life, either on account of the demands of their parents or profession, or for neurotic reasons, such persons realize too late that they need marriage and a home. Some are fortunate enough to secure a suitable partner although aware that they have missed some of what marriage has to offer. Others marry unsuitably or not at all. It is small comfort to people in this predicament to point out that they could have avoided this trouble by an early marriage. In our experience, the success of treatment depends, among other things, on the absence of this type of frustration and deprivation.

Occupational achievement is also sacrificed at times to the care of parents. This is particularly true for professional occupations, when a career may be spoiled by refusing a post away from home. This type of difficulty, however, seems to be relatively unimportant in the histories of our neurotic patients.

The point that is being made in this chapter is that certain personal needs have to be satisfied if mental health is to be maintained. The individual needs to be sustained by the knowledge that he is secure in mutual affection with friends and other members of his family. Although marriage is usually the centre of this pattern of security, clearly it is not essential to it. Marriage is not needed by everyone, but loss of a partner by death, desertion or withdrawal of love can be an irremediable disaster for many. Secondly, each individual needs to have an accepted and acceptable place in his local community. Thirdly, he requires opportunities to express himself in work and to make himself required by the community. Naturally these needs are linked together; it might be more true to suggest that they are different expressions of a more fundamental need: to have and to know one has a place in the world. Men who undertake lonely occupations are nevertheless sustained by the knowledge that their services are essential. True social isolation—not to be needed by anyone—is probably incompatible with mental health.

Old people and especially widows are in grave danger of this type of social isolation. Cut off by bereavement from friends and family, unable through age to work, they realize with some bitterness that they are useless and a burden to others. It is no surprise that the statistics of suicide and mental illness are high in this group. When these states of deprivation are found—and at this stage it is unimportant whether they have been caused through misfortune or a faulty pattern of living—every effort must be made to make good the social deficiencies. Occupation is the most satisfactory answer, especially for the younger widow. Social clubs for old people go some way to providing an answer, but in each locality there is ample room for individual initiative in coping with this growing and distressing problem.

7

Functional Psychoses

It was said earlier (page 19) that there are mild forms of illnesses from the group called psychoses in which the patients have not lost insight and are therefore not psychotic in the sense of being overtly irrational. This situation causes much confusion and nowhere more so than in regard to depression. The confusion is made worse by the prevalence of different usages of the same terms and has probably been intensified paradoxically by the fact that varied treatment approaches to depression all have much to offer in cases which may seem identical. A brief account of the major classifications of depression may enable the reader to tolerate these complexities without being discomfited. If so he will have the chance in practice to experience some of the satisfactions of using his clinical skills on a common problem which has many different and interesting patterns.

ENDOGENOUS DEPRESSION

The student or doctor may find himself exposed to diverse alternative terms like endogenous and reactive, psychotic and neurotic, unipolar and bipolar depression. These have arisen from different attempts to classify depression. To make their consideration easier the pattern of what has been called endogenous depression will first be described.

Even a cursory examination of patients who complain of

anxiety and depression shows that there are many whose symptoms and history cannot be satisfactorily explained in terms of neurotic psychology and social stresses. These discrepancies fall roughly into three groups.

Previous personality

The previous personality may give little indication of the previous neurotic character traits. It has been said that he is a poor psychiatrist who cannot discover some psychopathology in those he examines; conversely, many neurotic patients may give an account of themselves which carefully, although unwittingly, avoids those topics in which their neurotic behaviour shows itself; yet, bearing all these points in mind, the general practitioner may often be puzzled in finding overt psychiatric disorder in a patient whom he has known intimately for many years as being free from neurotic behaviour. It is difficult for any man or woman to pass the age of thirty-five without being subject to emotional stresses of the type which easily precipitate neurotic illness. When the psychiatric illness occurs for the first time in middle life, and especially when previous emotional stresses such as bereavement have already been surmounted easily, it is hard to escape the conclusion that some fundamental change has occurred in the patient's personality which has brought about an alarming increase in emotional instability.

A careful history of the illness

This may also fail to demonstrate the adequate emotional stress which is found universally in neurotic illness. Of course the patient may not be telling the truth: it took one patient six months before she revealed that the cause of her inexplicable illness was an extramarital love affair. Other patients, without being deliberately untruthful, contrive to give the wrong impression. An illness which, from the patient's account, occurs spontaneously is revealed by the husband as no more than an acute exacerbation of a long-continuing neurotic state dating from the patient's last confinement. Yet, even when such examples have been excluded, there still remains a large group of patients who open consultation with the words: 'I should be the happiest person in the world ... ' and the family confirms the complete absence of stress. Even when emotional difficulties can be demonstrated, it is hard to explain why this stress, and not a previous one, has brought about the illness. In cases where there is long-sustained emotional stress, such as business worries, it is also hard to explain why the breakdown has come now, and not five years ago.

Here it is worth noting that depressive illnesses also result from certain physical agents. Head injury, especially if moderately severe, may be followed after some months, when recovery seems to be almost established, by the onset of depression. Quite often viral infections are followed after a few weeks by a phase of depression. This is particularly common with infective hepatitis and with some epidemics of influenza. Drugs such as reserpine and hypotensive agents may provoke depressive reactions. Similar episodes occur also in the first week after childbirth. A careful consideration, both of the premorbid personality and of the events leading to the onset of this illness, points therefore to the possibility of pathological processes in psychiatric illness other than neurotic. An examination of symptomatology confirms this hypothesis.

Pattern of endogenous depression

At the start of this chapter it was emphasized that depression, anxiety and allied symptoms can be produced in a number of ways. That is true. However, certain symptoms are more likely to be found in association with certain conditions than others, although at the best this is no more than a statistical correlation to which there are always exceptions. It is very rare in psychiatry for a symptom to be pathognomonic of a certain condition. The symptoms of the endogenous depression tend to differ from the neurotic in the following ways.

1. *Weight.* Loss of weight is common at the outset of neurotic illness, but it is rarely sustained or serious. It is not uncommon for depressives to lose up to two stones in weight,

and this loss continues until the patient begins to recover.

2. *Sleep.* Sleep is disturbed in every type of psychiatric illness, but in the depressive the major disturbance is a contraction of the amount of sleep needed, so that the patient wakes early, whether or not he has had difficulty in falling asleep.

3. *Diurnal variation.* In neurotic patients, as in normal people, anxiety and tension tend to increase with fatigue towards the end of the day. This occurs also in depressives, but they often also suffer an increase in symptoms on first waking which gradually diminishes as the day progresses until the onset of fatigue.

4. *Retardation.* Almost all patients with psychiatric illness complain of lack of energy and concentration. In neurotic depression this difficulty is subjective and testing reveals no significant impairment of intellectual performance. In depressives there is often a real decrease in ability to concentrate which can be objectively demonstrated.* The 'serial sevens' test is useful for this purpose. In well-developed examples of the depressive syndrome, a general slowing-up or retardation can be shown in movement, speech and thought, but in earlier cases this appears only as a difficulty in thinking and lack of concentration.

5. *Loss of interest.* In endogenous depression this is allied to retardation, but may also occur in patients who are tense and agitated. Zest is lost as well as pleasure in normal activity and pastimes. Nothing is enjoyable, nothing is worth doing and even a beloved grandchild raises no smiles. Both work which used to be enjoyed and normal pleasures are affected by persistent feelings of apathy. This is one of the most important changes which confirms the presence of psychiatric illness. In mild cases it may be the leading feature of the illness.

6. *Depression.* Depression is a universal experience; in the depressive syndrome it is marked by its extension, depth and quality. In the normal and neurotic person depression occurs in short spells, reacts favourably to pleasant changes of

---

* A similar result is also found in brain-damaged patients.

environment (for example, the arrival of a friend), and has an element of self-regard and self-pity. In the endogenous depression, the lowness of spirits is relatively unremitting and relatively uninfluenced by environmental changes. It frequently shows the diurnal variation described above. It is often associated with feelings of despair, hopelessness and self-reproach. The depressive will often have the feeling that he is at fault and is the cause of his condition, which is not a point of view that neurotic patients find attractive.

7. *Delusional ideas.* In severe depressives morbid ideas may arise with delusional force; these are never found in neurotic patients. Amongst the more common are delusions of guilt, unworthiness and poverty. Hypochondriacal fears are common in neurotic patients, but in depressives more irrational hypochondriacal delusions are found which cannot be influenced by reassurance: 'It is cancer, isn't it, Doctor?'—'My bowels are completely stopped up'.

8. *Mood swings.* In a few cases the patient is at times excessively cheerful, even elated and hypomanic, then he becomes depressed; or depression may be followed by states of elation. These states of elation are known as *mania* or *hypomania* and are described in Chapter 18. Although rare they are important because this pattern of alternating depression and elation constitutes a recognizable syndrome which is, to a considerable extent, autonomous.

For these reasons, therefore, many psychiatrists believe that there is an endogenous pathological process of depression which is probably physiological rather than psychological in nature. In fact, it seems likely that there are several types of *biochemical* or *neurophysiological* disturbances which separately or together contribute to the development of patterns of depressive illness. The proponents of this view point to the clinical differences noted above and to the fact that ECT (EST) appears to have a specific therapeutic effect on such conditions, while making neurotic patients worse. Other psychiatrists, pointing out the practical difficulties in assigning many cases clearly to one diagnosis or the other, regard depression as a continuum reaching from melancholia to neurosis, with no clear dividing line. There is much to be said for both points of view.

We suggest then that it is helpful as a working hypothesis to assume the existence of an endogenous pattern of depression, with clinical features described above. This may occur spontaneously or as a reaction to physical or psychological trauma. It may occur in stable or neurotic personalities. It may coexist with a neurotic illness, in which case there will be a residuum of neurotic symptoms requiring treatment after the endogenous element has been dealt with. On the other hand, it is to be expected that if an endogenous illness occurs in a neurotic personality, many neurotic symptoms will be produced as a response to the stress of the depressive illness. When that stress is removed by antidepressant treatment the neurotic symptoms may be expected to clear of their own accord. In such cases, the neurotic symptoms are no more than the spray thrown up above by the ground swell of depression—eye-catching, but unimportant; but the anxiety may be so extensive that the signs of the underlying depressive illness can be almost completely obscured except to careful examination.

We feel it is important to distinguish the reactive depression which is a neurotic response to environment and the depressive reaction which is an endogenous response precipitated by an environmental stress. The former is a true neurosis which will clear only when the psychological problems have been resolved or the environment has been changed. When an endogenous depression has been produced it will continue after the environmental stress has been removed until either it improves spontaneously or the appropriate treatment is given.

In many cases it is reasonable to make an estimate of the relative weight of endogenous and reactive (or neurotic) features. Thus one may describe a depression as mixed endogenous and reactive but more endogenous than reactive or vice versa. This discussion inevitably requires a further word about terminology. It is worth pointing out that the words *retarded* and *agitated*, which qualify particular types of depression, imply the term *endogenous*. *Neurotic* depression is often employed as an alternative term to *exogenous* or *reactive* depression. This is reasonable since, as we have shown, neurotic mechanisms are frequently extremely important in the development of reactive depressions; and they distinguish neurotic depression from endogenous depression without necessarily suggesting that stress does not provoke endogenous depression. However, there are also many essentially normal people who in the face of appropriate stress develop reactive depression. Neurotic depression would not cover this group and so has a slightly narrower but very useful connotation.

What has been described so far is a fairly standard British and often a European and sometimes a North American approach to the diagnosis and classification of depression. In North America there is however a greater tendency to use the words 'neurotic depression' for those illnesses in which there is no break from reality such as would be manifested by delusions, hallucinations, severe withdrawal or serious suicidal thoughts.

Psychotic depression, a controversial term, is used particularly in North America to refer to depressions in which there is a break from reality severe enough to be called psychotic where there is no previous history of severe depression or of cyclothymic mood swings. Such depressions have precipitants and mechanisms resembling neurotic depression. The label may be wrongly applied however to bipolar or recurrent depressive illnesses (see below) presenting for the first time. The writer's preference is to use the terms *endogenous depression*, *reactive depression* and *neurotic depression* in the meanings commonly employed in Britain. The term *psychotic depression* is avoided altogether. The student or practitioner will encounter alternative usages and should not be uncomfortable with them provided he has some notion of the way in which they are being employed.

PRIMARY AND SECONDARY AFFECTIVE ILLNESS

Another approach altogether to the classification of depressions is popular in America and presents useful scientific features. This approach distinguishes affective illnesses, that is, those with anxiety, depression or elation, as either primary or secondary. Primary depressions are those which arise in people who have been previously well or whose only past psychiatric illnesses were depression or mania. These primary depressions are divided into unipolar affective illnesses and bipolar affective illnesses. In a first attack of depression without previous depression or mania, or in recurrent depression without previous mania, the illness is called unipolar. If the first attack of illness is mania, or if mania and depression have both occurred the illness is bipolar. This classification has been shown to be genetically and therapeutically relevant; bipolar cases have more bipolar near relatives and do better with lithium treatment. The pattern of depression in bipolar cases is also usually marked by biological ('endogenous') features. The kernel of this approach is thus to identify those illnesses resembling manic-depressive illness in older classifications and use them as a cornerstone of the diagnostic system.

By contrast the secondary affective illnesses are those which arise in patients who have other psychiatric conditions, for example schizophrenia, alcoholism, chronic anxiety. In the latter case they are usually depressions. Secondary affective disorders are also often associated with systemic illness or drug reactions, for example endocrine disorders, reserpine, amphetamines and steroids. A few secondary disorders due to drugs may be manic and even bipolar.

One disadvantage of this classification is that it may require hindsight for correct diagnosis. Another is that it does not regularly utilize the occurrence of the important data about patterns which may guide treatment. Its advantage has been to encourage systematic research and although it is not a definitive diagnostic tool (Klerman[37]) it is reasonably intended as a step towards describing multiple diagnostic groups. These varied systems present the reader with the problem of choice. A number of psychiatrists identify unipolar depression with endogenous depression but that is not strictly correct. However bipolar depression will always resemble endogenous depression and unipolar depression will do so most of the time. Secondary depression and neurotic depression will tend to label comparable cases but some unipolar depressions will be equivalent to neurotic depressions.

No matter how carefully clinical observations are made and diagnostic terms are defined, it must be admitted that difficulties remain. Antidepressants such as imipramine can on occasions bring relief to illnesses which would seem to be typical anxiety states. Forensic psychiatrists report that when a severe illness has led to murder, there are some cases in which the commission of the crime has been followed by a complete remission of the psychiatric symptoms. It may be that a lingering dualism clouds our thinking when we try to separate endogenous illnesses believed to arise out of a biochemical disturbance from reactive disorders in which the cause is thought to be psychological. It seems more probable that both the psychological and the physiological disturbances represent observations at different levels of the total pathology of depressive illness. The starting point for the illness may lie in events which can be most conveniently described in psychological terms or in events of a physiological nature; the end point of depression is the same.

Aetiology

It is worth noting at this point that the aetiology of depression is linked to disturbances of brain amine metabolism. The principal amines considered are the catecholeamines (epinephrine and norepinephrine) and 5-hydroxytryptamine (serotonin). Deficiencies of either catecholeamines or 5-hydroxytryptamine in the diencephalon are thought to be present in depression. It is not known if a single deficiency can cause depression or whether combined deficiencies or maldistribution of amines within the central nervous system are responsible. The most likely speculation is that several different patterns of amine disturbance may be involved in depression. Depressions which are clinically similar might be caused by different amine changes; and depressions which are clinically dissimilar might nevertheless have an identical biochemistry. There is a little evidence to date that two types of depression may be distinguished by CSF amine changes, but the phenomenology (that is, the clinical syndromes) has not been separated out. The relevance of this to drug treatment is considered later (see p. 393).

Notwithstanding the biochemical evidence it is also known, as we have remarked, that significant psychological events may cause, and skilful psychological management may relieve, depression. Thus irrespective of the events leading to the illness, most patients will benefit from pharmacological support to the biochemical systems and relationship support to the psychological systems; essentially these are palliative treatments. Full recovery probably involves the activation of homeostatic mechanisms, both physiological and psychological, whose nature is still obscure.

The concept of neurotic depression implies that only the 'psyche' is disturbed and that physiological processes are left unchanged. It must be true that in some patients there are no significant physiological disturbances; but the other cases who make a complete recovery with psychotherapy may be those who have a physical disturbance but whose homeostatic mechanisms are especially responsive to psychological stimuli. Until we possess trustworthy means of detecting the presence of physiological disorders it will be difficult to distinguish between the patients who are simply unhappy and those who are truly depressed but who are responsive to a psychological approach. Thus it may be that there are some patients whose symptoms are alleviated by antidepressants but in whom full recovery must await a significant change at a psychological level.

Difficulty often arises when a patient gives a previous history of psychiatric illness. Although there may be evidence of neurotic difficulties in adjustment, it must also be remembered that the endogenous depression tends to recur. A careful history may reveal the circumstances of each illness, but the memory of patients is not always reliable. A previous history of recovery with ECT (EST) or a particular antidepressant may be a useful clue as to the nature of the illness. Fortunately, patients with recurrent illnesses rarely change the pattern.

The natural history of this type of endogenous depression is not easy to determine. It may recur in regular episodes with a periodicity varying from six months to over ten years, it may occur as a single episode in later life, or unpredictably. Occasionally attacks of depression may alternate with, or be followed by, periods of elation, an observation which led to the concept of manic-depressive insanity. Endogenous depression does occur in children, although it is uncommon until the third decade of life. Attacks of endogenous depression which occur for the first time in the postclimacteric period are sometimes referred to as a special category of involutional depression. This is mainly because they tend to show rather often a pattern of agitated behaviour with marked hypochondriasis which is often delusional, and sometimes schizophrenic-like hallucinations. Current opinion, as a result of systematic investigation, holds that these illnesses are not a distinct affective disorder. They may well take their pattern from the pathoplastic effects of age in influencing symptoms. Some writers use the label 'affective disorder' which covers all the syndromes of endogenous depression without expressing a firm opinion as to whether these syndromes are nosologically distinct. Thus a puerperal depression is an endogenous depression which occurs in the puerperium. There is a strong likelihood of recurrence after succeeding confinements, but otherwise it shows no important diagnostic differences from other depressions in the same age group.

Personalities prone to depression merit some consideration. They fall into three groups. Obsessional personalities (*v.s.*) are very prone to depressive reactions, and most obsessional neuroses are accompanied by a disturbance of mood. The rigid, perfectionistic traits of this personality are found very commonly in those patients who suffer their first attack of depression in the involutional period of life. Other authors point out that inadequate and self-effacing personalities are also especially prone to involutional disorder. More well known, though actually less common in current clinical practice is the cycloid temperament described by Kretchmer. This may manifest itself either in a dour, pessimistic and retiring disposition or in a buoyant, energetic and optimistic character ('the life and soul of the party'), or in the cyclothymic temperament where the two moods alternate with a regular and predictable rhythm. It is obvious that morbid depression and elation are pathological caricatures of this temperament, which often seems to occur in men of superior ability.

SCHIZOPHRENIA

Clinical diagnosis

The depressive syndrome discussed in the last section is not the only endogenous mechanism that has to be considered. Especially in younger patients, early schizophrenia also presents a diagnostic hazard.

At the start of such an illness, and perhaps for many months, the clinical picture differs considerably from the established cases of chronic schizophrenia. The patients usually complain of an insidious depression, often with physical symptoms such as headaches and hypochondriacal fears. Careful examination shows a number of features which are not typical of either neurotic depression or the endogenous depressive response.

The initial impression is often that of a neurotic illness. The patients are usually in their twenties or early thirties, which is a favoured age for the start of a neurosis. The personality of the patient before his illness often shows neurotic character traits and signs of emotional inadequacy in personal relationships. Once the suspicions of the clinician have been aroused by the history, he will find his doubts supported by the behaviour of the patient; instead of the dependent, clinging attitude of the depressed neurotic patient, the doctor is faced with a curious lack of interest towards his examination and therapeutic suggestions. He may gain the impression that the patient is so wrapped up in his illness that a discussion of treatment seems irrelevant.

Once the diagnosis of neurosis is questioned, the doctor may then consider whether he is not dealing with the endogenous response of depression. Again his enquiries fail to establish the expected facts: no weight loss, no early waking, no diurnal variation, although morbid ideas of unworthiness, self-reproach and suicide are often present. Sometimes the doctor is impressed by a curious anomaly in the emotional tone of the patient's personal relationships. This change, which is difficult to describe, has been noted by many clinicians. Unfortunately, the appreciation of this change depends upon the subjective response of the examiner, and it is not a reliable sign on which to base a diagnosis. The blunting of emotional responses which is correctly described in accounts of schizophrenia may mislead the reader into believing that the schizophrenic lacks emotion and feeling. Of course, poverty of feeling is not infrequent, but more often the schizophrenic patient is at the mercy of strong and violent feelings which can occasionally lead him to uncontrolled outbursts of rage or savage suicidal acts.

The pathognomonic disturbance of feeling is more subtle than this. Quite simply, other people seem to matter less. On entering the room one misses the reorientation of interest and feeling with which non-schizophrenic patients greet a visitor. At the end of an examination, most psychiatric patients have manifestly changed in their feelings towards the doctor. The resentment, indifference or even hostility, which is the first reaction of so many patients, gives way to feelings of trust and confidence. This sort of change is so little shown by schizophrenics that the physician complains that he has not been able to establish rapport with the patient. Even if the schizophrenic turns with feeling towards the doctor, one is left with the impression that such attitudes are fleeting and unreliable. The patient's family, if perceptive, will have noticed similar changes. It must be stressed that this type of emotional coolness becomes apparent only when one tries to make a personal contact with the patient; the schizophrenic may talk of people who are not present with a normal emotional warmth. This lack of rapport which is found with a schizophrenic must not be confused with the tense and guarded behaviour of a hostile neurotic patient. In spite of a façade of blank indifference, the latter will be found to be vitally concerned with the doctor's response to him, although his concern may be shown only by an occasional glance out of the corner of his eye towards the person who is asking the questions. In a similar way a very retarded depressed patient may unwittingly simulate schizophrenic coldness. With these patients it is very difficult to explain why one feels that the lack of emotional response is due not to an emotional aloofness but to an inability to project feelings in words and gestures. Of course, the history and clinical signs point unmistakably to the correct diagnosis when the illness is well developed.

The acute onset of schizophrenia also rarely presents problems in diagnosis. In the first few words the patient usually reveals serious abnormalities in his state of mind.

Disorders of thinking are frequent in schizophrenia. In early cases which present with depression this may be no more than the inability to control the sequence of associations and thoughts. After a short conversation the examining physician finds himself confused and far away from the point after which he was enquiring. The relatives may have noticed a real impairment of the patient's ability to accomplish mental work. In acute cases, thought disorder can show itself in a more striking fashion, with a bizarre use of words and an eccentric approach to intellectual problems which eventually may lead to a complete disorganization of the patient's thinking.

Ideas of bodily disease and disorder are commonly found in schizophrenic depression. Sometimes they are so bizarre as to leave no doubt about the diagnosis ('My blood is going round the wrong way'), but usually they are more vague and nondescript, lacking the entrancing detail with which hysterics describe their complaints.

The question of paranoid ideas deserves more discussion. The adjective *paranoid* is widely and sometimes loosely used by psychiatrists. It really has two distinct meanings. In the first of these it is used to describe states of mind in which delusions are prominent. A delusion is defined as a false belief which the patient holds and which would not be accepted by other members of his own subcultural group. Delusions occur in other illnesses besides schizophrenia but paranoid schizophrenia is that form of it in which delusional thinking or delusional beliefs are major features. Very often these beliefs include the idea that other people are hostile to the patient; inevitably many patients with delusions find that others object to their views. These patients thus readily tend to feel that others are persecuting them. From this a second use of the word (paranoid) has developed to imply feelings of suspicion and hostility or of being aggrieved or persecuted. Paranoid in this use may refer to the aggressive neurotic patient with a chip on his shoulder who misinterprets the reactions of other people to his own hostile behaviour; it may apply to the timid virgin, uneasily aware of her sexuality, who feels that she is the cynosure of all eyes when she first walks across the ballroom floor: both attitudes are neurotic exaggerations of normal experience and are open to reason and reassurance. Indeed, the patients concerned often have intellectual insight into the irrational nature of their feelings. Patients with a depressive illness also not uncommonly exhibit persecutory fears, but in this case they are experienced as the inevitable response of others to their guilt, unworthiness and sin. 'They're coming to take me to prison' is only another way of saying that one is too wicked to be left at large.

In contrast to these situations some delusions of the schizophrenic are primary and cannot be demonstrated as contingent on other psychopathology, although they often follow a period of uneasy feeling in which others seem to show a spontaneous hostile interest in the patient. In such primary delusions ordinary objects are endowed with an additional significance or a changed appearance to the individual. Thus the captain of a submarine saw his vessel 'all silver' and gleaming. Frequently, the patient is at a loss to account for this change, but consistently misinterprets everyday events as personally relevant to him in some obscurely threatening way. This delusional state of mind may persist for some time or may crystallize out in explicit delusions of persecution which 'explain' these sinister happenings to the patient. So he believes he is being 'watched' (not 'looked at'—which describes a neurotic sense of embarrassment), his conversation and perhaps even his thoughts are being recorded on tape; newspapers, wireless and television make guarded but unequivocal references to his 'case'. In hospital he doubts the authenticity of his fellow patients, wondering if they are not members of the hospital staff (or worse) spying on him.

Frequently, the suspiciousness of the depressed and paranoid patient will also be shown in his attitude towards the examiner. Hostility may be shown more openly, as in a refusal to submit to an examination. Although patients with a neurotic or depressive illness may be reluctant to submit to an examination, they are sufficiently appreciative of the demands of the routine social courtesies to cooperate unwillingly. A blank refusal or a precipitate exit from the consulting room in defiance of social conventions should at once raise the suspicion of schizophrenia in the mind of the examining physician. On the other hand it is surprising how often patients will speak freely about their ideas of persecution once the topic is raised. Frequently, their behaviour is ill-assorted with their ideas: believing themselves to be persecuted they seek the solace of a medical consultation instead of complaining to the police or consulting a solicitor. One characteristic sign of schizophrenia is this incongruity among thought content, emotional response and behaviour. Such patients may show a surprising cheerfulness although preoccupied with what would be thought-distressing and peculiar ideas.

The presence of persecutory ideas or delusions should not by itself be regarded as evidence of schizophrenia. The delusions should be primary, having the characteristics outlined and they should occur in clear consciousness, and other signs of schizophrenia should be present. Patients suffering from organic cerebral impairment which causes delirium (Chapter 18) or dementia (Chapters 8, 13) may also show delusions; manic patients may have delusions about their ability and powers, and become hostile when frustrated, leading the inexperienced to diagnose paranoid or excited schizophrenia. Some patients have gross hallucinatory, persecutory or depressive symptoms but do not show the pathognomonic signs of schizophrenia. They can usually be regarded as having a schizophreniform psychosis with a different (better) prognosis than classical schizophrenia. Occasionally patients are encountered who have a psychotic breakdown under stress which may look to the uninitiated—and sometimes to the experienced—like a case of schizophrenia. These psychoses are rare. They occur most often in patients with both hysterical and sociopathic characteristics. In Britain they are called psychoses in hysterical psychopaths. In North America they are often called 'borderline states' and are assimilated without justification to schizophrenia. Culturally conditioned delusional illnesses especially in patients of rural background with relatively poor education (for example, some West Indians) should also be considered when appropriate and not necessarily diagnosed as schizophrenia. The psychoses of subnormal (retarded) patients likewise often lack typical schizophrenic characteristics and should be simply called psychoses in the retarded unless they do show the classical signs of passivity and alienation to a sufficient extent. It is noteworthy, however, that there is a modest but definite increase in subnormality amongst those diagnosed as having schizophrenia.

The leading signs which permit a generally acceptable diagnosis of schizophrenia are passivity feelings. The fundamental nature of this experience is for the patient to feel that his mind and occasionally his body are under the influence of some outside force. This is most often ascribed by the patient to. hypnosis, and a complaint of being hypnotized almost always has this significance except for the occasional patient who has consulted a medical hypnotist. Passivity experiences are sometimes known as alienation experiences since in them some part or function of the individual seems to have come under external control, as happens with feelings of influences affecting the body or other persons reading the thoughts or whispering in his ears. 'Thought control' and 'thought transference' are also common expressions used by such patients to describe feelings of passivity. It is extraordinary how such phrases when used by a physician are meaningless to non-schizophrenic patients, but are immediately understood by schizophrenics who have experienced feelings of passivity. This immediate understanding by patients of the language of schizophrenic existence is widely used by psychiatrists in the diagnosis of schizophrenia.

Another well-known term in the schizophrenic vocabulary is *the voices*. Hallucinations, like delusions, do not occur only in schizophrenia. Other psychotics, some hysterics and even perfectly normal people in states of drowsiness may have very vivid hallucinations. Moreover, contrary to what might be expected, it is not so obvious why schizophrenics speak of the voices, although they often mention them. Only in florid cases does this term have the same meaning for normals as for schizophrenics. Then indeed the patient is shouted at, sworn at, mocked as if loudspeakers were invisibly placed around the patient. But this is not the common experience in the early stages of the disease. The so-called voice may be no more than an autonomous train of thought which presents itself to the patient as if it came from another person. So one patient while in the act of purchasing some clothes was startled by the thought: 'You'll never need these'. 'It was', she explained, 'as if somebody had whispered in my ear.' These experiences differ from the compulsive thoughts in an obsessional neurosis or indeed from the stray thoughts which are found unpredictably in the minds of all of us from time to time by one salient characteristic: they feel as if they do not belong to the patient. This characteristic shows itself in a number of ways; they occur unexpectedly and usually are unrelated to his conscious stream of thought so that the patient is startled by their presence and not infrequently shocked by their content, which may be obscene or accusatory. They are not under his voluntary control and can be neither suppressed nor encouraged. Frequently, they are intrusive and have a stronger claim on his attention than the demands of his environment. In the deepest sense of the word, the patient feels that they do not belong to him. This is in contrast to the obsessional neurotic patient who has to admit that the compulsive thoughts do arise from somewhere inside his own mind, however distasteful they may be. These hallucinatory thoughts have a strange and unaccustomed feeling: they are so clearly alien to himself that the patient at once disclaims ownership, rather in the same way as when one picks up the wrong coat after a party. It is obvious at once that the coat belongs to someone else, although it may take a careful inspection before the point can be proved. Such hallucinatory experiences can of course occur when consciousness is clouded, perhaps by drugs or simply in the twilight state of falling asleep or waking up, when their significance is usually trivial; their occurrence in clear consciousness, however, almost always indicates the presence of schizophrenia.

Similar dogmatic assertions cannot be made about hallucinations in other sense modalities, but these are usually unformed and inchoate: a bright light in the room, a blue flame above the heads of others, and so on. Visions, in which the image of a person occurs, often speaking but without moving, are more commonly found in hysterical personalities and, indeed, if the hagiographers are to be believed, in persons whose sanity was beyond question. In any case, such experiences can be shown to be lacking in the characteristic independent quality of schizophrenic hallucinosis, so that frequently they reflect the dominant trends in the subject's affectivity. Hallucinations of taste, smell and enteroceptive feeling also occur in schizophrenia, but are also sometimes associated with abnormal electrical activity in the temporal lobe, and on their own do not command the diagnosis of schizophrenia.

These then are the characteristics of schizophrenia. Those which are thought to be pathognomonic have been called first rank symptoms; they include the range of passivity experienced. Before such signs ever appear suspicion is aroused either by the fact that the clinical pattern of the illness does not fit easily into that of neurosis or depression or, perhaps, by the unexpected failure to respond to appropriate treatment. The suspicion deepens when it is noted that only a faulty rapport is obtained with the patient, and on enquiry pathognomonic signs of schizophrenia are elicited: thought disorder, primary delusions, passivity feelings, auditory hallucinations. In recent years joint international studies, especially between the United States and the United Kingdom, but also including other countries, have led to an increasingly conservative attitude towards the diagnosis of schizophrenia. It is now only diagnosed in many centres after careful demonstration of the presence of passivity and alienation experiences. The American Psychiatric Association, in accordance with some Scandinavian thinking, currently recommends that schizophrenia should only be diagnosed in those who have shown signs of the illness for at least six months. To the present writer this is illogical but at least it errs on the side of caution. If that practice is followed illnesses resembling schizophrenia but of lesser duration have to be called schizophrenia-like.

The distinction between schizophrenia and endogenous depression is sometimes difficult. A mood of depression is not uncommon in schizophrenia, as has already been explained, and does not affect the diagnosis. On the other hand, cases are found in which classical signs of both endogenous depression and schizophrenia occur together, and it can be almost impossible to allot diagnostic precedence to one or the other. Such cases are often labelled *schizo-affective* disorders. The final outcome of these cases usually resolves the problem one way or the other, but it may be extremely difficult at the outset to predict what is going to happen. A very different nosological problem is the occasional patient in the involutional period of life who presents with unequivocal signs of schizophrenia, but who responds to treatment and has a good prognosis in a manner identical with the depression. There is reason to think that such patients are better treated as cases of manic-depressive (bipolar) illness with lithium and/or antidepressants rather than with neuroleptic drugs like phenothiazines. Very occasionally, however, a patient may require both types of treatment.

Schizophrenia is also described in four syndromes having regard to which clinical features predominate. In the first, simple schizophrenia, often the only sign of the disease is a blunting of the emotional responses. Those with this form of the illness are prone to become drifters in society, tramps and human flotsam sleeping indifferently on London's Embankment or the park benches of other cities. Further reference is made to these cases in the section on chronic unemployment.

In the second type, catatonic schizophrenia, there are serious disorders of volition, which are most commonly shown in negativism. In this condition the patient automatically carries out the opposite of any request or command. He falls silent when asked about his complaints, but breaks out into speech when the doctor rises to leave; when asked to close his eyes he opens them wider and so on. This naturally leads to difficulties for those responsible for his nursing care. In other cases the patient will spend long periods in fixed postures; often these are accidentally chosen and he seems unable to initiate normal positive actions. In chronic cases the limbs hang immobile with cyanotic extremities. When the examiner alters their position, perhaps to some bizarre posture, they may stay in it indefinitely. Such patients tend to speak little and seem inaccessible but on recovery may give a complete and precise account of events that occurred around them during the time of their immobility. At other times they may burst into phases of excitement and this sometimes produces a psychiatric emergency. Catatonic schizophrenia with its famous waxy flexibility in which the patient's limbs remain in unusual positions, as arranged by the examiner, is now extremely rare in Europe and North America. Catatonic immobility may also occur as a result of organic lesions, for example, of the midbrain.

The third main, conventionally described type is the hebephrenic or 'foolish'. This is characterized by massive disorders of thinking; in it blocking of thought and incongruity of affect—perhaps with fatuous grimacing—are notable; it is frequently accompanied by passivity experiences, delusional ideas and mannerisms and antics.

The fourth type is the paranoid, and this merits further attention. The occurrence of delusional or paranoid ideas has already been described, and these may be present in all types of schizophrenia but when they dominate the picture the condition is called paranoid schizophrenia. There is also an important group of patients, generally over the age of thirty-five, who develop paranoid illnesses but without the general deterioration, disintegration, flattening or withdrawal characteristic of the other schizophrenic syndromes. In these patients there is an organized system of delusion, at times associated with hallucinations. Some writers include these conditions in paranoid schizophrenia, others distinguish them as paraphrenia and still others call them merely paranoid states or paranoid psychoses. Since these conditions all shade into each other the use of one particular term rather than another is less important than recognition of the different trends which predominate—whether to disintegration of the personality or organization of delusions. It is probably simplest to call these cases paranoid schizophrenia so long as schizophrenic characteristics are discernible in them; the others may be called paranoid states or psychoses. At the same time it must always be noted whether there is disintegration or preservation of the general personality structure. In the latter case it will often be possible for the patient to remain outside hospital despite the presence of firmly held delusions so long as these do not lead to antisocial behaviour or suicide.

In limited respects these four syndromes may be of help in assessing prognosis or planning treatment, and they represent convenient ways of noting the four common clinical pictures. Their value, however, scarcely goes beyond that. A patient's symptoms may change from one syndrome to the other, or contain elements drawn from more than one of the syndromes.

In a few cases schizophrenia or an illness closely resembling it (schizophreniform psychosis) appears to be the result of brain disease. Routine skull X rays are reported to have revealed an unsuspected cerebral tumour in 1.4 per cent of schizophrenic patients, a proportion much higher than in the general population.[40] Schizophrenia also occurs more frequently than expected in cases of epilepsy, general paresis, narcolepsy and head injury. The psychological disorders found in this group of patients are indistinguishable from those of other schizophrenics.

Management and treatment

The difficulties in the diagnosis of schizophrenia are only the beginning of the doctor's problems. It is easy to lay down the principles of treatment: the major tranquillizers and ECT (EST) will control the more florid symptoms; depot neuroleptics are frequently needed for those who will not take medication and have been unequivocally shown to be effective; hospital care but not admission is almost always desirable; and early rehabilitation in a work environment. But this simple prescription reckons without the patient's family. Almost all families are deeply involved in the patient's emotional disturbance, and this is especially true if the patient is young and unmarried. Serious emotional problems, such as the patient's behaviour and illness, are glossed over in an unrealistic demonstration of understanding which Morris and Wynne called 'pseudomutuality'.[61] The doctor, therefore, may find it very difficult to persuade the parents that the young person is ill and in need of treatment; at a later stage the family may 'rescue' the patient and remove him from hospital against medical advice. At other times the family will suddenly reject the patient and demand his immediate admission to hospital. Attempts to rehabilitate the patient into an independent existence will be foiled by their efforts to keep him at home.

Although there are many studies of the families of schizophrenics which amply confirm these clinical impressions,[11] the importance of these observations is far from clear. One school of thought[41] holds that schizophrenia is the only adjustment open to patients who are subject to the emotional pressures engendered in such families, but it can be argued with equal force that the family disturbance represents their failure to cope with the developing illness of one of their members. Much more has been written than proved in support of the first point of view. There is certainly evidence that the onset of schizophrenia is associated with emotional stress. Eitinger[20] showed that the prevalence of schizophrenia in refugees in Norway after the Second World War was nearly five times that of the indigenous population; in more settled conditions Brown and Birley[12] demonstrated that life changes and crises frequently precipitated the acute onset, relapse or exacerbation of schizophrenic states. It has further been shown that patients exposed after discharge from hospital to family members who frequently express criticism of them are more likely than others to relapse.[77] On the other hand, the writers have sometimes observed the conflicts and tensions of the family resolve once the schizophrenic member has been successfully treated and rehabilitated. More important, the families of children with Down's syndrome may show comparable disturbances. There is probably no need to choose absolutely between the rival hypotheses: the failure of the family to adjust to the patient's difficulties even prior to the frank onset of symptoms will necessarily mean that the family atmosphere will become pathogenic rather than a helpful influence. However, the frequent suggestion that patients with schizophrenia have developed their illness because of stifling treatment in their families is a wounding assertion which lacks scientific evidence. Nevertheless on any formulation it is seen to be necessary to rehabilitate the majority of unmarried schizophrenics away from their families.

Faced with these complexities it is hardly necessary to urge that specialist advice is necessary for the management and treatment of schizophrenia. It is the gravest of all functional psychoses and even with modern methods of treatment its prognosis is uncertain. However there has been considerable improvement in the prognosis since the introduction of ECT (EST) and phenothiazines together with active programmes of rehabilitation, job-finding and the provision of hostel accommodation. In about half those affected a symptomatic recovery can be obtained, secured if necessary by the use of long-acting depot injections of fluphenazine and a recent thiaxanthene drug flupenthixol or yet another preparation, fluspirilene; in the remainder there will be some deterioration of personality and emotional responses leading perhaps to a degradation in their occupational status. Long-term follow-up suggests that repeated attacks are liable to occur requiring hospital treatment, although now only a small percentage require the permanent shelter of the long-stay wards of a mental hospital. Preservation of emotional responses is perhaps the best prognostic sign, but even in these cases perhaps one-third will have further attacks; in the remainder the proportion of cases which relapse may rise to two-thirds.

8
Physical Illness and Psychiatric Disorder

So far in our discussion of psychiatric pathology we have considered the psychological difficulties of the neuroses, the complicating effects of social factors and the quasi-physiological disturbances of the endogenous illnesses of depression and schizophrenia. The last and by no means least important process which often has to be reckoned with in the final formulation is the effect of frank physical pathology in the central nervous system.

BRAIN DAMAGE

The physician comes across the problem of brain damage in a variety of ways. Sometimes there are atypical features in a depressed and anxious patient which lead to hesitation; sometimes it is the failure to respond to psychiatric treatment which indicates an omission in the provisional diagnosis. All such cases clearly involve a neuropsychiatric deficit of a chronic nature; more acute interruptions of brain function lead to the typical syndromes of delirium which is discussed in Chapter 18, or of dysmnesic states which are described in Chapter 14. Chronic diffuse brain damage leads to a widespread disturbance of psychological functions which is called

dementia when it develops in adult life. It consists princi-
pally of an impairment of intellectual function, powers of
judgement, reasoning and memory. Such loss of function can
also be due to more localized disease and may be quite specific at times, for example on occasion the loss may only be
for constructing simple designs in two or three dimensions or
for reading but not for writing. Sometimes also these impairments are reversible, even if chronic, as in some cases of
general paralysis of the insane (GPI) after treatment.

The characteristic clinical syndrome results from the fusion
of two different psychopathological processes. In the first
place there are the psychological signs of brain damage which
are virtually the same no matter what the underlying pathology is; second, there are psychological symptoms which are
determined by the basic personality of the patient. A man,
therefore, who is liable to react to stress with depression will
experience a sharp depression if his nervous system is assaulted by the *Treponema pallidum*. The signs of brain damage
will distinguish this depression from one which results only
from a psychological stress. The syndrome of depression and
brain damage will be the same whether the pathology is infective or space-occupying; as a rule only the neurological
signs and other investigations will distinguish between the
different physical pathologies, the psychological signs of
brain damage usually being produced in common by all
pathologies. This point is of some importance in that, for
example, it is often assumed that GPI is accompanied by an
expansive euphoria, but this is true in only 50 per cent of
cases. The remainder are depressed or show symptoms remi-
niscent of neurosis or schizophrenia or simple dementia.
What is probably nearer the truth is that the type of man
who is most liable to contract syphilis is a happy-go-lucky
extravert who is not averse to casual sexual contacts. Brain
damage, which produces a caricature of the personality,
parodies his natural *bonhomie* in a foolish elation.

The characteristic psychological deficit which results from
brain damage is the impairment of the ability to respond to
new situations with intelligent behaviour. Naturally this
affects all aspects of behaviour, and the resulting syndrome
is termed *dementia*. Such a patient can be distinguished from

one with subnormal intelligence by the fact that the life history of the demented shows evidence, for example, in his occupational history, of abilities superior to his present condition; the subnormal patient presents a consistent history of below-average ability. Psychological tests can demonstrate that the patient's present ability to learn and reason are inadequate for acquiring the information and knowledge which he in fact possesses. Therefore, his past level of ability was superior to the present level, and some intellectual deterioration has taken place.

At first, these changes are very subtle and may be noticed only in the most complex discriminatory functions. The judgement of the businessman becomes unreliable, and he begins to lose money; the papers of the research worker are not up to his usual standard. Disturbances of interest and concentration can later be demonstrated. Partly due to lack of attention, memory begins to be faulty especially for day-to-day events. Although impairment can be demonstrated in retention, memory for events of long ago is often surprisingly well preserved.

Social insight is almost always damaged, so that the patient often becomes self-centred and demanding, quite oblivious of the effects of his actions on others. This may allow surprising lapses of behaviour, such as urinating in public or sexual perversions. Brain damage must always be considered when a hitherto respectable man commits an uncharacteristic act of indecency or antisocial offence. Another frequent emotional change is lability of mood in which tears and laughter can be too easily provoked.

In some cases insight is lost, so that the patient has no appreciation of the extent of the changes which have occurred to him. He may not be able to appreciate, for example, that he has lost his job because of increasing inefficiency at work. It is generally believed that loss of insight is more commonly found when the neurones are attacked directly by the disease process (as in degenerations or in GPI). When the brain damage is secondary to vascular disease, insight is more often preserved and the condition runs a fluctuating course.

Amongst signs which are sought as carefully by psychiatrists as neurologists are aphasia, and in particular the simple difficulty in naming objects, and constructional apraxia which is the inability to reproduce simple designs especially from memory.

It will be expected that not all the signs will be present in every patient, and an isolated finding is of doubtful significance. Many patients with retarded depression or schizophrenia will show serious lapses of interest and concentration, and this may lead to memory difficulties. This, however, will not progress to disorientation in time and space, which is almost pathognomonic of brain damage. Difficulties in concentration and memory in excess of what might be expected from the level of depression often indicate an underlying dementia.

The demonstration of the exact nature of the physical pathology usually depends on neurological and laboratory findings. Although a full discussion of the various types of lesion involved is outside the scope of this book, it may be helpful to indicate those which are most commonly encountered in psychiatric practice. From the age of fifty-five onwards, cerebral arterial disease and Alzheimer's disease (which refers to progressive degeneration both in the presenile and the senile) are the most common causes of brain damage. Although each can present a characteristic clinical picture the conditions overlap more often than by chance. About half the elderly demented patients have Alzheimer's disease at post-mortem, less than one-third have signs of cerebral softening from infarcts and about 10 to 20 per cent show both types of pathology. The prognosis is overall rather bad; in one series 75 per cent of patients who were admitted to hospital with these conditions died within two years. However this may not represent the prognosis of patients outside hospital. Occasionally degenerative conditions similar to senile dementia occur in younger age groups (the presenile dementias) but apart from Huntington's chorea, it is hard to predict the type of degeneration from clinical signs alone. Neurosyphilis used to rank high in the causes of dementia, but is now rarely encountered. Frequently, the physical signs amount to no more than a tremor of the tongue and hands with the characteristic pupillary changes. Head injury, anaesthetic anoxia and other trauma account for a small percentage of cases.

The delineation of some cases due to a transmissible 'slow' virus, usually with additional signs of disease such as extrapyramidal involvement, muscle wasting or spasticity is a notable scientific advance. The patients with these features mainly correspond to the Jakob-Creutzfeldt syndrome and are relatively rare.

In the case which presents routinely in the surgery with a suggestion of dementia the practitioner should think first, even in older people, of a space-occupying lesion. Amongst older patients vascular and degenerative conditions are much more common but even here a search should be made for treatable organic diseases. A common pitfall is the easy assumption that signs of dementia in an elderly patient are the result of cerebral vascular disease, until a colleague demonstrates papilloedema. Another problem in treatment occurs when there are signs both of depression and dementia in elderly patients. The presence of depression often exaggerates the signs of brain damage, so that if antidepressant treatment is given (drugs, not ECT (EST)) the improvement in mood leads to a regression of the 'dementia'.

Apart from the possibility of treating depression it is also important not to miss the possibility of treating some cases of true dementia which are due to organic disease and which can at least be partly recoverable. It used to be held that confusional states implied remedial organic disease but dementia reflected an irreversible process. This is no longer always so in regard to dementia. The distinction between confusional states and dementia is that in the former there is a fluctuating level of awareness. In the latter there is a static or progressive loss of one or more intellectual abilities, for example, memory, problem solving, learning ability. Treatable conditions which may cause such impairment include myxoedema, pernicious anaemia, hypoglycaemia, porphyrinuria, extreme dietary neglect, uraemia and normal pressure hydrocephalus. The last of these conditions is one in which fibrosis around the basilar cisterns may give rise to a progressive internal hydrocephalus which is relatively easy to relieve neurosurgically by shunting. Such relief is often followed by considerable improvement. For these reasons specialist psychiatric or neurological investigation is indicated in suspected cases of dementia.

Decisions about dementia can be helped at times by specialized psychological testing (psychometry). This is rarely available to the general practitioner, but it will be found sometimes in the investigations reported to him by psychiatrists and others. It may be useful, therefore, if we mention briefly the main features of such tests.

The use of psychological tests in current practice depends upon the assumption that children and adults in a given community have a similar degree of common experience so that tests can be employed using questions on, say, the meaning of words or the use of a pillar box without one person being unfairly handicapped in relation to another because of his lack of opportunity to learn. Such tests have been shown to predict academic and vocational skills with considerable success, often better than teachers could do. They lead to the notion of intelligence as a potential to acquire skills or solve problems. We discuss this further in Chapter 15. For practical purposes some intelligence tests can be divided into a part which depends mainly on verbal skills and a part which depends upon spatial, constructional and performance skills. The most satisfactory test in clinical use is the Wechsler Intelligence Scale (Wechsler Adult Intelligence Scale, and Wechsler Intelligence Scale for Children), and this has a verbal scale and a performance scale on which patients and others can be measured.

Previous test results are rarely available in patients with dementia. However, some estimates of probable previous levels can be made. A successful businessman with three shops is unlikely when well to have had an IQ of less than 100 on either the performance or verbal scales. Similarly, a university professor or lecturer is unlikely to have had an IQ of less than 120. A marked fall from such levels would probably be highly significant. Moreover, a big discrepancy between the two scales would also be likely (although not certain) to indicate brain damage. Most often such a discrepancy is associated with a lowering of the performance scale relative to the verbal scale. The latter depends more on established knowledge in older people, whilst the former tends more to indicate ability to solve new problems. Accordingly, it declines faster in the presence of brain damage.

Differences between hemispheres, the effects of dysphasia from a dominant hemisphere lesion or loss of spatial ability from a minor hemisphere lesion can also influence the results and their interpretations. Further, depression and anxiety may impair an individual's performance. Bearing these points in mind, however, it can be said that intelligence testing may serve to support or confirm a clinical impression of dementia as the explanation of a behaviour disorder or a memory disturbance. More specific tests of memory for retained material and of new learning and memorizing are also available.

In conclusion, it should be noted that subtle small changes in personality which are often the first signs of a dementia may be evident before intelligence tests can demonstrate any change. His normal life may subject an individual to a far more varied series of tests than can be compiled in a standardized procedure, and life is thus often the most telling way of demonstrating a man's adjustment or the lack of it.

Epilepsy

The modern view of epilepsy holds that it is essentially a threshold phenomenon. Nearly everyone will have a fit if given ECT (EST). Others are liable to have fits in unusual circumstances, for example hypoglycaemia or anoxia. Still others have fits in response to flickering lights and a few have frequent spontaneous fits. In every case the degree of liability depends to some extent upon inherited predisposition. In some cases, an inherited dysrhythmia will be the sole or major factor in the aetiology of the disorder. In a second group, acquired organic disease will play the principal part. This is the group in which psychiatric disorders are more common. It used to be thought that the inherited factor contributed both to epilepsy and to 'insanity'. Paradoxically, it is now evident that genetic factors in epilepsy are least associated with psychiatric illness whilst the organic factors show a close relationship. This is because many cases which used to be called idiopathic epilepsy have now, as a result of intensive combined clinical and electroencephalographic study, been shown to be due to brain damage; so that a group of cases which used to be regarded as the result of inherited defects is now established as attributable to brain damage.

In the light of these electroclinical studies epilepsy can be divided into two main classes. First, there is centrencephalic epilepsy in which the hereditary factor is dominant. This type of dysrhythmia is generated in the diencephalon and affects the cerebral cortex symmetrically. It is associated with childhood *petit mal* and with *grand mal* when there is no evidence of a focal disturbance. The second main group is acquired or symptomatic epilepsy which is associated with cerebral damage and which may cause minor disturbances of consciousness, psychomotor fits and *grand mal*. Cases with an aura or with focal disturbances (even minimal ones) fall into this group as do all cases of psychomotor fits. In accordance with this classification *grand mal* may be either centrencephalic or symptomatic. *Petit mal* or the occurrence of 'absences' in children is usually centrencephalic and so-called *petit mal* in adults is nearly always a minor form of symptomatic epilepsy.

The psychiatric complications of epilepsy are varied. Patients who are liable to epileptic fits show very great anxiety or discontent at their illness. Such a disability can be very grievous and will precipitate a neurotic response in some patients as inevitably as trouble at work, at home or in other aspects of their lives. When patients are upset in this way or by any other cause of stress they are then liable to have more fits. Worry and tension are factors which promote and increase the risk of epileptic attacks. So much is this the case that their effective treatment may abolish bouts of fits which have not responded to correct doses of anticonvulsants. In this respect psychotherapy may be more effective than an additional anticonvulsant. We give an example of emotional change benefiting epilepsy in Chapter 2. Alternatively, diazepam, which is only a weak anticonvulsant when given orally, may be helpful because it reduces tension. In this connection it is probably worth mentioning that antidepressant medication can reasonably be used with patients with epilepsy. Such medication carries a slight increased risk of provoking fits. That risk must be balanced against the probably larger risk of fits becoming more frequent because of depression or anxiety.

Another neurotic disturbance which is associated with temporal lobe epilepsy is the occurrence of hysterical conversion symptoms. Conversion symptoms, as previously mentioned (p. 41), have a special association with central nervous system disturbances. This is well marked in connection with temporal lobe epilepsy, and although gross conversion symptoms are normally very rare they may be found in at least 3 per cent of patients with temporal lobe epilepsy. Like other neurotic symptoms including depression, they seem to occur when the anticonvulsant dose is too high. Clearly the management of such infrequent events requires specialist attention, but their theoretical significance makes it appropriate to mention them here. If, as is the case, hysterical symptoms can come or go with a change in the level of serum phenytoin there are important implications for any theory of hysteria.

Apart from the foregoing there are three other main groups of psychiatric disorders especially associated with epilepsy. Almost invariably these are found with acquired or symptomatic epilepsy due to damage to the temporal lobes.

The first group consists of acute delirious states which may follow an epileptic fit or be caused by a continuous electrical discharge in the temporal lobe. These conditions present as emergencies and are dealt with in Chapter 18. Second, chronic schizophrenic conditions commonly of a paranoid type are found in association with temporal lobe epilepsy. While some of these psychoses may benefit from anti-epileptic treatment, others appear to be made worse by a more effective control of the epilepsy. Finally, there are personality changes which are associated with epilepsy. These have been described for a long time and have been ascribed to the bad effects of institutionalization and to bromism; nevertheless they are still seen although epileptics are now cared for in the community and bromides are no longer used. Some may be attributable to unsuitable anticonvulsants. The most important of these personality changes are: an extreme and sometimes catastrophic lability of mood, so that a patient may swing from normal cheerfulness to suicidal depression in the space of an hour; retardation of thinking, which is accompanied by a circumlocution of speech which can be infuriating to the listener; a shallow, sentimental and sometimes sanctimonious attitude which convicts the patient (perhaps unfairly) of insincerity with those around him. These patients are difficult, stubborn and egocentric and are as unpopular at home as they are in hospital, and a suitable solution to their social difficulties may be very hard to find.

This type of personality change is usually related to brain damage to the temporal lobes, although of course a neurotic pattern is also involved here and the objective difficulties of the patient may well contribute to his behaviour. Some special centres for people with epilepsy have been set up lately with the intention of providing a combination of medical care and rehabilitation to relieve the fits, the personal difficulties and the employment problems of some of the most handicapped but recoverable individuals. These centres are still, however, in an experimental phase.

SYSTEMIC CONDITIONS AND PSYCHIATRIC DISORDER

As well as the physical diseases which produce psychiatric symptoms directly through their action on the central nervous system, there are two further aspects which require attention: psychiatric disorder can also be precipitated by, or complicated by, physical illness.

Almost any physical disease can serve as a precipitating factor to psychiatric disorder in the predisposed individual. Abdominal operations and especially hysterectomy are noteworthy in this respect, as are virus infections. The psychiatric disorder which most often follows is the endogenous depressive illness, but schizophrenic syndromes can also occur. Younger patients will sometimes give a history of neurosis which began with a physical illness, although a careful history will usually show some signs of neurotic disorder prior to the illness. There is no doubt, however, that a serious illness, especially if it involves hospitalization and an operation, is a very potent factor in producing a decompensation of the patient's emotional adjustment and overt neurotic symptoms.

The fact that the highest incidence of psychiatric illness occurs in the latter half of life when the incidence of physical disease is also highest should warn the practitioner that a double diagnosis of both physical and psychiatric disorder must not uncommonly be made. Myxoedema and anaemia have already been mentioned. Hypertension used to be a common condition associated with depression. *Rauwolfia* derivatives, used to treat hypertension, were often responsible for this depression. Such a mood change with hypotensive drugs now seems to occur sometimes with alpha-methyl-dopa.

However, depression and hypertension together do present a problem in treatment because of the antagonistic actions of antidepressants and many hypotensive drugs (p. 389).

Double diagnoses are so common that the practitioner must not relax his vigilance even if a competent examination for physical disease has a negative result; unequivocal signs of physical disease may appear only later in the history, perhaps hastened by the debilitating effects of the psychiatric disorder. It is a good rule to review the physical state whenever symptoms persist despite seemingly appropriate psychiatric treatment. Deafness in old people is often thought to predispose to psychiatric illness. Deaf people are sometimes prone to be suspicious and misinterpret half-heard remarks; this tendency can on occasion be so developed that a paranoid psychosis results. Loss of sight would appear to be less damaging in this respect although cases are occasionally reported in which blindness may facilitate a visual hallucinosis. Profuse visual hallucinations can be a normal occurrence (Galton[25]). Clinically, we find them most often in association with visual impairment (for example, cataracts, glaucoma) and in the presence of anticholinergic drugs for Parkinsonism.

In spite of the hypochondriacal fears of neurotic patients, complicating physical disease is less common in them, perhaps because of their comparatively younger age. However, anaemia and thyrotoxicosis are two disorders whose early symptoms may be obscured by a severe anxiety state.

It was mentioned earlier (page 45) that chronic pain due to physical illness is a potent cause of depression. Patients with chronic pain often become anxious and depressed and indeed irritable. They are aware of both the reasons for their depression and the fact that in many cases they were stable persons previously. Those with neoplasms inevitably are fearful at the portent of their pain. Their treatment calls for suitable understanding as well as the use of antidepressant medication and phenothiazines in addition to recognized analgesics.[52]

The physiology of reproduction in women has a special relationship to psychiatric disorder. K. Dalton[17] has drawn attention to the changes in behaviour which occur before menstruation: 49 per cent of female prisoners commit their offence in the premenstrual period, and in a study of schoolgirls the incidence of rule-breaking doubled in that period. Suicide attempts, as well as urgent psychiatric admissions, also occur more frequently in this phase. Some women, perhaps 20 to 30 per cent, report symptoms of nervous tension, irritability, anxiety, depression, bloated feelings in the abdomen, swelling of fingers and legs, tightness and itching of the skin, headaches, dizziness and palpitations. This is the premenstrual syndrome and is relieved by the onset of menstruation. The nature of this syndrome is still uncertain. Some cases are in fact neurotic women who appear to complain too much of a normal premenstrual discomfort. In others, it consists of a premenstrual exacerbation of a concurrent psychiatric illness. There are some cases, however, in which the woman is perfectly normal outside the premenstrual phase and cannot be regarded as having a neurotic personality. In these cases, the onset is sometimes precipitated by a confinement or a physical illness, and neurotic symptoms may develop at a later stage, as a result of continuing distress due to the physical condition.

The aetiology of this condition, and therefore its treatment, is controversial. Some authorities believe it to be the result of a hormonal imbalance. Herzberg and Coppen[30] reported that some women were helped by the oral contraceptive. Headaches and swelling were unrelieved. Others have advocated progestogens in larger doses than for contraception (norethisterone 10 to 20 mg daily during the menstrual period), and testosterone has also been advised. More recently, progesterone has been tried in large doses. Diuretics and fluid restriction relieve the swelling but not always the psychological symptoms. Tranquillizers such as diazepam and antidepressants such as amitriptyline also help some patients. No method of treatment is universally successful, and there is probably a disturbance in more than one physiological system. As the menstrual cycle is still imperfectly understood, the treatment of the premenstrual syndrome remains empirical.

The timing of the complaints suggests that hormonal imbalance must be important in some cases. But we find hormone treatments to be the least helpful.

This perhaps may be a convenient point to discuss the psychiatric disorders associated with childbirth. Pregnancy is surprisingly free from psychiatric disorders, and some of our patients have even claimed to have felt improved during this time. Nevertheless depressive and schizophrenic illnesses as well as neurotic disorders may begin during pregnancy. Clinical experience suggests that at least they are not more frequent than in other women of the same age who are not pregnant.

Nevertheless the termination of pregnancy on psychiatric grounds has often been canvassed both with reference to the current effect of a pregnancy and in regard to the outcome for the patient subsequently. The British Act of 1967 envisages that termination can be performed on one or more of the following grounds:

1. The continuation of the pregnancy would involve risk to the life of the pregnant woman greater than if the pregnancy were terminated.

2. The continuation of the pregnancy would involve risk of injury to the physical or mental health of the pregnant woman greater than if the pregnancy were terminated.

3. The continuance of the pregnancy would involve a risk of injury to the physical health of the existing child(ren) of the family of the pregnant woman greater than if the pregnancy were terminated.

4. There is a substantial risk that if the child were born it would suffer from such physical or mental abnormalities as to be seriously handicapped.

In Canada, since 1969, abortion has been permitted for the sake of the health of the mother, as well as her life. The procedure must be carried out by a qualified medical practitioner in an approved or accredited hospital and must have the approval of a committee of three qualified medical practitioners appointed by the board of that hospital. In the United States a Supreme Court ruling forbids a state to prohibit abortion before the fetus becomes viable in the 24th to 28th week of pregnancy. The state may prohibit abortion thereafter. Clearly in all three countries there has been an increasingly permissive trend towards legal abortions.

There are doctors, mainly Roman Catholic, who on religious grounds cannot countenance termination of pregnancy. A larger number feel uneasy at the ethical consequences of the ready practice of termination. They feel that an ethical barrier against the disregard of innocent human life has been broken down. Further ethical objections have been raised against termination of pregnancy on the third grounds quoted, since this involves intervention on social grounds.

There is no difficulty in applying the criteria of the British Act to women who have a history of previous psychiatric illness following childbirth. There are also women in all social classes in whom it is evident that the last child has already drained their meagre resources of mothering. It is certain that too many children are an important cause of child neglect. There remain many cases in which the practitioner is in doubt, especially in married women whose families are not necessarily large.

Because of the wide current practice of abortion, it makes better sense clinically to try to decide which women would be harmed by the operation. In the first place, there are women who do not want an abortion but are under pressure from anxious relatives to have it done. Although they will firmly demand an operation, a careful enquiry will discover whose idea it was in the first place. These women will often show obvious relief when the operation is refused. Second, there are women who have changed their mind. The actions of these women demonstrate clearly that they were seeking pregnancy, for example, by ignoring the need for contraceptive measures, but are appalled by the fact of pregnancy when it occurs. It would seem as if these women are in unconscious conflict over their need to be pregnant. Termination will frustrate their need to have a baby, but a confinement will wreck their plans. One patient like this had a history of both previous psychiatric disorders and three wrecked marriages. The pregnancy occurred in a stable relationship with a man with whom she was living. She was desperately anxious to make a success of this relationship, and after much discussion she decided to go on with the pregnancy.

Unfortunately one does not always have time to help the patient work out her problem.

An unsatisfactory result from termination is rare. When this occurs it is usually because a choice had to be made between two evils. One woman who had an insecure marriage became pregnant by her lover to whom she was very attached. Continuation of the pregnancy would have wrecked her marriage, but after the operation she became depressed, mourning the sacrifice of her baby and of her lover for the sake of her marriage. Although doctors are loath to admit it, they are social agents, and their practice reflects the demands of the society they live in. Their professional responsibility is to make sure that the patient is not harmed.

However, the way in which changes in abortion laws have altered medical practice has had much influence on the discussion of medical ethics. Since the existence of a fetus may be so readily abolished the traditional code of the physician to preserve life has been disrupted and seriously challenged. Many doctors could accept the idea that preserving the life of a woman might require the death of her fetus, and even that there would be some hard cases where the decision was marginal. The choice between two lives was at least arguable to them. When the fetus is sacrificed for social or economic convenience or to avoid the chores of child-rearing it seems to many that a humane code is being violated. No consensus has emerged yet on this topic.

Psychiatric disorders in the puerperium are not essentially different from those occurring at other periods of life. Depressive reactions are common, and although they often respond slowly to treatment this is true also of endogenous depressions in young patients who are not pregnant. Some authorities believe that puerperal schizophrenia has an especially poor prognosis, but this has not been our experience and it has yet to be confirmed. Acute delirious states are not uncommon and usually settle in a very satisfactory way with adequate medical treatment and tranquillization. One interesting aspect of these puerperal psychoses is that they come on some days or weeks after the confinement, when the patient appears to be making good progress. In contemporary practice they do not seem to be related either to sepsis or obstetrical complications. Neurotic disorders often begin after a confinement, but this is rarely a complication of the puerperium.

A very important point in these puerperal conditions is the risk to the patient's children. The law recognizes that women in this period may be particularly unstable and even liable to kill their progeny. For this reason such an act within twelve months of the birth of the child is classed as infanticide—a less serious offence than murder. Sometimes the woman may seek to kill the child and then herself—an occasional happening in other types of depressive psychosis as well. To help prevent such tragedies careful psychiatric assessment is essential for all cases where there is any suspicion of puerperal mental illness; and, regrettably, segregation of the mother from her baby may be necessary.

9

General Principles of Treatment

It is the aim of this book to help the practitioner to think clearly about his psychiatric cases. Without this clear thinking rational and effective treatment is difficult. Before details of treatment are discussed it may be helpful to summarize some of the important points which have been dealt with in the previous chapters.

Who is the patient?

In Chapter 6 it was pointed out that the patient who presents (or is brought) for treatment is not necessarily the person in whom the disturbance is located. An effective psychiatric formulation begins by locating the emotional disturbance, whether it be in the patient himself, some other person or shared between the patient and another as is the case in some married couples or between mother and child.

What is the nature of the disturbance?

It was pointed out that there are four basic pathologies which produce psychiatric illness:

1. Emotional disturbance which arises out of a distorted emotional development reaching back into childhood. This may show itself equally in the psychological symptoms of a

neurosis, the physical symptoms of a psychosomatic disorder, or the disturbed interpersonal relationships of a behaviour disorder in a young person or a marital problem.

2. Social stresses and misfortunes.

3. The endogenous illnesses of depression and schizophrenia.

4. Physical illness.

It was further pointed out that more than one (perhaps all four) of these pathogenic mechanisms may operate together.

Having decided which mechanisms are operating, the physician must then place them in a hierarchy. The first that must be dealt with are the endogenous illnesses; attempts at profound psychotherapy are usually fruitless when the patient is endogenously depressed. Moreover, personal problems which may seem to be insuperable in a depressed person often shrink to a minor place when a normal mood is restored.

The treatment of depression

There are three main points to be dealt with here.

1. *Antidepressant treatment.** Many drugs are now available for this and provide the first line of treatment in most cases. Tricyclic antidepressants like amitriptyline have pride of place here, but it must be remembered that only trial and error may establish the best antidepressant for a particular patient. It should be noted that these provide a *symptomatic* treatment. It must be stressed that many patients with neurotic symptoms complain of severe depression, although there is no clinical evidence of an endogenous depression, and they can sometimes be helped by antidepressants. When the mood disturbance is controlled in this way, psychotherapy may be more effective in helping these patients in coming to terms with their psychological problems. Being a symptomatic treatment, antidepressant drugs have to be continued until the depression clears spontaneously. If they are stopped

---

* Only types of drugs are dealt with in the text; details and schemes of dosages of the different members of each group, and their side effects, are given in Appendix 1, Drug Treatment.

before this time, the symptoms return in full force. As the depression clears, the doses can be slowly reduced.

ECT (EST) is still the method of choice in severe depressions. If the depression does not clear quickly or satisfactorily on drug treatment or if the patient is severely depressed with suicidal thoughts, referral to a psychiatric clinic is necessary.

2. *Rest.* Depression always produces difficulties in concentration and a reduction in the output of mental work. Except in the mildest depressions, reduction or relief from mental work is essential. Physical bed rest at the outset of treatment is occasionally helpful in severe depressions, but most depressed patients are best up and occupied with tasks which compromise between providing some interest and demanding little concentration. A severely depressed patient may attempt little more than a jigsaw puzzle, but improvement brings with it the ability to cope with tasks which are more demanding. Many such depressions can be treated at home (unless the risk of suicide or the need for ECT (EST) makes hospital treatment necessary), but housewives with depression will never rest at home and inpatient treatment is often desirable for this reason alone, and for agitated patients it is essential. Patients with depression, especially the endogenous pattern, are often worse on holiday and at such times as Christmas. They think they should be enjoying themselves and they become still more keenly aware of their sad mood. By contrast news of some public disaster gives them some feelings of justification for their morbid state. After recovery from depression holidays may be appropriate but such patients are often happy to resume ordinary life without a vacation.

3. *Sedation and tranquillization.* It is important to secure a good night's rest for depressed patients. As a rule the best way to do this is to give part or all of the daily dose of tricyclic antidepressants at night together with nitrazepam if the latter is required. Barbiturates and glutethimide are known to interfere with the action of tricyclic drugs and should be avoided for this reason and also because of the risk of addiction or at least habituation. Such a risk does not exist with the action of tricyclic drugs and is probably much less with nitrazepam. A relatively sedative antidepressant such as

amitriptyline or trimipramine will normally be found to be the most helpful if there is a difficult sleep problem, but the dose needs individual adjustment from person to person. Phenothiazines may also be used but some can make depression worse. By day diazepam and other benzodiazepines like chlordiazepoxide, oxazepam and medazepam can be of great value.

It is a matter of some concern that lethal quantities of drugs are supplied to depressed and potentially suicidal patients. In all cases it is wise to give the drugs in charge of a relative. Drug addition is extraordinarily rare in this type of patient even with those drugs which carry a slight risk of dependency, because as the depression clears so does the need for drugs.

ECT (EST) remains an important standby in the treatment of resistant and severe depressions of the endogenous type. It is normally a hospital procedure albeit one often given to outpatients, but the practitioner needs certain information in regard to it. ECT (EST) is essentially an empirical treatment found to work best in patients with the endogenous type of depression. Fits were first induced in patients with schizophrenia in the incorrect belief that schizophrenia and epilepsy were biologically antagonistic. They were found helpful in some patients with schizophrenia and even more so in patients with this type of depression. The original agent used was cardiazole by injection. Cerletti and Bini introduced the use of electric shock which has been widely adopted.

In the standard procedure of modified ECT (EST), the patient is anaesthetized with intravenous hexobarbitone and then receives succinylcholine or a similar muscle relaxant. After insertion of an airway and insufflation with oxygen a gag is placed between the teeth and an electric shock of low amperage but of some 60 to 120 volts passed through electrodes either bifrontally or unilaterally via frontal and mastoid placings. Ordinarily a generalized convulsion, modified by the muscle relaxant, follows. In the absence of a muscle relaxant there is an increased risk of fractures and of imposing an excessive strain upon the heart and circulation. The treatment needs to be repeated about twice a week for two or three weeks in most instances and in a few cases up to 20 or 30 times. It is extremely safe causing only about one death in 28 000.[4] Most deaths reported have been in patients with preexisting heart disease. The main complication is a transitory impairment of memory for current events. A generalized convulsion is required to produce a therapeutic effect and the degree of recovery is proportional to the amount of cerebral epileptic discharge.[62] This is an important scientific proof of the efficacy of convulsive treatment compared with placebo procedures. Memory disturbances are greater after bilateral than after unilateral ECT (EST) and also are proportionate to the quantity of electricity used. Unilateral ECT (EST) to the nondominant hemisphere, using a measured dose, is thus the least traumatic form. It may also work because the hemisphere which is non-dominant for speech appears to be dominant for affective change. Bilateral ECT (EST) with a measured dose is also less harmful to the memory than bilateral ECT (EST) given without the dose measurement. However, bilateral ECT (EST) of either sort is somewhat more effective than the unilateral form.

4. *Cognitive therapy.* An approach to the treatment of depression which contrasts with the physical methods is provided by cognitive therapy. This starts from the assumption that depression is caused by false cognitions or ideas which have become established in the individual on the basis of a negative view of the self, the world and the future. Individuals who for insufficient reason see themselves as inadequate or unsuccessful and have a systematic bias against themselves may be persuaded by appropriate revision of their attitudes to view differently their lives and attainments. This is done by detailed attention to the false cognitions and by systematic instruction in handling these cognitions in a less self-critical and self-damaging way. For example, a patient who maintains incorrectly that he is a poor workman may be made to record, and remind himself of, the many jobs which he has undertaken satisfactorily. A manufacturer with a small business who because of some wrong decisions (which had been corrected) saw himself as a 'total failure', was given a series of tasks which successfully challenged this assumption. [71]

Impressive results have been obtained with this approach in some depressions (as well as in anxiety states and some other conditions). In particular, there is one controlled trial in which cognitive therapy was more successful than imipramine.[67] Severe depressive illness should not be treated by cognitive therapy unless physical methods are not available. Delusions are not known to respond to cognitive therapy. In one sense it might be described as a deliberate combination of suggestion and auto-suggestion; this is not a reason for rejecting it and it has a place in the management of depression, particularly for individuals with depressive personality traits. The selection of cognitive therapy as the principal treatment for depression is at present a matter for specialist judgement. Family practitioners and others interested in this approach may refer to Beck's book.[6] Unsystematic cognitive therapy is often used by both psychiatrists and others as part of their treatment of patients, often without defining their approach as such or recognizing that it has been given a formal structure.

Schizophrenia

The other major functional endogenous psychosis is schizophrenia. In our opinion these cases should be treated in consultation with a psychiatrist, owing to their uncertain prognosis. The treatment of choice is at present the phenothiazine tranquillizers, but ECT (EST) is helpful in some cases.

Physical illness

It is important to attend to the physical health of the patient at the very outset of treatment. Although a depressed patient with myxoedema will often not recover with thyroxine treatment on its own, yet clearly the response to antidepressant treatment will be unsatisfactory until the thyroid deficiency is relieved. Similarly, the social disability of a patient with an anxiety state will be exaggerated if a concurrent anaemia is left untreated. It cannot be over-emphasized that a considerable minority of elderly psychiatric patients are likely to have a concurrent organic disorder which requires attention. Major psychiatric illness is also associated with a high incidence of physical illness[19]. The social and psychological problems cannot be correctly assessed until adequate treatment has been instituted for the endogenous and organic components of the psychiatric illness. Quite frequently patients will exhibit an unsuspected resilience in coping with their sociopsychological difficulties once these matters have been dealt with, and problems which at first appeared intractable will disappear when the patient is physically fit and no longer depressed. On the other hand, hypertension may be greatly relieved by the successful treatment of agitation and mental tension.

Changing the environment

Chapter 6 points to the real needs of patients which can be frustrated by an adverse social environment. Once treatment has been instituted for both endogenous and physical illness, the physician must then turn his attention to the patient's social problems. Suitable occupation is often the most important single factor. Its value in helping the schizophrenic patient is discussed further on, but it is equally important in all psychiatric illnesses, especially those which follow widowhood. Financial stress, loneliness, uselessness, boredom and idleness, all these problems are cleared away when a suitable job is found. Many married women with neurotic illnesses improve remarkably when they find a suitable part-time employment. Unsuitable occupations are often important in the emotional disturbances of adolescence, and sometimes in adult men.

In Britain, under the Disabled Persons Employment Act (1944), a special officer (Disablement Resettlement Officer) is available through the local Employment Office, and patients with occupational problems should be encouraged to seek his advice. In younger patients courses of rehabilitation and training for new jobs are all available under the Act. Remploy provides employment for some who are permanently disabled, but it is not often suitable for the psychiatrically disabled. Many adult men take time off work at the start of their neurosis, but will readily return to work when so advised. In our experience failure to return to work is allied to poor prognosis in neurotic patients. On occasion, promotion has improved or even cured neurotic symptoms. This is especially true of the second-in-command, whose loyalties are divided between his boss and other colleagues. The effect of a destructive boss on the mental health of a group working with him can be disastrous, and the remedy here may not lie in the doctor's hands. It seems probable, however, that work in itself does not produce breakdown unless the patient has an emotionally disturbed attitude towards it.

Follow-up of schizophrenics discharged from hospital shows that the prognosis is better in those who live away from their parents in hostels or satisfactory lodgings. The anxious parents of such patients are often hard to convince that this is the case, but the evidence is impressive. Return to work is equally important, and even patients who appear not to have responded very favourably to physical treatment may begin to show marked improvement if they can be persuaded to start work. Many mental hospitals now have workshops for the rehabilitation of schizophrenic patients, and every effort must be made to find work for them on discharge from hospital. It must be expected that for some patients there will be a drop in their occupational status, but this is unimportant compared to the fact that they are working regularly. General practitioners can be of great help in persuading sceptical families that it is in their son's best interest to let him live in a hostel and undertake work of an inferior status if he so wishes.

Loneliness can be a difficult social problem. For many it is solved at work, but especially for old patients who do not easily make friends it is sometimes very hard to graft them into an acceptable social group. We are convinced, however, that clubs for old people do valuable preventive work in psychiatry, and many psychiatric hospitals run social clubs themselves to meet this need.

The relief of material needs also must not be forgotten. Depending on the country, state or province, and on the circumstances, the Social Security or Welfare Office or Unemployment Insurance Commission Office or Workmen's Compensation Board should be approached when the man is not working. In North America the municipality is the first line of approach for welfare and then the state or province. Assistance is also available under certain conditions in Britain and

Canada for people who are employed or partly employed. Further, charitable funds exist which are anxious to help people in need. Where the need arises out of poor management as much as from inadequate income the Family Service Units which exist in some towns in Britain and Family Service Associations in North America are very helpful.

Many patients blame their illness on to poor housing conditions, and while it is true that house removal is one of the more common precipitants of psychiatric illness, in our experience the search for better housing conditions rarely produces the benefit for which the patient hopes. It would appear that the stress of removal in itself is more important than the adequacy or otherwise of the dwelling.

It is often tempting to advise patients to move away from other disturbing members of their family, and while this occasionally may be successful the point must be considered as to why the patient did not think of this for himself without prompting from the doctor. In such cases there is usually a childish dependence on the family which is not improved by the mere fact of geographical separation. A change of attitude must come first, and once achieved will often lead to a more independent existence without further advice. Indeed in such matters it is usually unwise to give advice at all. We prefer to help the patient to grasp his problems clearly so that he can see what he has to do. The same considerations apply to young single adults who remain mother-bound at home. It is obvious that they would be a good deal better if they could detach themselves from the symbiotic existence, but the fact that they are unable to do this is not improved by them being told that that is what they ought to do. Help consists not only in pointing out the way but enabling them to get started on it.

PSYCHOTHERAPY

It will be evident from what has been written so far that the only satisfactory solution to many psychiatric problems is a change of attitude, if not a change of heart on the part of the patient. Only when the patient revises his ideas of what others expect of him and of what he requires of them, only when he responds with different feelings to his recurring personal problems will the anxiety and tension diminish. Psychotherapy is the art of inducing such a change of heart.

The word *psychotherapy* itself is simply misleading. It suggests a special skill and the medical reader naturally assumes that it is a skill similar to those which he was taught as a houseman, such as administering an anaesthetic. The essence of nonpsychological treatments is that the practitioner is in control of the situation. At every step he knows what to do next. The aim of his training is to ensure that the procedure is correctly carried out on each occasion. The indication for the treatment procedure, its success and limitations can be demonstrated in controlled trials.

By these criteria psychotherapy is not a treatment. It has proved practically impossible to demonstrate unequivocally that it is effective and techniques of different practitioners vary widely. Psychotherapy is either a waste of time or it is a skill of a very different order from the other skills of medical treatment. Let us look again at clinical experience.

In consulting a doctor, a patient is asking for help, but he is usually not clear at this stage what sort of help he needs. In response to the doctor's sympathetic enquiry, the patient discloses an unordered stream of symptoms and anxieties, distress at his life situation and complaints. Some worries are plainly stated, some hinted at.

The doctor will then not only be aware of the symptoms and emotional disturbances which bring the patient for treatment but by paying attention to the situations which bring on the symptoms will be alerted to the fundamental difficulties of the patient. So, for example, the patient's recurring difficulties with father figures (the boss, teachers, and the like) will indicate basic difficulties with his father although the patient may not be aware of it himself; a girl's constant difficulties in sexual situations such as engagement and marriage should outweigh her denial of sexual worries; constant nagging and criticism of a spouse may be an outlet for unacknowledged hostility to a parent. A survey of the patient's childhood situation will often indicate the origin of the neurotic difficulties of later life, unless a refusal to face the facts of emotional life has led the patient unconsciously to gloss over his earlier difficulties.

At this point the doctor must provisionally decide if his patient's problems are likely to be resolved by medication and advice. If that is not the case, a delicate confrontation takes place. A simple explanation of the physiology of anxiety or the symbolism of body language, for example, 'a pain in the neck,' leads to the translation of symptoms into personal anxieties. Although the nature of these anxieties will not yet be clear to either the patient or the doctor, the coincidence of symptoms with certain life events often gives a clear hint to both sides as to where the problem should be sought. A proposition is then put to the patient that these problematical areas of his life would be worth discussing. At this point either the patient will assent and accept the challenge and psychotherapy has started or he will demur and return to complaints about symptoms. If the patient is adamant that he is only seeking a pill to alleviate his discomfort, we are sure that at this stage it is wiser to prescribe a tranquillizer and keep the situation under review. Sometimes this confrontation does not occur until medication and simple advice have been tried and found wanting. Sometimes patients arrive with their minds made up that they are seeking an opportunity to discuss their problems.

We do not believe that psychotherapy is the 'treatment of choice' of 'neurotic illness' (to use medical jargon). *We believe it refers to the doctor's response to the admission on the part of the patient that he has personal problems which are causing him distress and with which he can cope no longer.* It is thus an automatic accompaniment of medical work. The problems are those which the doctor believes he cannot touch through the prescription of drugs or a change of environment. They are often first formulated by the patient as difficulties in his relationships with other people.

The first point to be made is that the patient is helped more by what he says than by what the doctor says. The doctor's task is, therefore, mainly one of listening, but this is a special type of listening. A patient remarked to one of the writers that he was not treating her as a person. She was right. The doctor was concerned with making the diagnosis of epilepsy and was therefore paying careful attention to parts of her history which had significance only for him. She needed him to pay attention to what was meaningful for her. This means that the control of the interview, and the direction it takes, is largely out of the doctor's hands. Many doctors find this difficult to accept. They exclaim at the end of an interview, 'What shall I do next?' and are put off by the reply 'Wait and see what the patient brings.'

Much of psychotherapy is, therefore, a silent waiting while the patient unfolds his story, not in the chronological convenience of a medical history, but with the inner logic of feeling. Thus a painful deathbed scene reminds the patient of other broken relationships, of loves who have let him down and friends who have deserted him.

It is not clear why this recital of painful events should be so helpful. Probably it is because the anxiety and distress which accompany these memories are comforted by the reassuring acceptance of the doctor. When the unpleasant feelings have died down, the memories are no longer troublesome. Patients often object that psychotherapy cannot change the past. This is true, but it can change the way we feel about the past, which is more important.

Even a single interview can be of great help to a person in distress if it is conducted along these lines. But often what troubles patients is not only what has happened to them but their continuing propensity to provoke attack or misfortune, such as repeatedly taking up enterprises which fail, or friendships in which they are disappointed. They feel they ought not to have such feelings.

In the section on the Neurotic Predicament, it was pointed out that the unpleasant feelings of anxiety and guilt will prevent a patient from acknowledging his true feelings. In a psychotherapeutic relationship therefore the physician aims at creating an understanding and accepting atmosphere which will assuage these unpleasant feelings and make it easy for the patient to talk about distasteful topics. The patient reveals something about himself of which he is ashamed and fails to elicit the expected reactions of censure from the therapist. Taking his cue from the therapist, the patient gradually learns to accept the unpleasant aspects of himself, as the therapist accepts him. The noncensorious attitude of the therapist shows that there is no longer any need to feel guilty. More happens than this however. Most patients are very shy at expressing their deeper feelings for fear of criticism or ridicule. When the patient has learned that there is no need to fear an adverse reaction he will often find himself pouring out to the therapist feelings which he had hardly realized were within him, checked as they had been by his guilt and anxiety. As his intelligence becomes less constrained by fear, the patient finds that new understandings about his problems rise up unbidden and become clear in his mind. This is a very different experience from the insight given by an intellectual explanation. The latter may be compared with an exposition of the workings of a machine to a layman, while the former is a grasp of a new perspective in which the old problems no longer seem to exist. It must not be thought that these processes are separate and distinct operations in psychotherapy; they are better understood as different aspects of a single experience. The relationship of care and concern which the therapist extends undermines the effects of anxiety and guilt. Where unpleasant feelings are held in check, these are released in an abreaction. Where the patient has castigated himself he learns to accept his impulses and feelings as an essential part of his nature.

The role of the therapist has been described so far as one of silent reassuring acceptance. But there are occasions on which he must intervene. Patients often find difficulty in putting their feelings into words. For example, a patient who begins a session by recounting incidents in which other people were angry may be seeking (unconsciously) an opportunity to speak about his own angry feelings. By noting the sequence of topics one can often grasp the unconscious drift of what the patient is getting at. Sometimes when a patient speaks, for example, of a spouse, one can catch an echo of a similar feeling which he expressed about a parent. It can be very helpful to draw the patient's attention to such a link.

There are other ways too in which the therapist may become aware of what is going on inside his patient. It sometimes happens that for little reason the therapist is aware of an inexplicable emotion during the interview. At first he is tempted to blame his irritability or boredom on himself, but with experience he begins to realize that he is responding to a hidden affect on the part of the patient. So he neither voices his irritability nor disciplines himself; he asks the patient: 'I wonder why you are feeling angry.' The therapist's sense of boredom is likewise an indication that the patient is emotionally uninvolved in what he is saying. At this point he draws the patient's attention to the possibility that an important topic is being avoided.

These remarks will indicate that the fundamental activity of a psychotherapist is to be open to receive what he can from his patient, using his feelings as much as his intelligence. But observation must not be neglected: many a woman has betrayed her anxieties about her marriage by fiddling with her wedding ring.

In the course of the treatment, and sometimes after the first few interviews, the doctor becomes aware that he is playing a different part with his patient compared with his other patients who are not in psychotherapy. It is difficult to write about this change in the relationship in a concrete fashion, although occasionally it may be signalled by an objective event such as the bringing of a present or being late for an appointment. Most commonly, the patient becomes more dependent on the doctor and more anxious that the doctor should think well of him. It is vital that the doctor should comprehend the meaning of this change. In many instances the patient's behaviour is transparently that of a child towards his parent, but on some occasions, such as the bringing of a present, the patient's motive is unclear. On such occasions it is important for the doctor to discuss this event, and its meaning, with the patient. To fail to do so is tantamount to receiving a letter from the patient and leaving it unopened.

Any change of behaviour on the part of the patient is a communication, the meaning of which must be defined. This will entail the doctor discussing with the patient the nature of the relationship between them. Many psychotherapists find this difficult at the outset of their career, but this perhaps is the one outstanding characteristic which distinguishes psychotherapy from other professional relationships. Almost always it is found that this change of relationship has occurred because the patient has come to think of the doctor as a parent, and has transferred the unsolved problems with the parents of his childhood on to the doctor. This gives the psychotherapist an immense opportunity of correcting the mistakes of the parents of the patient. The patient who never dared talk about sex to his parents can now do so with safety.

A patient, after a mildly scandalous revelation said: 'I looked to see if you were shocked.' She was learning not to be afraid to talk about sex to her mother (curiously the sex of the psychotherapist is irrelevant). The patient who never dared rebel against his parents can now (safely) appear to have a row with the doctor. It is necessary, of course, for the new parent-surrogate (the doctor) to be more understanding than the original parents, so that the patient is aware that he continues to be accepted no matter what he says—and this includes personal (verbal) attacks on the therapist. Eventually the patient learns that he no longer needs to be afraid of his feelings: he has grown up. Depressed patients can be very difficult in psychotherapy. They often feel deprived in childhood and it may take a long time for the doctor, playing the part of mother, to convince them that they are cared for.

In this way, a problem of long ago between the patient and the parents of his childhood becomes a problem of the here and now between the patient and the doctor. The patient is offered a second opportunity for his emotional education. If it were not for this, the problems of many neurotic patients would indeed be insoluble.

This, however, is not the only therapeutic mechanism of psychotherapy. So much of the anxiety and tension of the neurotic state arises from the struggle not to pay attention to unacceptable thoughts and wishes. To have these thoughts put into words by the empathic intelligence of the psychotherapist at once affords relief; the cat has been let out of the bag, so to speak, and the patient no longer needs to pretend to be other than he is. In the same way, feelings that have long been held in check by fear may come pouring out in an emotionally exhausting catharsis called *abreaction*. These are both important mechanisms, but not as basic as the emotional relearning offered by the transference experience. However, there are some patients in whom transference plays a small or negligible part in their treatment. Such patients require help mainly in putting their feelings into words, so that they can gain a greater emotional honesty. When dealing with patients it is important to avoid technical terms such as *aggression* (even *anger*), *depression, rejection*, and the like. 'Fed up', 'resentful', 'left out of it', feel like crying', are the sort of words and phrases that mean much to patients.

A more difficult step in psychotherapy involves offering some challenge to the patient's behaviour or attitudes. This is sometimes necessary with patients who adopt a pattern of retreat or destructive nihilism to the world about them. The drug-taking adolescent for whom everyone else is at fault or the babyish adult with hysterical symptoms may be helped by being confronted with some of the ordinary consequences of their behaviour. Such procedures ought to be attempted only by the experienced therapist and then only in the context of complete acceptance of the patient. They can be extremely useful, but except in expert hands they are liable to be disastrous. However, every doctor must be able to indicate firm albeit gentle dissent from a patient's attitudes. Obviously, acceptance of the patient does not mean that one accepts his views of either, say, the value of marijuana or the harmlessness of promiscuity. Such dissent should be stated only pragmatically, not as grounds for criticism of the patient nor for moral persuasion. Criticism and conversion are not the function of the therapist.

It should be clear by now that much of what goes on in interviews does not count as psychotherapy. Giving the patient an explanation of his illness, for example, is only of limited value. It is true that any explanation to an anxious person is helpful; it is reassuring to know that the disturbing symptoms have got a rational basis. Such explanations do not, however, dispel the trouble. Most of us when in the grip of a bad temper, for example, have perfect intellectual insight into our behaviour, its causes and consequences, but that does not make us less irritable or unpleasant to those around us.

Many beginners in psychotherapy complain that they feel 'inadequate'. This usually means that they fear that they fail to offer constructive help in the face of their patient's need. Believing that the essence of psychotherapy is to foster the patient in constructing his own solutions to his problems, we would advise that at least at the outset the psychotherapist should interfere as little as possible. He should watch for the movement of the patient's feelings, clarifying them and translating them into words whenever the patient appears to be in difficulties. The danger for the beginner is in speaking too much rather than too little. Instead of attempting to inculcate 'insight' we would advise that the doctor wait for the patient to uncover his problem.

It is a temptation for the doctor with his clearer insight into the patient's life to direct the discussions straight into the problem areas, but this is probably a mistake. In the first place it is very important that the task of psychotherapy should be conducted with the greatest humility; we may believe that we understand the pattern of the patient's life, but the subsequent course of the treatment will always bring some revision to the preliminary formulation of a patient's problems. To stick rigidly to a predetermined plan of treatment courts the risk that vital points that arise in the course of the treatment may be ignored because they were not considered in the initial formulation. This, however, is not the only hazard of a psychotherapy which is directive and self-assured. The therapist may be quite correct in believing, for example, that unacknowledged hostility to a parent is the main cause of the trouble, but there is nothing to be gained by forcing the patient to talk about it until he is ready. The patient who has an internal cause for fear (for example, his feelings of uncontrollable anger) has to approach the matter delicately. Too brusque an assault on the problem may meet with a flat denial, perhaps even with the patient terminating the treatment.

The difficulties of psychotherapy consist mainly in being perceptively alert as to the state of the patient's feelings. The complexities of psychotherapy are concerned not so much with what the patient talks about but rather of what he doesn't speak; what is only implied 'in between the lines' or by his actions or, perhaps, altogether excluded by repression from the interview. The skill required is in helping the patient to overcome his reluctance to face his feelings. It follows, therefore, that while the patient is talking freely with appropriate feeling and is improving not only in his symptoms but in his relations with other people, the doctor need not worry unduly about the value of his treatment even though he may not fully understand all the dreams and memories which the patient brings to the interview; in fact difficulty in understanding a dream is unimportant compared with the failure to recognize the suppressed hostility of an overpolite patient. This type of feeling with the patient (empathy) is in part a natural gift, but grows with experience and training. Silence can also be a serious problem in some patients. In almost all treatments short periods of silence will occur at times, and the doctor must be prepared to learn to tolerate them. If, however, the patient repeatedly fails to speak or declares that he has nothing to say, it is likely that his treatment will need extra skill and experience.

Much has been written about the psychotherapeutic relation from the doctor's side, not all of it helpful. Some writers suggest that the psychotherapist is cool, neutral and detached. This is not true. A successful therapist is a warm person, deeply involved and deeply caring for his patients. In one review of psychotherapy it was concluded that successful treatment occurred when both patient and therapist were deeply committed to each other. This has been our experience also. Yet the relationship is different from that which we have with our friends. The psychotherapist is emotionally detached in the sense that he needs no emotional return from the patient. This allows him to pull out from the relationship and regard it objectively so that he can reflect on the significance of the patient's speech and behaviour. Without this type of detachment the therapist is liable to be offended by the patient's attacks, gratified by the patient's affection, forgetting that the patient's feelings are probably directed not personally at the doctor but at the parent he represents. If the patient's relationship with the doctor is the basic stuff of psychotherapy, then it is essential that the doctor should be able to view it scientifically rather than personally. On the other hand, to be aloof or distant towards the patient will prevent a relationship from forming, and psychotherapy will never start. (One cannot call an intellectual discussion on psychology any form of therapy.)

Psychotherapy therefore is a special type of relationship which a doctor has with a patient. Its characteristics can be summed up under three headings:

1. The doctor is concerned with the emotional problems of the patient.

2. He is able to relinquish his controlling role.

3. He has the capacity to reflect upon the emotional interaction between the patient and himself, and the courage to comment on it.

This type of relationship can arise in the middle of a routine consultation when the doctor suddenly becomes interested in listening to the patient as a person rather than as a case. At the end of a single interview the patient may have obtained sufficient relief not to need to come again. Other patients clearly need and expect to attend again, perhaps for as many as twenty or thirty sessions spread over a year. However, there is a law of diminishing returns in psychotherapy. After that length of time few patients make major gains although many may still require supportive treatment. There are a few, however, for whom a more experienced therapist or a different approach may lead to further advances. As the patient improves, his dependence lessens, and the interviews become more spaced out. A natural break in the treatment, such as holidays, is often the occasion when patients realize that they no longer need regular appointments but can fend for themselves. Nevertheless, patients are grateful for occasional follow-up appointments. Most patients continue to improve after their treatment has finished.

There is minor psychotherapy as there is minor surgery, and as the hazards of some operative procedures demand the most experienced skills so there are many neurotic patients whose resistances will defeat the beginner in psychotherapy. For the general practitioner who has not had a special training or who has no access to an experienced psychotherapist for consultation there are a number of warning signs that must be obeyed. Difficulties in speaking and failure to respond within a reasonable time have already been noted. Patients who disturb others at home or at work by threatening or attempting suicide or some other type of disruptive behaviour can be a great anxiety to the therapist.

Finally, the most important warning sign is when the doctor's own equilibrium is disturbed. He may lose his objectivity and passionately take sides against the patient's 'enemies'; he may become oversolicitous in an anxious compulsion to help his patient and comply with unreasonable demands for attention; the patient may provoke feelings of anger, irritation or sexuality in the doctor to an uncomfortable degree. In all these instances, the doctor is in danger of losing his judgement, and therefore his ability to help. Caring for people is not the same as being identified with them. Naturally all psychotherapists care for their patients, but the ones who are effective do not feel guilty if their patients fail to improve nor do they feel elated at a successful outcome of treatment. They seek no personal gratification from the patient's recovery and do not look for gratitude. They realize that the successful outcome of treatment depends on the good use which the patient makes of the doctor's understanding and insight; it is not a question of exerting an 'influence' on the patient.

Naturally, doctors vary a good deal in their ability to help patients on a personal level. Moreover some who are excellent in caring for patients of one sort such as angry, hostile people, are much less effective with others, such as anxious, dependent individuals; and the converse is true. Techniques of intensive psychotherapy may be appropriate for some personality disorders and less frequent interviews cast in a different mould will suit others. There are also many variants of psychotherapy. The pattern just described owes most to the findings of psychoanalysis, and moves from supportive interest to interpretation and revision of the individual's feelings and attitudes. If a doctor finds by experience that he can help people in this way, he should be encouraged to go further, although on the alert for danger signs. The advice and help of a psychiatrist experienced in psychotherapy should be sought whenever possible.

Supportive psychotherapy

Supportive psychotherapy is a type in which most general practitioners are more skilled than they realize. Many neurotic patients are faced with unalterable and unfavourable environmental situations. Because of age or other reasons it is unlikely that they will respond to analytical psychotherapy by revising their attitudes and emotional responses. This unpromising situation can often be greatly helped by the longcontinued friendly interest of the doctor. We have many patients whom we see for twenty minutes every two or three months. Their symptoms continue unchanged, but they make a better adjustment to their illness. The men continue in work, the housewives go on cooking. We advise such patients 'pretend to be well', while acknowledging the suffering caused by their symptoms. Although not encouraging facile optimism, we do not allow them to lose hope. 'I wouldn't be at all surprised if you were not improved by this time next year' is a useful phrase in this connection. We encourage their aspirations to reach out after a more normal way of life by applying for better jobs, joining social clubs or taking up hobbies. Although this is the least dramatic of psychotherapies, it is one which is economical of the doctor's time and most rewarding in its effects.

This type of management is most needed when patients refuse specialized psychiatric help or else have attended a clinic but have been discharged as unsuitable for intensive psychiatric treatment. It is easy for the clinic staff to banish such difficult patients by not giving them further appointments, but the general practitioner is constantly reminded of them in his surgery. Rather than lose patience and hope that they will transfer to a colleague's list, we would suggest that the general practitioner offer them supportive psychotherapy, if possible with planned appointments. The advantage of an appointment is that the patient will often wait until then, so economizing on the doctor's time. If the next consultation is left to the patient he will attend the surgery with increasing frequency to display more dramatic symptoms in an effort to capture the doctor's attention. As with demanding children, one must meet the patient halfway by freely offering him some of the attention he seeks.

Marital and family therapy

The joint treatment of spouses is known as marital therapy.

This is one form of family therapy which may be defined as the treatment together of two or more members of a family. Marital therapy in general is somewhat different from individual therapy; however, some family therapists consider that intervention with one member of a family alone might be family therapy inasmuch as it changes relationships within the whole system of a family. Family therapy is less concerned with the sexual adjustment of the parents and more with the interaction between the family members, including the children. The outstanding difference from other psychotherapy lies in the view of the family as a system. This view is concerned with the networks of power, alliance and emotion within the system and the way in which disorders of the system may be remedied. Individual pathology is seen as a symptom of the disturbed system.

Several formal theories of explanation and practice exist for family therapy but perhaps the simplest version of treatment is based on drawing the attention of members of the pair or family to their recurring patterns of dealing with each other. Further interpretations may encompass the ways in which individual expectations are reflected in the demands made upon other family members. This is much like the application to a group setting of the notions discussed above in regard to psychotherapy in general. But in family therapy more than one person is at liberty to comment on the therapist's observations. There is thus a more pressing need for the therapist to be perceptive and skilful, although obviously such attributes are desirable for any form of treatment. Some family therapy proceeds along the lines of mutual contract making. Jack will do A which Jill appreciates and Jill will do B which Jack desires and so on. Family therapy also tends to involve more active responses on the part of the therapist. The family tends to set up a demand for therapists to take sides and give advice. Family therapists have recognized that they must guard against their own value judgements in therapy, and must reflect to the participants what is taking place. It is conceivable that some value judgements are in fact introduced by therapists. It was mentioned earlier that this could occur in individual treatment (p. 141). The chance of it occurring in family therapy is much higher.

It is unwise to attempt family therapy without either previous experience or advice and guidance from a suitable specialist who is readily available. Although somewhat unpredictable in their outcome, family therapies are a form of treatment which can deal successfully with both acute and chronic problems of maladjustment and many of these chronic problems are unlikely to respond to any other approach. Some cases of psychosis, where the patient's psychosis is made worse or even provoked by the attitudes of members of the family, may also be dealt with in this way. Family therapy is currently popular in North America and increasingly popular in Europe. Its successes are being measured against alternative methods of treatment such as individual counselling, and the findings are positive so far, but not conclusive. It is a promising and important area of development in current psychiatric treatment.

Cognitive therapy

The principles of cognitive therapy have been briefly mentioned in relation to the treatment of depression (p. 126). There is a tendency to assimilate cognitive therapy with the behaviour therapies which are discussed next, on the grounds that what the patient reports is part of his behaviour and the management of those reports is a behavioural skill. This is a justified view. As our discussion of behaviour therapy indicates, however, the standardized arrangements which form a part of behaviour therapy and cognitive therapy procedures such as making programmes of de-conditioning, or re-learning or training to act upon a topic or experience it differently, all involve a personal relationship with the therapist when they are well conducted. This relationship is perhaps more evident in cognitive therapy than in some other forms of behavioural management. The sympathetic support of the cognitive therapist in depression is clearly an essential part of the procedure which helps the patient to feel different.

The essence of cognitive therapy, as has already been mentioned, is to train the patient to take a more positive view of himself/herself, to drop unjustified thoughts which negate that view and to adopt others which uphold it. In the example quoted earlier from Shaw and Beck [71] (p. 126) a man had made some mistaken business decisions. He became severely depressed, but despite his company's moderate recovery he continued to experience depression and ruminated almost continuously about his errors and current indecisiveness. He was asked to keep an activity diary and record mastery and pleasure experiences and initially his claim that he was 'totally inadequate' was tested by an 'experiment' in which he was asked to wash and dry his clothes. Despite a constant stream of negative predictions the patient was able to see the results of his effort. This was the first of a number of tasks used to challenge his belief of 'total inadequacy'.

Another example [70] is of a woman who experienced intense suicidal wishes after having broken up with her boyfriend. She stated that she could not get along without a man but questions about her life history led her to realize that she had done well at one time acting in opposition to her ex-husband's views. When she thus recognized the fallacy of her idea, her attitude about herself changed, she became more independent and ceased to be suicidal.

As mentioned earlier (p. 127) the employment of cognitive therapy as the sole treatment of depression may be a matter for specialist judgement, but there is no reason why a practitioner should not use the principles of this approach, at least as a supplementary measure, in his management of depression.

The range of cognitive therapy includes the treatment of depression, anxiety and some, so far limited, work with chronic pain. Other conditions have been suggested including hysterical symptoms but the indications there seem less strong. The writer has not employed cognitive therapy as a first line treatment but considers that it deserves a trial at least in some instances. But it will normally only be chosen at present after other well-established methods have been tried or considered inappropriate. The cognitive therapy approach is also immediately available as an adjunct measure. Patients whose views of themselves are too negative should be encouraged to develop the recognition of their successes, moving from minor, seemingly trivial instances to more important ones.

Group psychotherapy

The psychotherapy techniques so far described are all suitable (with modifications) for use outside psychiatric clinics. It is felt, however, that group psychotherapy is unsuitable for general practice, and in any case requires a doctor who is already experienced in individual psychotherapy. A group of about eight patients with emotional problems are invited to meet weekly in the presence of the psychotherapist. The meetings last about one and a half hours. The principles underlying this treatment are identical with those relating to individual treatment, in the same way as bringing up a family corresponds to bringing up an only child: there are advantages and disadvantages with both methods. Most psychotherapy clinics employ this method to a major extent as a means of offering adequate psychotherapy by a limited staff to the largest number of patients. Many patients who have had experience of both prefer group treatment. Most neurotic disorders are suitable for treatment in groups except severe depressive reactions and antisocial behaviour which would not be accepted by the group. The quality of improvement after group psychotherapy would seem to be not inferior to that after individual treatment.

BEHAVIOUR THERAPY

The name behaviour therapy has been given to some methods of treatment which developed increasingly during the last decade. These methods aim to provide an approach to the cure of neurotic complaints based upon principles derived from learning theory and experimental psychology. The value of these methods and their significance are the subject of much discussion but a place has been established for them in at least some respects. One method—the use of a pad and bell in the treatment of enuresis—is already available in general practice, and other forms of behaviour therapy are in regular use in a number of hospital centres. The practitioner may, therefore, wish to have some knowledge of principles which have been thought to underlie behaviour therapy.

The theory of behaviour therapy generally assumes that

neurotic symptoms are a form of habit produced accidentally in people who tend to be anxious. The way in which
such accidents might arise can be illustrated in one case. This
was a young married woman who was referred because of a
fear of worms. She recounted that at the age of seven she had
unexpectedly trodden with her bare feet on a worm on the
beach. The fright that she had received never left her, so that
at the time of the referral some twenty years later she was
continually preoccupied with watching out for worms. She
dared not go out in wet weather when worms might be
expected to be more numerous, and she dared not visit the
outside lavatory of her house at night for fear that she trod
on a worm in the yard. In all other respects she appeared to
be a happy and well-adjusted young woman, and there was
no evidence of neurotic traits in her character. She realized
that her fear of worms was irrational but nevertheless it continued to cripple her life out of doors.

In a case like this the theorists of behaviour therapy would
be likely to hold that an original primary unpleasant stimulus
gave rise to a maladaptive pattern of reaction—regular withdrawal from worms or any place where they might be found.
The pattern would be held to be developed and strengthened
(technically 'reinforced') because each time panic was aroused
by the possibility of a worm being near the panic was abated
and relieved by withdrawal from the unpleasant situation.
Thus the patient was fostered in her habit of withdrawal
although it became increasingly awkward to her in other
respects.

Now it is evident so far that the theory of behaviour
therapy, like the psychodynamic theories which we have
already described, seeks to explain the patient's symptoms as
an acquired misfortune. So far also, however, it is more ready
to accept the worm as a primary unpleasant stimulus than to
seek an answer, which psychoanalysts would inevitably
require to the questions: 'Why was the worm so unpleasant
for this particular woman?'; 'Why was the original stimulus so
frightening when objectively it presented no danger?'. Yet in
such cases as the above behaviour therapy has been held to
offer more chance of improvement for the patient than
psychoanalysis and it was thought worth while to try its

effects. Behaviour therapy was, therefore, undertaken for her by a psychologist colleague. His procedure began with a careful history so that he could draw up a hierarchy of situations ranging from those in which the fear produced was minimal to those in which it was intolerable. He then arranged for the patient to be exposed to the least disturbing of these situations until encouraged by his reassurance she learned no longer to feel fear. When this step had been accomplished she then proceeded to the situation next on the list. So, for example, the patient could be seen with her therapist learning to walk past twigs which resembled worms, then past dead worms, and finally past ones which were moving. At the end of thirty sessions the patient declared herself to be free of symptoms and at follow-up twelve months later there was no significant relapse.

This is a typical example of behaviour therapy in which patients learn healthy responses in place of neurotic behaviour. It is very possible that the personal relationship of the patient to the therapist played a major part in her improvement; it is also possible that the therapist did no more in training the patient than many mothers do with their children through common sense alone. Yet there may be more than one mechanism through which the therapy influenced the patient and the empirical methods of common sense can be improved by the insight of scientific understanding so that the principles which underlie behaviour therapy deserve some fuller consideration. Some of these principles may be considered by reference to the above case.

In the first place it was noted that the fear-producing stimulus of a live worm underfoot extends to include any worm-like object. This is called *stimulus generalization* and was first demonstrated by Pavlov who showed that his dogs would exhibit the learned (conditioned) response of salivation to signals which differed from the original stimulus. Naturally, the more remote the signal from the original stimulus the weaker would be the response. In the process of *desensitization* it is obvious that the situation of weakest stimulus value must be tackled first, where the patient can most easily learn not to respond with anxiety to the fear-producing object. If this is done repeatedly, the neurotic response of apprehensiveness is gradually extinguished in the same way as Pavlov's dogs ceased to salivate if the unconditioned stimulus of food failed to follow the conditioned stimulus of the bell on a sufficient number of occasions.

Many authorities believe that the simple process of extinction is insufficient to account for the disappearance of anxiety in the process of desensitization treatment. In the case just quoted, lack of an anxiety response when faced with worms was rewarded by the therapist's approval as well as by a rise in the patient's self-esteem. These experiences, it is thought, tend to reinforce an emotional response to worms which was the opposite of anxiety, namely self-confidence. This is the principle of *reciprocal inhibition*, in which an emotional response antagonistic to anxiety is learned by the patient in face of the original stimulus to fear. It will be seen that the treatment of impotence described in Chapter 12 makes use of this principle. Another important example involving the same principle occurs when we advise a timid patient to assert himself instead of feeling frightened. It is our belief, too, that the simple extinction of fear responses through repetition is not enough and that the patient needs to learn a healthy emotional response which displaces that of fear and anxiety.

Another, and rather different example of conditioning treatment is the use of the pad and bell apparatus in the treatment of nocturnal enuresis. With this apparatus, the voiding of even a small quantity of urine completes the circuit for an electric alarm which wakes the enuretic sleeper. The theory suggests that the stimulus of a distended bladder becomes conditioned to the response of waking rather than of micturition, and indeed this usually happens at first, with the patient waking to empty his bladder. Soon, however, the patient sleeps through the night, neither waking nor wetting the bed, which is not predicted by the theory.

The use of desensitization has been extended by the attractive expedient of arranging for patients to practise imaginary situations which provoke anxiety. Thus instead of constructing a hierarchy of real increasingly unpleasant situations, some of which may be difficult to realize in practice and with which the patient has to make contact, it is possible to construct a hierarchy on which the patient simply reflects. In this case too, of course, the patient starts with the least disturbing and proceeds to the most disturbing. As with desensitization in contact with the external stimulus each step in this *desensitization in imagination* is accompanied by reinforcement from the knowledge that the anxiety has been confronted and overcome. A number of reports indicate that desensitization in imagination may be facilitated by small simultaneous intravenous injections of barbiturates (for example, hexobarbitone).

Paradoxically, a wholly opposite technique known as *flooding* or *implosion* is also credited with success in the behaviour therapy of anxiety. In this case the patient is exposed not to minimal increasing doses of the unwelcome stimulus but to a maximum presentation of that stimulus. Provided that the patient tolerates the experience without untimely withdrawal this too leads to the reduction of anxiety on subsequent occasions. The occurrence of recovery as a result of this procedure naturally indicates some revision or qualification of the basic concepts of behaviour therapy.

The use of planned methods of thinking in behaviour therapy has led to possible useful treatments of sexual difficulty. Patients wishing to change an abnormal sexual inclination may be encouraged to reflect on material appropriate to the normal aim. Male homosexuals wishing to alter to a heterosexual pattern are encouraged to take an increasing interest in attractive females by associating them in imagination or in visual material with pleasure situations. At the same time satisfaction from homosexual material is discouraged. Sometimes the latter procedure is combined with aversive stimulation of which more will be said later. Although these techniques are not invariably successful they appear to offer a useful approach for a proportion of homosexuals who wish to adopt a heterosexual state of behaviour and feeling.

This approach clearly requires that material which is sexually stimulating in undesirable ways has to be avoided for these patients. By the same token it could be argued that the general distribution of pornographic material may predispose normal individuals to alter attitudes and to indulge in sexual experiences from which they might otherwise have refrained. We do not know of any appropriate systematic investigation which has shown this, but nevertheless there are grounds for considering that sexual material which arouses abnormal erotic interest or perhaps excessive normal hetero-sexual interest ought not to be too readily available. This is a long way from saying that the publication of such material should be banned since such a decision involves many other issues. However, patients who have a sexual problem have occasionally been known to us to suffer because they were encouraged to take some opportunity to do things which later they regretted and would have wished to avoid. We think it wise to counsel patients who wish to change not to enjoy aberrant wishes even in imagination; they should avoid material which promotes aberrant fantasies or activities.

The wide range of symptoms now treated by behaviour therapy also includes stammering and obsessional symptoms. Obsessional ruminations may be treated by 'thought-stopping'. When the patient signals that the rumination is present the therapist intervenes by shouting 'stop'. Compulsions may be treated by response prevention, for example, hand-washing after contamination is deliberately blocked. Previously in-tractable symptoms have been shown to yield at times to these techniques (as well as responding at times to some anti-depressants).

From what has been said so far it will be evident that in the desensitization technique whether gradual or by flooding, patients learn not to respond to certain situations with an anxiety which forbids efficient functioning. In the aversion methods an unpleasant affect is aroused which discourages the patient from carrying out some undesirable behaviour. In the aversion treatment of alcoholism (Chapter 16) the patient is conditioned to respond with nausea to the taste, smell or sight of drink, and experiments in similar methods have been tried in sexual deviations, writer's cramp and other condi-tions. In writer's cramp and tics electric shock is most often used, and this type of aversion therapy is apparently quite successful in some cases.

Aversion therapy is not always discussed objectively. Many doctors dislike it because the infliction of distress on the patient is understood to be an integral part of the treatment and not an undesirable side effect, as is the case with other

types of medical and surgical treatment. There is the dangerous possibility that the patient may gladly accept the treatment from morbid motives such as the wish to be punished
or because of (unconscious) sexual gratification. The doctor
is placed in the powerful position of believing he can mould
the emotional and motor responses of his patients. In *behaviour modification* techniques are deliberately employed to
achieve such purposes. For example, subnormal (retarded)
patients may be rewarded for specific actions or achieve-
ments like not being dirty or following particular rules. The
rewards tend to take the form of tokens which may have
some internal value within the institution. Occasionally
aversive treatments have been used to try and induce very
retarded patients not to damage themselves or their clothing.
These situations approach the technique of brainwashing.
The evidence for the value of these treatments has, therefore,
to be scrutinized with more care than usual, and in the selection of patients it is important to make sure that the patient
is not under the duress of a probation order or the demands
of a domineering family. In the case of aversion treatment of
retarded patients the balance of advantage and discomfort
has to be clearly in the patient's favour and decisions about it
should be the responsibility of more than one consultant.

The exact place of behaviour therapy remains to be established for a variety of conditions. Currently it has a leading
role in the treatment of single isolated fears known as *monosymptomatic phobias,* for example, cat phobias and other
fears of specific objects and situations. In these rather rare
conditions, it is more effective than psychotherapy. It is
less easy to apply to generalized anxiety but the limits of its
usefulness remain to be defined. The reader is referred to one
of the more comprehensive texts for a fuller exposition,
Meyer and Chesser[54], whose book gives an excellent balanced
account of the principles and application of behaviour therapy.

In the first years of behaviour therapy its advocates, who
were often clinical psychologists, tended to stress that their
theories, unlike those of psychoanalysts, were based on
experimental data and complied with scientific principles in
regard to both theory and the testing of hypotheses. They
also pointed out that many neuroses which psychotherapy

claimed to help could recover spontaneously. However, the theories of behaviour therapy are still not established nor are its results. The same is perhaps true of psychotherapy, but there is little doubt in our own minds that both approaches contribute usefully—and can be shown so to contribute— both to psychiatric theory and to treatment. In fact there is evidence in the literature for such a conclusion. Some notable examples are the better response of single phobic symptoms to behaviour therapy than to psychotherapy and the relief of some obsessional compulsions by behavioural techniques such as thought-stopping.

PSYCHOTHERAPY AND LEARNING THEORY

The conflict between psychotherapy and behaviour therapy no longer troubles many people, and the current tendency is for psychiatrists to combine the use of both disciplines. If psychotherapy is a learning process in emotional maturity, then it is reasonable to assume that the same principles of learning theory would apply to psychotherapy as to behaviour therapy. With this consideration in mind it might be worth while to examine some of the points on which behaviour therapy and psychotherapy appear to conflict.

The first concerns anxiety. Many exponents of behaviour therapy suggest that if the overt neurotic symptom is treated on behavioural lines, the anxiety which psychotherapists believe to be the cause of the symptom will also disappear and not produce further symptoms. There is no doubt that in some cases this is true, for example, the pad and bell apparatus for the treatment of enuresis. This perhaps finds a parallel in the mild cases of neurosis which are completely relieved by a tranquillizer; with supportive psychotherapy the tranquillizer can be withdrawn after a time without a relapse of symptoms. It seems likely that in many such cases the continuance of the symptom is in itself the major cause of the anxiety, and that the original precipitating factors have long since withered into insignificance. The symptoms may then aptly be termed a residual habit for which behavioural therapy is almost certainly the treatment of choice.

This point of view has led some behavioural therapists to

assert that 'there is no neurosis underlying the symptom, but merely the symptom itself. *Get rid of the symptoms and you have eliminated the neurosis.*'[22] This is a reasonable point of view. All investigators, whether psychologists or psychoanalysts, would agree that a neurosis is a learned maladaptive reaction, an extreme variant of the normal, without a nosologically distinctive pathology as is the case with GPI and, perhaps, too, in schizophrenia; they would agree that when the patient's behaviour proved acceptable the neurosis could be pronounced cured. The difficulty comes in defining what is meant by symptom. The majority of accounts of behaviour therapy are concerned with the symptoms for which the patient seeks help, but this by itself is a naïve and restricted view of neurotic disturbance.

The husband of a frigid woman may well count her lack of sexual response a minor trouble compared with her irritability and scarcely veiled hostility. These surely must count as symptoms, even though the patient herself may (truthfully) be unaware of them. This involves another point of conflict between behaviour therapists and psychotherapists: the necessity for postulating 'unconscious mechanisms'. If by unconscious is meant a different order of mental events relating to conscious experience in a manner analogous to the relation between biochemistry and physiology, then the point may be ceded. In Chapter 5 it was suggested that patients may have a seemingly wilful lack of awareness of what must clearly be important for them, so that patients may not only deliberately withhold their most pressing problems but even not be clear themselves as to how their difficulties should be formulated. This point is surely crucial for any therapy, behavioural or otherwise. One cannot plan a strategy of treatment with which the patient can cooperate unless the vital problems are clear to both patient and doctor. Moreover, this lack of awareness was thought to be due to a purposive but unconscious avoidance of the hurtful problem. This type of inner psychological behaviour is strikingly paralleled by the behaviour of rats in Miller's[55] experiments, in which he trained the animals by means of a strong shock to escape from a white compartment with a grid floor into a black compartment without a grid. Subsequently the rats, without any further electric shocks, learned a new habit of manipulating a simple device in order to open a closed door so that they could escape from out of the white compartment. Like Miller's rats, our patients learn to avoid the unpleasant topics which they associate with fear, without requiring additional reinforcements of fear. It is suggested here that repression is similarly a conditioned avoidance response. It follows, therefore, that the first task of any therapy is to extinguish this avoidance response; while the patient continues to run away (literally, in the case of a street phobia) he has no opportunity to check his fears with reality and to unlearn his morbid response of anxiety. Furthermore, each act of turning away again reinforces the danger of the anxiety situation.

A further difficulty is that although neurotic anxiety may appear to be focused on the external environment, this may in fact be a projection. A more candid statement of the patient's position might be: if they knew what was in my heart, what would they do to me! Naturally, the patient tends to avoid such insights. In such a situation desensitizing the patient to the external object of fear is clearly unhelpful. Wolpe* described a case in point in which he treated on behavioural lines a woman with social fears without success for twenty sessions before she revealed a distressing marital situation in which, for example, her husband would not let her drink alcohol.

We can now attempt an analysis of neurotic phenomena in terms of learning theory. In the simplest case a highly unpleasant experience conditions the patient to avoid that situation in future. The stimulus of approaching that situation awakens the response of anxiety in exactly the same way as the bell caused Pavlov's dogs to salivate. The patient responds by taking avoiding action, which he has learned will result in a reduction in the strength of the acquired drive of anxiety. Where danger is objectively present (for example, a bull) this pattern of behaviour has obvious biological value. However, two developments may turn it into a nonadaptive (neurotic)

---

* Unpublished observation.

response. In the first place, through stimulus generalization, related but essentially harmless objects (cows) may be almost as effective in arousing the response of anxiety. Second, when the patient learns that he can reduce the level of anxiety by taking avoiding action, this response is hard to extinguish for the simple reason that the patient never stays there long enough to find out if the unconditioned stimulus (of danger) is still present. This is well shown by the patient who was badly scared in childhood by being pecked by a parrot. Through stimulus generalization she soon came to fear all birds and learned the response of avoiding them at all costs. Her friends tried to break her fear by physically holding her in a place full of birds: she nearly fainted with fright. They did not appreciate that as well as teaching her that there was nothing to be afraid of, she first had to unlearn the habit of running away.

The majority of clinical material is unfortunately not as straight-forward as this case, but it will be seen that the same principles can also be applied to the description of the neurotic predicament in Chapter 5. To suffer rejection by one's parents (by indulging in forbidden impulses and feelings) is surely a traumatic conditioning, more devastating than a parrot's peck.

Much of the psychological treatment advocated in this book can be easily assimilated to the principles of learning theory. Earlier in this chapter the example was given of the patient who expected the therapist to be shocked. In this case the fear of the scandalous revelation took the place of the fear of worms, and the understanding of the therapist was equally reassuring. This may explain why a relatively permissive and nondirective technique is essential in psychotherapy: if the therapist insists too brutally on discussing anxiety-provoking topics the patient will exhibit the panic response known as resistance and much time will have been wasted. It will now be understood why transference phenomena are so important in psychotherapy. During the course of psychotherapy the patient comes to value the therapist as if he were a parent and begins to recreate between himself and the therapist the strains and conflicts which were left unsolved from his childhood. Instead of talking about what happened long ago, the problem has recreated itself here and now. The skilful therapist does not lose this opportunity to extinguish the original responses of fear and guilt elicited by parental figures and to encourage new habits of assertion and self-confidence on the part of his patient.

Reviewing this discussion, it would seem that both behaviour therapy and traditional psychotherapy are alike in their efforts to teach neurotic patients more acceptable emotional and motor responses. Where the object arousing anxiety can be clearly located outside the patient, treatment on behavioural lines may sometimes offer help not otherwise available. Care must be taken, however, that the proffered symptom is not a decoy to lead the attention of both patient and therapist away from the real problem. Much patient psychotherapy on analytical lines may be needed to expose clearly the real objects of fear. All too often these are found to be located inside the patient, in guilt-producing images of the parents or ungovernable affects. Although the behavioural principles of systematic desensitization and reciprocal inhibition may be held still to apply, they have to await the unpredictable development of a transference situation or the emergence of hitherto unacknowledged feelings before the crucial relearning can take place.

In conclusion it may be said that probably the most important contribution of learning theory is that it focuses attention on an experimental approach to psychological treatment. It suggests new lines of treatment and sharply criticizes the speculation of some psychotherapists. This experimental attitude must not, however, be allowed to obscure the necessity for clinical acumen and perception in understanding the emotional needs and anxieties of patients.

THE USE AND ABUSE OF SEDATIVES AND TRANQUILLIZERS

Earlier in this chapter the part played by these drugs during antidepressant treatment and in schizophrenia is described. It remains to discuss their use in patients suffering from acute or chronic neurosis as well as those personality disorders of a more long standing nature which may be revealed following the alleviation of depression.

Drugs which produce sleep are known as *hypnotics* and the same drugs, for example, nitrazepam, may also be used to calm the patient, in which case they are generally known as *sedatives*. Sedatives of this type inevitably tend to cause some drowsiness. When a drug, chlorpromazine, was introduced which produced a calming effect with significantly less drowsiness than the sedatives it was called a *tranquillizer*. The name has stuck and is now applied to all the phenothiazine group of drugs. Others such as diazepam, meprobamate, chlordiazepoxide, which do not help in schizophrenia are known both as sedatives and as minor tranquillizers, as well as similar preparations which have since become available.

Many doctors express concern about the amount of sedatives and tranquillizers which is prescribed. Undoubtedly, there are cases in which this concern is justified. Nevertheless, sedation or calming in our opinion constitutes an essential element in the management of many cases of neurosis.

The action of these sedatives can be defined as the relief of the physical and psychological symptoms of anxiety, fear and tension. It is essentially a symptomatic treatment which does not solve any of the patient's problems. It is an abuse of drugs, therefore, to prescribe them as an alternative to formulating and dealing with the psychological problem involved. In such cases the danger of addiction arises; if the neurosis becomes chronic, so does the prescription of tranquillizers.

However, we feel it is necessary to supply adequate sedation or tranquillization at the onset of an acute neurosis. The experience of anxiety can be so frightening that this in itself will produce a secondary anxiety, the fear that the anxiety attack will be repeated. Adequate sedation cuts short this vicious circle. This was well shown in the last war, in which it was demonstrated that adequate sedation at the onset of the anxiety state often allowed an early return to unit.

Once the acute stage of the neurosis has passed, continued sedation may be required during the period in which the patient is struggling to improve his adjustment. We have many patients who could not continue with outpatient psychotherapy without such help. Nevertheless, the patient must realize clearly that the tablets are no more than a crutch to help him over a difficult period. Once he begins to regard them as a definitive treatment, then it becomes very difficult to persuade him that he needs to improve his adjustment to life. This is where the danger of habituation is very real. In the successful management of these cases, the need for sedatives should diminish as readjustment is achieved. The continuing or increasing need for tablets is a danger signal that the treatment is not proceeding satisfactorily, and, perhaps, a consultation with a psychiatrist is required. Many patients prefer to cope without sedatives, and this aspiration should be encouraged unless their behaviour causes pain to other people. There is no virtue in eschewing drugs if the patient becomes impossible to live with.

An instance where a patient should not be allowed to discontinue drugs too readily is where he appears to be rejecting medication after trying something only briefly, because of a morbid belief that he does not deserve to get better and ought not to be having medication for a failure in his own character. Such views are common in depressive patients and particularly relevant to their use of antidepressants, which they need to be encouraged to take scrupulously, rather than allowed to discontinue from a nihilistic or pessimistic attitude, itself the result of the illness. On the other hand, troublesome side effects may sometimes reasonably lead patients to abandon medication in which case the reason should be carefully sought. These considerations may apply particularly in illnesses which look superficially like neurosis but turn out to be responsive to antidepressant medication. It is important when prescribing to discuss the doses of drug and the effect which can be anticipated and to enlist the patient's own active cooperation in working out the appropriate amount. The dosage of antidepressants should be that which will produce the minimal side effects, thus showing that the drug is being absorbed in significant amounts. We see very little justification for going above such a level since that merely increases the risk of toxic consequences and causes extra discomfort without clear benefit to the patient. Indeed there is evidence that unduly high doses of antidepressants are counter-productive therapeutically; it is possible that high doses of antidepressants may block the transmission of nerve impulses whereas lower doses may facilitate them.

There remains a residue of cases in which an improvement in the social environment is impossible and an adjustment in the patient's attitudes equally improbable. Marital disturbances in middle-aged couples often provide examples of this. In such cases continued medication may be unavoidable, but care should be taken to make this as harmless as possible. Barbiturates and amphetamine are especially to be avoided because of the danger of addiction. Similar considerations apply to night sedation. The onset of a neurosis is often accompanied by sleeplessness and a little night sedation is often helpful to support common sense advice. If there is a risk that night sedation may become a permanent feature of the patient's life it is sometimes useful to suggest that hypnotics be taken two or three nights a week. This prevents an accumulation of fatigue due to sleeplessness and yet avoids the habit of a nightly sedative.

If the decision is made to use sedatives by day then the benzodiazepines are the drugs of choice. Diazepam like its congeners is exceptionally safe where there is a suicidal risk, since enormous overdoses, upwards of sixty times the average therapeutic dose have been taken without fatality. The phenothiazine group, although very valuable in the treatment of psychoses has less place in the treatment of neurosis; they often give ineffective sedation in such conditions but may occasionally be valuable because they do not appear to carry any risk of addiction.

OTHER PHYSICAL TREATMENTS

The outstanding physical treatment in psychiatry is ECT (EST). This has already been discussed in detail. Here it is important to mention that it is of considerable use in a variety of states of agitation whether associated with depression, mania or schizophrenia. It is similarly helpful in patients with retarded depression and some forms of schizophrenia such as catatonic and paranoid. Its main use was and still is for patients with an endogenous depressive type of illness. The kindest thing that can be said about non-medical attacks upon it is that they are based on ignorance. The main disadvantage in some cases where it would otherwise be superbly useful, is that it may need to be given repeatedly. Therefore medication, although less quick to work and a little less effective, is often a more practicable treatment despite the fact that its overall risks are probably higher than those of ECT (EST).

Leucotomy

Leucotomy involves ablation of certain areas of the prefrontal cortex or, more often, the isolation of these areas by cutting white fibre tracts travelling, probably, from the cortex to the thalamus. There is a wide divergence of views on the value of this procedure. The original standard operation provoked disfavour on account of the deficits of personality (lack of initiative, emotional flattening) which were too frequently the sequel. More recent modified operations reduce this hazard to an acceptably low incidence. Whilst some authorities are perhaps overenthusiastic, it is probably true that the modified operations could be performed more often with benefit. Currently, there is interest in selective leucotomies which are more precisely placed and in which the lesion is defined by stereotactic procedure. These affect relatively few patients, but in general, are free from undesirable side effects. Adequate rehabilitation and after-care services are essential if the best results are to be obtained. While opinions vary, severe obsessional illness, long-standing tension and anxiety and intractable depression are the most widely accepted indications. Chronic schizophrenia is sometimes regarded as an indication, but the results of operation are rather poor. For some authorities, the type of illness is not as important as the type of personality: a conscientious obsessional personality with a high level of drive is thought to benefit especially. All authorities agree that leucotomy should be withheld until all other less irreversible treatments have been explored. In North America, probably because of adverse social and political influences, leucotomy is exceptionally rarely used.

Deep insulin coma treatment for schizophrenia has now been abandoned, since it has been shown to lack specific therapeutic value. *Modified insulin* treatment, in which the dose of insulin is adjusted to induce no more than drowsiness, was widely employed in any psychiatric patient with anxiety neurosis or in whom a gain of weight was to be desired. The concurrent improvement in the patient's mental state may be due to no more specific action than a placebo effect, but at least it gave both doctor and patient two or three weeks to reconsider their problems. It is now little used. It is best regarded as a descendant of Weir Mitchell's 'rest cure'. *Deep narcosis* is also used occasionally, its role being to calm very agitated patients whilst other forms of treatment such as ECT (EST) have time to take effect. More often heavy sedation with antidepressants and phenothiazines serves the same purpose.

HYPNOSIS

Hypnosis is of very little regular use either in psychiatry or in conditions for which it is sometimes recommended such as asthma, pain in childbirth and dentistry. However, because it is a psychological technique, because its complications are psychological ones and because it is sometimes used in psychiatric treatment and may be employed in general practice it deserves some consideration. Further, it is of great historical interest and has latterly been the subject of research which clarifies the effects attributed to it.

Hypnosis is commonly regarded as 'a state of heightened suggestibility' and throughout the centuries such states have apparently occurred in many subjects who have shown trance phenomena. In the eighteenth century it was thought to be the result of an animal quality comparable to magnetism and was then called Mesmerism after its principal practitioner. After vigorous controversy in the nineteenth century, it became accepted as a natural phenomenon which does not depend on any occult or supernal powers. Finally, it has become clear that it is not ordinarily a sleep state as the name would suggest. Hypnotic subjects remain in contact with some parts of their environment and do not show the physiological changes in their EEGs which are customary during sleep. Rather it appears that it is a state in which the attitudes and expectations of the subject are so altered that he behaves and feels in ways which would not normally be the result of conscious intention. A brief description of the phenomenon may help to make this more clear.

Techniques in inducing hypnosis vary greatly, and perhaps the only essential elements are the doctor's confidence in his ability and the patient's confidence in the doctor. Hypnosis certainly cannot be induced without the fullest cooperation. Most techniques insist that the recumbent patient should fixate his eyes on a point above his head, should breathe slowly and deeply and consciously relax his muscles. Suggestions are then given that he will go to sleep: 'Your eyes feel heavy, and they are slowly closing. You can't keep them open any longer ...', and the like. If the patient is susceptible to hypnosis (and a proportion of patients are not susceptible, especially if they are anxious, angry or tense) he will close his eyes in about five or ten minutes. This is the first stage of hypnosis. Suggestions are then given that the sleep is deepening, the relaxation is more profound. In the second stage of hypnosis the patient accepts suggestions that he cannot control his muscles voluntarily. A convenient way to test this is to give the suggestion that one arm is rising from the couch. As this suggestion is repeated, the arm will rise slowly into the air. At this point the suggestion can be given that the arm has gone stiff, when the patient will find that he can no longer move his arm until told to do so. This level of hypnosis is suitable for most treatment. The third stage of hypnosis is the somnambulist, in which the patient can walk about although still hypnotized. It is at this stage that some of the more curious phenomena can allegedly be observed. This level of hypnosis is only found in a minority of subjects.

When the second and third stages of hypnosis are reached psychogenic paralyses, amnesias, anaesthesias and even hallucinations or false beliefs may thus be induced or abolished. Posthypnotic suggestions may also be given and, like suggestions offered during the hypnotic session, may be acted upon; they are particularly used to make subsequent inductions easy.

It is imprudent to hypnotize a patient of the opposite sex without the presence of a chaperone. Many patients have unconscious sexual fantasies about hypnosis, and these may lead an unstable female patient into making scandalous accusations against the doctor who has been trying to help her.

In the practice of hypnosis one further very important condition must be observed. If a hypnotic state is induced the doctor must be very careful to remove the hypnotic suggestions given before waking up the patient (apart from any that had a therapeutic or experimental purpose). Thus having told one of our first patients that his eyes would want to close and having subsequently woken him up without saying that his eyes would cease wanting to close we were embarrassed by his complaint next day that he felt continually sleepy and could not keep his eyes open. Again it happened with another patient, who like the first one mentioned was a hysterical personality, that having used arm levitation for the purpose of induction we found that as he went to sleep each night in the ward his arm rose and floated in the air for a considerable period despite his efforts to bring it down and despite the fascinated consternation of his immediate neighbours. The practitioner must, therefore, be careful before terminating any hypnotic session to remove any unwanted posthypnotic effects. The possibility of such effects has a further bearing on the use of hypnosis, since they may arise not just as an accidental consequence of the technique employed but as a logical outcome of its use to remove symptoms; this is particularly relevant for psychiatric conditions.

When psychiatric symptoms, and the like, are produced they usually have the characteristics of hysterical ones; for instance, in a paralysis of an arm both agonists and antagonists can be found to contract and the distribution of the paralysis will correspond with the patient's ideas rather than with the facts of neuromuscular segmental innervations. It has been claimed that some curious physical and vascular changes can ensue from hypnosis, for example, removal of warts, the improvement of ichthyosis and the alteration of limb temperatures. Moreover, it has long been widely believed that major operations could be performed under hypnosis without a hint of pain. Whilst the phenomena cannot be elicited in everyone and whilst some subjects are only susceptible to a minimal degree there is no doubt that induced paralyses occur and that subjects believe in the reality of their own loss of control and in the occurrence of symptoms in accordance with the hypnotist's statements. This must be quite sufficient to justify the truism that hypnosis is a state of heightened suggestibility, but it leaves us with the problem as to how it is established. An impressive analysis of how this takes place has been provided by an American psychologist, T. X. Barber.[3] In a wealth of studies and experimental investigations Barber has provided impressive evidence of the following conclusions which we accept.

The historical accounts of the operations under hypnosis make it seem likely that the majority of subjects experienced some pain. The same applies to an analysis of reports of the attempted relief of pain of childbirth by hypnosis. Few subjects appear not to give some indication of having pain. For example, it was reported that when investigators questioned women after so called natural childbirth they related the experience of a good deal of pain during the procedure. Some of these women had in fact denied pain when asked about it by the doctors responsible for their direct treatment. When confronted with the discrepancies they said words to the effect that 'Oh but he is such a nice man ... I did not want to disappoint him'.

When strong suggestions without hypnosis are used to diminish pain experimentally this is just as successful in relieving pain as when hypnosis with suggestion is used. Physiological changes occurring under hypnosis are paralleled by those which can be obtained by suggestion without hypnosis.

There are, further, no reliable reports of hypnosis producing physiological changes other than such as might be produced by suggestion without hypnosis. Hypnotic suggestions are only followed when the subject connects them with the laboratory or clinical setting. They cease to have effect otherwise.

From these and related observations Barber concludes that the prime factor in the behaviour of hypnotic subjects is their expectation of what will follow. They accept a role, comply with its requirements and report on their own behaviour and experience in accordance with what they think they should say. Moreover, the phrasing of questions about their experiences has a direct bearing on the way in which they then comment on those experiences.

It follows from Barber's work that there is no special trance state which we can call hypnosis, and this is supported by the negative results of neurophysiological investigations in hypnotized subjects. There are no electrophysiological changes in hypnosis except such as may be attributed to altered attention in the normal waking state. Even studies of evoked potentials at the scalp indicate the same result, and physiological changes or reduction of the pain of noxious stimulation are not more than can result from suggestion or emotional change without the necessity to believe in a special trance state.

In reviewing this topic we have elsewhere defined hypnosis as follows:

> Hypnosis is a manoeuvre in which the subject and hypnotist have an implicit agreement that certain events (for example paralysis, hallucinations, amnesias) will occur, either during a special procedure or later, in accordance with the hypnotist's instructions. Both try hard to put this agreement into effect and adopt appropriate behavioural roles and the subject uses mechanisms of denial to report on the events in accordance with the implicit agreement. This situation is used to implement various motives whether therapeutic or otherwise, on the part of both participants.[50]

From this analysis we hope it may be accepted that after a long and fascinating career hypnosis has been placed in a niche which is a tribute to human imagination and to the power of suggestion but not one belonging to a mysterious or superordinate power. After that, what is its use? For the practitioner who accepts this argument hypnosis becomes the less attractive the more it seems to be a double bluff in which both the subject and hypnotist deceive themselves about the proceedings. We, therefore, do not recommend it ourselves for any treatment as a routine practice. Yet those who still believe in it as a special procedure can exert a useful influence with it on transient symptoms. For chronic illness it is rarely helpful. The exception where we still use it ourselves is the removal of conversion symptoms. Other methods of persuasion, encouragement, or psychotherapy are often useful, but occasionally when they fail or when patients already have the idea that hypnosis can help them it is helpful to go through the motions of hypnosis which enable the patient to relinquish the symptom which he or she wishes to lose. If, however, the patient is not ready to recover, then he may not lose the symptoms even though deeply hypnotized, that is, even though he is acting in a state which would suggest that he will follow the most remarkable suggestions.

If we suppose that many symptoms solve a conflict it is clear that their removal may present the patient with a difficult problem. The woman who has a hysterical paralysis of her legs because she does not wish to nurse her mother or because she fears intercourse with her husband is protected from the realization of her unconscious fears by her physical symptoms. The man who has lost his memory for his wife and family may be brought to face a desperate domestic crisis when his memory is restored. In such cases it is conceivable that the use of hypnosis will abolish the presenting symptom and pitchfork the patient back into a major personal difficulty. Depression, even suicide, could follow such a *dénouement*. Hypnosis should, therefore, generally not be used until the practitioner is satisfied that he can persuade the patient to accept the situation which will follow from the removal of the symptoms or knows how to cope with it.

A second and equally important reason for being cautious in the use of hypnosis is that it may serve to gratify unconscious wishes on the part of either the doctor or the patient. To use hypnosis is to exercise a special power, one which both for the doctor and the patient may have a sexual significance. At least the doctor gets a lift to his ego from this miraculous and extremely personal action and the patient is liable to develop an attitude of undue dependence. It has already been mentioned that females should not be hypnotized without a chaperone being present, but apart from that the practitioner must beware of the special feelings which can arise in this treatment situation. These can present him with a most severe problem in the handling of the treatment situation. The problem is severe because the patient may impute correctly that it is the doctor's attitude which has encouraged his dependence, and it is severe too because the doctor himself consciously or unconsciously may recognize a germ of truth in the criticism and be troubled by guilt accordingly. When the patient then develops fresh symptoms or unwanted complications of treatment they are blamed on the doctor who is liable to feel helpless to alter them, as they grow out of his control, and at fault for having engendered them. This is one of the most acute examples of the sort of situation which we discussed in our first two chapters when we concluded that the doctor could be of most use to his patient by avoiding emotional involvement in the latter's difficulties. It will be seen how strong the case is here then for adopting that neutral uncommitted attitude which we advocated earlier; when one adds to this the knowledge that hypnotism itself is a somewhat illusory procedure the indications for its use become very slight.

PROGNOSIS

Recovery is very common in psychiatric illness of all types except dementia, where it only occurs in a small minority of patients. Whilst the basic personality may remain the same the acute illness frequently remits very satisfactorily and this is particularly the case in general practice. Nevertheless, there is a widespread impression that the patient's prognosis in psychiatric illness is worse than in other types of disease. This is partly because of a common fond expectation that psychiatrists should be able to modify people's characters for the better. Except in rare cases this is not realistic. Secondly, psychiatric illness is only fatal in a limited number of cases and thus the persistence of chronic cases is forced upon our attention; someone usually has to live with our failures. However, there is a very large number of people who have had a psychiatric illness and got better to pursue useful and happy lives and this is the first point which the practitioner should always remember in advising patients.

The second point to remember is that hope of a recovery should never be abandoned in psychiatric illness. The most unexpected pleasant surprises are known to occur. The doctor should, therefore, never commit himself to giving a hopeless prognosis. To err this much on the side of optimism will be forgiven; to err in the other direction will not. Moreover, a degree of cautious optimism helps both the patient and his family and is supported by the facts.

This much being true it is still unfortunately the case that the estimating of psychiatric prognosis remains more of an art than a science, in spite of a number of long-term follow-up studies. The prognosis for schizophrenic illness is briefly mentioned at the end of Chapter 7, and this section is concerned with the prognosis for patients suffering from anxiety and depression.

Where the illness consists almost entirely of an endogenous depression (and the same is true for mania) without any complicating factors such as neurotic personality disorders, social stresses, or physical illnesses, it can be said that recovery is the rule, with or without specific antidepressant treatment; the natural history of an untreated depression may, however, last several years. Provided that a depression is energetically treated so as to be completely free from symptoms for *at least two weeks*, relapse is highly unlikely. Unfortunately, many depressed patients finish treatment still suffering from minor depressive symptoms which leave the door ajar for a speedy relapse. Such a relapse is commonly produced by ceasing antidepressant medication before full recovery has occurred. Further, with attacks of depression severe enough to require specialist attention it has been shown that patients who cease antidepressants in the six months following recovery have a greatly increased risk of another attack during that time. In general, the longer the time since the last attack, the lower the risk of relapse, the rate of the latter falling from about 50 per cent in the first year to as little as 5 to 10 per cent in the fifth year. Following successful treatment, the patient's future is hard to predict. Many may have no further attacks, while others may get further attacks at regular intervals. A history of previous attacks may provide a guide insofar as depressive illnesses often occur at regular intervals. If the illness was provoked by a specific stress (influenza, childbirth or bereavement) then future attacks may depend on the recurrence of the specific stress. If the illness is associated with a hypomanic or manic upswing or if the diagnosis of recurrent unipolar depression is established, lithium treatment may have a very effective role to play in reducing future attacks by as much as 80 to 90 per cent. Specialist advice is appropriate in such cases.

It seems likely that the natural history of neurosis is also self-limiting in the majority of cases. In one study of obssessional neurosis (believed to be the most intransigent of neuroses), recovery or marked improvement had occurred in two-thirds of the cases after five years. In neurotic conditions, however, much depends on what happens to the patient. Whereas one illness may be precipitated by a bereavement, another patient may be freed from his neurotic burden by the timely death of a spouse. If the patient succeeds in gaining greater emotional maturity with or without the benefit of psychotherapy, an increased immunity to neurotic reactions may be predicted. A happy marriage or promotion at work may remove social stresses and frustrations with equally beneficial results. The successful treatment of an isolated symptom through behaviour therapy appears to have little danger of relapse.

The prognosis of any particular case will depend, therefore, on the assessment of a group of factors: the adequacy and maturity of the personality; the satisfactoriness of the social environment; the liability to future depressive responses and finally the unpredictable circumstances with which the future may endow or afflict any individual.

Part Three

Special Problems in Consultation

10

Psychosomatic Illness

We believe it is now generally accepted that emotional factors
help to cause organic disease or physiological dysfunction.
The description *psychosomatic* has been applied to such
effects. The term then covers equally the morbid anatomical
changes of eczema brought on by worry and the disturbed
bowel habit, without structural lesions, of the examination
candidate who develops a transitory diarrhoea. Many normal
phenomena such as blushing or trembling are psychosomatic
in this meaning of the word although it is not necessary to
regard them as signs of illness and we do not include them in
the definition of psychosomatic illness which we restrict to
physical disease or major physiological dysfunction in whose
origin emotional factors play an important part. They help
us, however, to understand the aetiology of the psychosomatic conditions inasmuch as the direct connection between
the state of mind and the paths of action of the nervous
system are readily comprehended in these latter instances.

It must be noted that while all psychosomatic conditions
are *ipso facto* of psychological origin, that is, originating at
least in part from emotional states, the word *psychosomatic*
is often wrongly applied to other bodily symptoms which are
not caused in the same way even though they may be due to
emotional causes. For example, in an hysterical aphonia or
paraplegia the physiology of the part or of the peripheral
nervous system is not disordered so as to cause the symptom.

In the extreme case it is true that hysterical paralysis may lead to contractures and hyperventilation to tetany, but in the first instance these changes, like those of dermatitis arte-facta, are the consequence of alterations in behaviour and may be so distinguished. Like the injuries sustained by some individuals, who have an excessive number of accidents, they are the result of a pathological pattern of action or inaction. It is true that some authorities have classified these latter effects as psychosomatic also, since they represent an effect of the mind upon the body, but we think that it is better to emphasize direct physiological effects as the touchstone of psychosomatic illness and to retain the word *psychosomatic* for them. This distinction may sometimes be made for a single symptom. Thus a man who has a precordial pain on the anniversary of his father's sudden death from cardiac disease in the absence of any evidence that he himself has angina or muscular spasm may be considered to have a symbolic and, therefore, psychogenic symptom. If we find that his blood pressure was temporarily raised, causing angina or a coronary thrombosis we could conclude that he had had a psychoso-matic illness.

Once the formulation is made that physical changes occur as a result of emotional factors, mainly operating through the autonomic nervous system, it becomes apparent that a wide range of illnesses may be attributed to the mental make-up of the individual and to his experiences. Many eczemas and cer-tain types of bronchial asthma, migraine, duodenal ulcer and menstrual disturbance are amongst the more notable condi-tions where we think a good case exists for such a proposi-tion and these are but a few of the numerous conditions for which worth-while evidence has been presented that psycho-logical factors are important in the aetiology.

Further, many regional muscular pains including the tight band of headache and many tachycardias and intestinal dis-turbances are undoubtedly due to tension or anxiety. In say-ing this, however, we would stress that it is out of keeping with modern concepts of disease to regard psychological causes as the only important ones even in those illnesses where their action is best validated. Indeed such an error is almost as bad as ignoring them altogether. Although we all rightly prefer not to make two diagnoses where a single one would cover all a patient's symptoms, we must nevertheless recognize that even a single diagnosis does not necessarily mean there has been a single cause for the illness. In infectious diseases the concept of 'the seed and the soil' is well recognized and important. The description of psychosomatic mechanisms is the description of some of the important constituents of the soil and should be so understood as, for example, in pulmonary tuberculosis where the immunological constitution of the individual and his state of mind both seem to have a bearing on the progress of the disease even in the presence of antibiotics. Allergic skin diseases provide another illustration of this phenomenon since many dermatologists would probably agree that even so 'organic' a reaction as nickel-sensitivity may only appear when the patient has been under emotional stress. We conclude, therefore, that the concept of multiple aetiology is essential to the proper appreciation of psychosomatic illness.

Attempts have been made recently to measure more accurately the significance of events which could predispose to psychosomatic illness. Accordingly research has concentrated on measuring the frequency and importance of different life events, for example, bereavements, divorce, change of employment, alteration in financial status whether for better or worse, which have preceded the onset of various illnesses in different people. It has become quite clear from this work that important changes in circumstances are often followed by illnesses of all types. In particular, Rees[64] has shown widows to have a much increased morbidity in the year following the death of their spouse. This notion of significant life events is accordingly one of the most impressive and reliable leading to the conclusion that physical illness may be provoked by psychological stress. Such life events have long been linked with psychological illness, especially depression. The recognition of the relationship of psychological stress to physical illness also derives from the observation that when people are ill with one condition they often tend to be ill about the same time with another. The 'cluster' theory of illness implies that several disorders may be provoked by one continuing cause, for example, emotional stress may first promote furuncles then attacks of headache and finally gastric haemorrhage as a result of the excessive use of aspirin. Although not all the effects of emotional stress are directly mediated by physiological pathways the interaction of psychological and physical factors plainly merits attention.

In any concept of multiple aetiology the question arises as to which cause is the most important. Current evidence tends to suggest that psychological factors are rarely the essential cause of any of the illnesses we are discussing. Although asthma may be provoked or exacerbated by anxiety it is much more often due primarily to allergic sensitivity or bronchial infection. The latter two are essential causes without which psychological factors do not usually come into play. However, factors which trigger off an illness can be as important as basic causes. It is doubtful if psychological factors are the essential cause of migraine, but there is no reasonable doubt that in some patients states of anxiety or depression are the main factor in provoking frequent attacks of migraine. When the anxiety is treated the migraine may abate substantially or even completely.

An important qualification which has to be made is that recognizing the psychological aetiology of a condition does not mean that it has to be treated invariably by psychological means. For example, thyrotoxicosis often follows an emotional shock but it nevertheless derives only limited benefit from the production of psychic calm compared with specific physical methods of treatment. But in other illnesses, as just indicated, psychological causes can be treated with benefit. However, we shall shortly say more on the treatment of psychosomatic illness. The first question which the practitioner will ask is how may he recognize psychosomatic disturbances and only after this what should be done about prevention and treatment.

One method of recognition would be to say that given a certain physical diagnosis, for example, asthma, hay fever, migraine, the practitioner may then assume that a psychosomatic illness is present. Clearly this is a risky method of work, and we would rather say that he should look for psychological causes to test the above assumption. The procedure then becomes very like that with other types of neurotic illness already discussed. Enquiry will be directed to the family history, the personal history, sexual relationships, unrealized ambitions and so forth. In many cases in general practice it will be very clear at the outset what has disturbed the patient. A detailed psychological analysis of the type of personality may not then be essential and the practitioner will be able to treat the patient by simple psychological and physical measures. The prestige of the doctor in understanding bodily disturbances, his willingness to help without condemning the attitudes of his patients and the advice he gives either on changing such attitudes or on altering the environment will usually be enough to provide an adequate resolution both of the illness and of its cause. These milder psychosomatic illnesses may well befall nearly all types of personality. It is obvious that in specialist practice the more severe cases tend to be seen. On the basis of such practice certain personality types have been described in association with psychosomatic illness as well as certain sorts of emotional difficulties. Thus sufferers from psychogenic eczema are often found to be worrying people, perhaps sensitive, and inclined to brood. Quite superficial current conflicts may cause illness in them although, like everyone else, they are not immune from deeper difficulties. Housing troubles or too many children for whom to care and similar problems, both conscious and readily expressible, may serve to provoke their skin disorder. Similarly patients with duodenal ulcer have been said to have a characteristic personality pattern more often than chance would allow. They tend to be tense, hard-working, conscientious, often driving and obsessional individuals and, like all other patients with psychosomatic complaints, have more than an average share of childhood difficulties followed by neurotic traits in later life.

Sufferers from intractable asthma likewise may be handicapped by feelings which they cannot express, whether towards parents, marital partners or employers. They may be liable to be conscientious and scrupulous in their own actions, but also ready to apply the same standards to other people. In their case the suppression of resentment or aggression and the evidence of impatience are prominent.

Descriptions of this sort imply the claim that there are

specific personality patterns which predispose to specific illnesses. There are considerable difficulties involved in proving
such an argument, unlike the significance of life events. The
measurement of personality characteristics is undoubtedly
difficult. This does not mean that it has not sometimes been
done well, but it does mean that there are very few studies in
which it has been satisfactory. There are two major problems
which cast further doubt on the validity of the personality
patterns said to cause certain psychosomatic illnesses. The
first is that inevitably most observation of the personality of
the sick has been undertaken with those sick people who
have presented for treatment at hospital centres. This means
that the patients concerned are preselected; the obsessional,
the persistent, the hypochondriacal, and the anxious in need
of reassurance are bound to be present in excess of their true
proportions, whilst the phlegmatic and serene will be found
less frequently than they occur. This is true also of general
practice. Problems of bias of this sort are rarely overcome. It
is a truism that psychological problems are important in the
patients whom every doctor will see. They may be less frequent in those, also ill, whom the doctor tends not to see.

Second, it is also a truism that physical illness, especially
if protracted, will bring psychological problems in its wake.
This point does not need elaboration. However, it is reasonable to suppose that many of the definite psychological
changes described in people with ulcerative colitis may result
from the suffering and indignity imposed by physical changes.
Similarly, there is reason to believe that few people with
chronic pain of physical origin (for example, with causalgia,
chronic postherpetic neuralgia, chronic rheumatoid arthritis)
fail to escape some increase in anxiety or depression as a
result of their organic troubles.

Despite these considerations it is still probably correct to
assume that patients with most of the classical psychosomatic
illnesses do have psychological problems which help to promote their condition and that they are in general more prone
to anxiety, depression and repressed emotional conflicts.
Specific patterns cannot, however, be safely attributed to
particular illnesses, and many changes are also likely to follow
from the physical afflictions. This being said it remains likely

that psychological factors are important in provoking or exacerbating asthma, migraine and duodenal ulcer. There is quite good systematic evidence that personality factors conduce to coronary artery disease.[23] In patients with pain related to physical disease psychological factors are important both in making the pain worse, and even sometimes in allowing it to occur, and emotional changes also result from pain caused by organic lesions. There are, however, two important conditions in which the importance of emotional causes has been increasingly challenged. These are ulcerative colitis and rheumatoid arthritis, and it may well be the case that the admitted changes in personality noted in patients with the latter two conditions are a consequence of the physical disease.

In looking at the psychological conditions which make asthma and other illnesses worse, an example may now be helpful. One man whom we treated illustrates the importance of suppressed resentment or aggression and also overt impatience. He was a teacher who had risen from working as an artisan by his own persistent efforts. The wife of his youth was, by contrast, consistently unreliable in her conduct of day-to-day affairs. She would contract foolish debts and lie to him about them even when she would inevitably be found out. His aspirations to run a solvent, respectable, modest white-collar worker's life were continually endangered by her shiftlessness. His wife bore him three children plus one whom he had some reason to believe was not his own. Prior to this he had had his first attack of asthma during the war when faced with the opportunity of being unfaithful with a more personable woman. Then as his socioeconomic level rose he had further attacks despite his attempts to reconcile himself to his wife's 'inferiority' which became increasingly evident and troublesome. Gradually he gathered the purse strings into his own hands and controlled his wife's expenditure rigidly. Their marital relationship became increasingly one of two companions who tolerated each other because they were yoked together by the children. Although testy and domineering at home the feelings he expressed were in no way as strong as those he contained, and any irritation, whether the inconsiderate behaviour of his brother-in-law or the dilatory and rapacious actions of a garage owner, would then exacerbate his wheezing. As with other neurotic symptoms, so here, too, antecedent causes could be found in his childhood, laying the basis for the adult personality which reacted so severely to these not uncommon frustrations.

With more explicitly neurotic complaints it was recognized that, while there are certain patterns of illness and types of individual, the boundaries between them are fluid. The same is inevitably true of psychosomatic complaints. After discriminating some pattern, whether hazy or precise, the basic problem is again one of recognizing the particular disturbed emotional relationship and discovering what may be done about it. We have noted already that even if an illness has psychological causes its best treatment may be physical. In general, and for all practical purposes, in a case like thyrotoxicosis if the cause is a single non-recurring one there is little more to be done by psychological means. Quite frequently, however, the individual may have been presented with a problem situation which is likely to recur, say an argument with his wife or a disappointment in business. In these circumstances, he may well wish to find a means of prevention for the future. The power of psychotherapy to assist in this respect has not yet been adequately proved, but it is at least logical to try and assist the willing patient to gain some further insight into the way in which his illness has been precipitated. It will often also be desirable, as we have emphasized, to consider the effects of the lesion upon the individual. Many patients are greatly comforted by an explicit recognition of this on the part of the doctor. People often need to be told that others are aware of their distress.

There are thus many patients with acute or chronic physical illness of psychological origin who may not obtain maximum or adequate benefit from physical methods of treatment alone. Our asthmatic patient already quoted is an illustration of this and it is probably true of others, as of him, that there may exist a personality disturbance which is sufficiently severe to deserve treatment even if it had never led to physical symptoms. In such cases psychological treatment is indicated; it may include temporary sedation but is most appropriate when it takes the form of sympathetic interviews aimed at releasing feelings, increasing insight and/or giving emotional support. There must be some cases where the general practitioner will feel able to attempt these measures. If he does, the basic principles of psychological treatment will apply here as elsewhere and, if he is wise, he will be careful to avoid getting himself personally involved in the patient's situation. This is particularly important because the first psychological 'improvement' may not produce any change for the better in the patient's physical state. In specialist practice it may take several interviews before the patient derives any benefit and indeed temporary exacerbations of the physical symptoms can, and have, been caused by the approach to emotionally painful material. The doctor should allow for this and be able to take it into account in his treatment of such cases. By being ready to ask whether psychological treatment has made the patient worse, and if so why, the doctor can often produce a notable advance both in his relationship with the patient and in the latter's appreciation of the causes of his symptoms. The patient will usually then see how the interview has disturbed him because it has touched on unpleasant topics or he will be able to relate some further cause for his trouble in his recent experiences. If the general practitioner does not wish to risk handling such problems himself he still needs to be aware that they may arise with patients whom he refers to psychiatrists. If he should feel and prove able to handle such cases effectively, they can be a source to him of great professional and human satisfaction.

11

Children and Adolescents

It is a common error to think of children simply as 'little adults'. They are not, and because of this child psychiatry has to differ from adult psychiatry both in its approach and in its concepts. The first major difference is that the child is always *developing* and changing, and accordingly must always be seen in the light of his developmental stage. Thus obstinacy in a two-year-old is a normal primitive method of self-expression at that age, but will be seen as stubbornness or anger in a six-year-old. Parental expectations are often out of line with the child's developmental stage, and this is a frequent source of presenting complaints. Furthermore, disturbing behaviour on the part of a child is much more likely to be an experiment in a new behavioural pattern than to be a relative 'fixture' as it would be in an adult, and therefore should more often receive a response of mild discouragement than a major therapeutic assault which, by its very nature, could set the pattern irretrievably. Much of child psychiatry, therefore, involves education and reassurance about normal development and since many of the disorders of childhood do not arise de novo but rather represent stages in this process where the child has become blocked, normal psychosocial development will be used as an organizing principle for most of this chapter.

A second major difference is that children are much more *dependent upon the family system* than adults, and therefore the family context becomes of crucial importance in interpreting and resolving problems of childhood. A child will almost always behave in such a way as to preserve (at least from his point of view) his position as a respected member of the family system and the more paradoxical his behaviour appears in the light of this principle the more carefully the explanation for the paradox must be sought within the family context. For instance, the seemingly self-defeating behaviour of sibling rivalry that drives the mother to distraction may sometimes have its true purpose elucidated by the observation that the mother's attention is drawn to this phenomenon at a time when she would otherwise be confronting her husband. The child's behaviour is thus designed to maintain the integrity of the family system upon which he is dependent, despite some personal cost in terms of frequent admonishments. Furthermore, a family has been described as a mobile, such that a change in the position or behaviour of one member necessitates an adjustment in one or more of the other members in order to preserve an equilibrium. Thus if a child's behaviour is simply 'corrected' without a corresponding change in one or more other family members it will often mean a high resistance to change on the part of the child, or another child becoming 'symptom-bearer' for the family. An elaboration of family system theories is beyond the scope of this chapter, but it is essential to note that the family context must be taken into consideration in any assessment, interpretation or treatment of a child.

Another essential point of difference lies in the fact that the primary mode of expression in childhood is through *action and play* rather than words, and it is thus much more important to note what a child actually *does* than to trust his verbal expressions. This is particularly true insofar as children recognize that their survival depends upon their preserving their essential relationships and they therefore tend to use a number of primitive defence mechanisms such as denial and projection with respect to any activity or behaviour they feel might meet with adult disapproval. This use of projection and displacement onto other objects, however, makes doll and puppet play a very rewarding approach for looking beneath the surface in children in order to determine their actual thoughts and feelings.

Because of the above differences and because of the child's relative unwillingness or inability to state directly what his concerns are, assessment must obviously be carried out in many areas simultaneously in order to obtain the necessary data to provide a correct interpretation of the nature of whatever difficulties are present. Biological, psychological, social, educational and familial factors must always be carefully examined concurrently for significant clues. This means that multidisciplinary teams are the norm in work with children, and the family practitioner should ideally know where to obtain help from other specialties when working with children.

Bearing the above in mind, then, we will first address ourselves to the basic relationships between child and adult, then to normal psychosocial development, thirdly to the common general patterns that can result from relative blocks in this development, and finally to some of the *specific* symptoms that can emerge in childhood, many of which will be found to stem directly from the general developmental patterns previously outlined.

OVERVIEW OF CHILD DEVELOPMENT

A child is born with certain innate drives and needs and the development of his capacity to fulfil these (first in the context of his family and later in the social world) is determined partly by other innate temperamental characteristics and partly by exogenous influences that are brought to bear upon him in his early experience with his environment.

Inborn factors in child development

Apart from certain survival instincts and basic drives (such as hunger and thirst) with which a child is born, he also has inherent needs for affection and achievement; and he has certain definable temperamental characteristics. The latter differ from infant to infant both in quality and strength. They include, for example, activity level, regularity, intensity of response to stimuli, the balance between tendencies to approach, or withdraw, adaptability to new situations, threshold of response to stimuli, degree of distractibility, and affective tone. Thus each infant, in a sense, comes into the world with a unique set of reactions. He also comes into the world with an innate capacity to develop along certain lines, for example, motor skills, perception, speech and language development, intellectual and cognitive abilities, and personal relationships. All the lines of development overlap and interrelate with one another so that delays or blocks in development in any one line will have effects on all others. The list at the end of this chapter gives a broad sketch of the stages of development through the course of childhood. Each biological line of development can be delayed or even arrested by environmental influences and alterations therein can effect major changes in a child who is not performing up to his or her potential.

Learned factors in child development

Certain very basic impressions about one's self and about one's relationship to others are formed in the first two years of life and they are largely pre-verbal or affective in nature. They are very broad and fundamental to the personality and although they can change with experience they are, nevertheless, very hard to alter later in life. It is more likely, in fact, that the individual will later seek changes in the world to conform to these early impressions rather than vice versa. These early impressions form the foundation stones for what is commonly known as 'personality', that is, a person's characteristic method or 'style' of coping with both intra- and interpersonal relationships. The process by which experience modifies temperament to become the ultimate 'personality' has four developmental stages.

Stage 1: Establishment of 'basic messages'

A 'basic message' is an impression that the child receives either about himself, his behaviour, or what he can expect from others, that is, about his existence. The earlier in life that the message is learned by the naive and totally dependent infant, the more likely it is to be accepted as an essential truth about the universe. He takes this as a given axiom or 'basic assumption' around which he subsequently believes he must organize his life. Examples are given here in cognitive style, but it should be recognized that they are often 'sent' in a non-cognitive manner and registered more as an unconscious affective tone than in the conscious symbolic form in which they appear here. Such messages include:

Statements of fact: the world is a safe/dangerous place; you are a good/bad person; you can/cannot trust your parents to look after you; you are/are not a competent human being.

Statements of values: using the potty is good; picking your nose is bad; your angry feelings are/are not acceptable.

Statements of conditions for continued acceptance: never cry when you are hurt; never object to parental injunctions but pretend you like them; strive hard to perform up to your parents' expectations regardless of your own motivation and abilities; sickness is the only acceptable way to gain extra attention.

Much could be elaborated about these early 'messages' and how they are conveyed. All that is needed for the purposes of the model presented here, however, is a general acceptance of the fact that such messages are received in early childhood as more or less accepted 'assumptions', 'facts' or 'truths' about existence, many of which are necessarily conflicting. Out of this morass of individual basic messages, conflicts and secondarily derived conflict-reducing mechanisms, the child develops a concept of how he should be ('ideal self'), who he actually is ('self-concept'), an expectation of how others will behave towards him under various circumstances, and hence a method of coping with the world as he now understands it.

Stage II: Internalization

The child internalizes the above basic messages and makes them into his own, because he learns them before he has developed the ability to be critical. They thus leave the realm of 'what someone else has said' where they can be subjected to continuing evaluation and become part of what the child says to himself about the way the world works ('internal dialogue') where they are thereafter used as 'universal criteria' for making decisions about the 'correct' way to cope or behave under any given circumstances.

Stage III: Generalization and projection

Once internalized, the basic messages then have a tendency to be both generalized to others (learning theory) and projected (psychoanalytic defence mechanism). For instance, an early message that it is unsafe to express anger towards mother or that one must be pleasing and charming to father at all costs may become generalized or 'transferred' to all other members of the same sex, especially members of high interpersonal importance such as a spouse. Such a belief, while perhaps valid in its original form, is likely to be invalid and maladaptive in its general form, for example, in a current school relationship.

Stage IV: Re-affirmation

The first three steps are finalized by re-affirmation. The question may be logically asked why this stage of personality development is so definitive and why these early basic messages are not subsequently subjected to reality testing so that those that prove to be still relevant, appropriate and adaptive are retained, while those that prove to be essentially inappropriate and maladaptive are discarded. Even without postulating that such processes as 'internalization' prevent the basic assumptions being available for re-evaluation there is a twofold answer to this question. Firstly, from a learning theory standpoint, the individual behaves in such a way as to prevent extinction and allow self-reinforcement. Behaviour is constantly emitted in accordance with the original basic message, which removes the potential for the 'assumed disaster' and this in turn reduces anxiety, which is self-reinforcing. For example, if the original learning implied that confined spaces were dangerous (claustrophobia), continued survival by avoiding confined spaces only proves the point and the individual never stays in the situation long enough to 'unlearn' the original belief.

Secondly, the individual tends unwittingly to 'create his own environment' in accordance with his learned expectations such that it re-affirms his original assumptions. For instance, panic behaviour of the claustrophobic individual when caught in a confined space is very likely to lead to self-injury and feelings of terror that serve to reinforce the original message. An anxious child or man striving to impress his fellows may be inept and thereby set up the very rejection he fears.

Thus behaviour in accordance with the original message not only prevents extinction and is self-reinforcing through anxiety reduction, but also, defiance of the original message tends to set up circumstances which produce the feared disaster. This basic process is augmented by the tendency of the organism to maintain a known equilibrium at all costs and not to 'risk' new behaviour, thereby also avoiding the mourning and depression consequent upon giving up an old belief or behaviour pattern, no matter how maladaptive or dysfunctional it was.

From the foregoing it can be seen that both inborn and learned factors combine very early in the life of the child so that he develops a self-concept and an understanding of the world and his relationship to others from which will develop, in turn, his characteristic mode of coping with both intra- and inter-personal relationships. Where the combination is adaptive and reality-oriented, he will be said to have a 'healthy' personality, but where some of the basic assumptions are erroneous or in conflict, symptoms will arise (cf. Chapter 5), sometimes in isolation and sometimes in characteristic clusters, depending upon the stage of development at which the maladaptive assumptions were incorporated. To understand these later stage-related clusters more clearly, it is necessary to look at normal psychosocial development in more detail.

NORMAL PSYCHOSOCIAL DEVELOPMENT*

Normal psychosocial development involves three separate but

---

* The authors are much indebted to the concepts of John Bowlby, Margaret Mahler and Erik Erikson in the development of this section.

mutually interdependent and concurrent processes: attachment, basic trust and separation–individuation. We will trace their development chronologically.

From approximately 0 to 3 months of age the child does not apparently distinguish between itself and the rest of the world. Even the infant's smile is thought to be reflex and not a social response. In this respect the child may be said to be in a stage of 'normal autism'.

From 3 to 6 months the infant begins to smile more selectively at facial stimuli. He can differentiate between self and non-self. By his behaviour he appears to recognize his dependency upon others and this stage is called 'normal symbiosis', as there is still some fusion with the 'mothering one'. The process termed *attachment* begins at this stage. Attachment can best be defined operationally as a relationship between an infant and the 'mothering one' within which the child appears secure and content. From this secure base he explores the rest of the world. He returns to it when frightened or anxious, and he protests with vigour, marked distress and anxiety about enforced separation from it. Attachment occurs most naturally between 3 and 12 months and is solidified primarily between 12 and 24 months although it remains fragile for a considerable period thereafter. Studies on attachment indicate that it is more than just a learned phenomenon and has some of the characteristics of an instinctive process. It seems to defy some of the basic laws of learning in that punishment or unpleasant experiences do not seem to deter it but can actually increase it. The absence or neglect of the mothering figure, on the other hand, may have a profound negative effect on attachment. Examples of such circumstances include emotional neglect by a parent, death of a parent, institutionalization, frequent changes of primary attachment figures as occurs in multiple foster placement, and hospitalization.

Attachment appears to be basic to the development of adequate self-esteem and subsequent interpersonal relationships, and anything which interferes with it appears to lead to a greater or lesser degree of pathology, depending upon the extent of the interference.

Between the ages of 4 and 7 months attachment becomes

more specific to a single mothering figure and during the early portion of this stage anxiety in the presence of strangers may emerge. The *quality* of response to the child's distress and the amount of positive *social* interaction initiated appear to be the most important variables at this stage in developing attachment rather than the absolute amount of time spent on routine caretaking functions, and hence, despite the short-term nature of memory retention at this age, there is no conclusive evidence to show that communal day-care facilities will interfere with the process.

The development of 'basic trust' is closely linked to attachment, but probably should be separated from it. While attachment has been called 'instinctive' and related to the ethological concept of 'imprinting', it is likely that the development of 'basic trust' is a learned phenomenon and reflects the *quality* of the process of attachment rather than the process itself. For example, a child who has become attached to an abusive parent may be strongly 'attached' but may totally lack 'basic trust'. The latter can best be defined as the degree of security and confidence which the child can place in his basic acceptability and desirability to the people around him, especially the primary attachment figure. The less 'basic trust' a child has, the more he feels he has to hide parts of himself (for example, his anger) and be compliant in order to please those around him so that he will not be abandoned, and the less he is willing to risk being open, honest and direct. The more 'basic trust' he has, the more he feels the environment will meet his needs. Thus, while attachment is probably necessary for the initial establishment of interpersonal relationships, it is 'basic trust' that determines the child's self-esteem and his subsequent way of handling those relationships.

Separation–individuation is the third major process that occurs in early development. It is initially dependent upon attachment having developed to some degree and occurs concurrently with it. It begins between the ages of 4 and 7 months as the child begins to differentiate himself from the normal symbiotic union with the 'mothering one', and is enhanced by the early development of locomotor ability between the ages of 7 and 10 months where the infant appears to be practising separation from his mother for brief periods of time. At this time, separation is not prolonged voluntarily for more than a few minutes, and the child frequently seems to return to the close proximity of the mother for what Mahler terms 'emotional refuelling'. This 'early practising period' is followed by the development of upright locomotion, and between the ages of 10 and 18 months the child takes longer and longer exploratory trips from the mother's side to indulge his curiosity about the rest of the world, often taking symbolic representation of the mother such as a blanket or a teddy bear ('transitional object') along with him to bridge the gap. The distance that the child is able to move from his mother in this late practising period appears to be directly related to the amount of basic trust he has been able to develop in the security of his relationship with her. It is as if the child were using his mother as an explorer's base camp from which he makes sorties to indulge his curiosity about the new and exciting world he is discovering around him. The more confidence he has that his base camp will be safely and securely awaiting him upon his return, the more confidence he has to take longer and longer trips into the surrounding terrain. It is essentially a testing period, and his elation in his 'love affair with the world' alternates with marked periods of distress ('anaclitic depression') as he suddenly becomes aware of his distance from his mother and rushes back to check on her continued presence. Towards the end of this stage, if it has gone well and all the 'tests' have been met, the child appears to develop an aura of grandiose *omnipotence* based upon his supreme confidence that his mother will always be there to look after him and do his bidding.

Between the ages of 16 and 24 months two very important and related events occur. The first is that the child suddenly becomes aware that his mother in fact is a separate individual in her own right whose continued nurture and support is voluntary on her part rather than a matter of the 'divine right of King Baby' as he had previously assumed. This is the very first awareness of the rights and needs of others—the first step beyond basic narcissism—and produces the so-called 'rapprochement crisis' where the omnipotence and elation of the previous stage give way to a sudden panic as the child rushes to 'reapproach' the mother to ascertain what conditions are necessary to ensure his continued acceptance. It is at this stage that many 'basic messages' are sent, assumed or received which will dramatically influence the future course of the child's self-image and behaviour. The 'conditions' may be non-existent, impossible, conflicting, or possible but very demanding or demeaning. In the normal course of events, however, the child is reassured that the conditions are possible, fair and tolerable and this prepares him for a period of rapid, assertive progress.

The second major event that occurs at this stage is that the child's ability to use mental and verbal symbols to refer to absent objects and people develops and, for the first time, he can now imitate a model which is no longer concretely present in his perceptual field. He is thus capable of maintaining an internalized representation of the 'mothering one', attachment and basic trust have become less dependent upon the constant presence of the person, his 'base camp' has become portable as it were, and brief separations are much more tolerable. This gives him the confidence, along with his increasing motor development, to proceed with more separation and individuation, to try out his new sense of independent self, and to risk some autonomy and expression of himself (including the defiance of the 'terrible twos'). His attachment and trust remain vulnerable and fragile, however, and will not withstand much stress for several years if they are not supported by enough cognitive understanding and ability to predict or to withstand frustration.

If the child has successfully resolved the mother-child relationship and is secure within the conditions upon which it rests, he is now free to explore further his own powers as an individual and the ages from 2 to 4 are characterized by the development of autonomy. He passes from the oppositional behaviour of the first part of this period to relatively cooperative behaviour based on parental models in the second part, developing a sense of autonomy and worth from their approval. Gender role is learned and adopted during this phase.

GENERAL PATTERNS OF
PATHOLOGICAL PSYCHOSOCIAL DEVELOPMENT

Many of the disorders of childhood owe their origin to blocks in the sequence of normal psychosocial development just outlined. These blocks may come from inadequacies in the parent, which in turn may come from inadequacies in that parent's background, or from inadequacies in the present family system. Or the blocks may come from unfortunate crises in the environment occurring at a crucial time such as illness, death, birth of a sibling and so on. Whatever their origin, these blocks produce an attitude about the self and the world that colours all of the individual's future interactions, beliefs and behaviour, and the blocks are the source of many future symptoms and syndromes. Some of the most important future consequences of blocks at given stages are outlined in the next part of this section.

Failure of attachment

Failure of attachment in the first six months of life may lead to later failure to develop close personal relationships. It may result from gross deficiencies in any aspect of development whether physical, neurological, linguistic or psychosocial. Examples of this are found with any physical disability which interferes with the parent's ability to nurture the child (for example, asthma or colic) or to play normally with the child (for example, congenital defects, physical illness with hospitalization, and so on). They occur also with any neurological or muscular disorder which interferes with the child's capacity to relate to the parent or to adequately explore his environment and develop a sense of autonomy and independence (for example, polio, cerebral palsy, perceptual defects such as deafness or blindness), and with psychosocial defects such as autism. Disrupted attachment may also result from separation such as occurs with the hospitalization or death of a parent, or rejection by the parenting figure, or from removal from primary attachment figures. Thus it may follow multiple foster placement or prematurity with a prolonged period in hospital where the mother has little early contact.

In the short-term the effects of disrupted attachment are seen in a characteristic pattern of responses. The infant at first seems to *protest* at the separation and exhibits gross distress for a few hours up to two or three days. He will then appear to give up in a phase of *despair* characterized by hopeless, apathetic withdrawal. This is next followed by what is termed *detachment*. The infant seems to settle down and become normal, but is minimally invested in relationships and when the mother returns, anger and rejection are displayed. This sequence is most severe between 7 months and 2 years. Following the return of normal parenting, the symptoms may remain. Usually, however, they will subside with time. The implications of these short-term effects are considered later in the section on Hospitalization.

In the long-term, early disrupted, distorted or deficient parent–child bonding can produce a serious deprivation and failure of attachment which leads to a spectrum of disorders known as the *withdrawal syndrome*. The most serious form of this early emotional deprivation can, despite good physical maintenance, lead to a psychological and physical withdrawal which first appears as a *failure to thrive* and which, if untreated, can further deteriorate to the point of death, a condition known as *marasmus*. Less serious degrees, at least in theory, can leave the child in the normal *autistic* phase of development where he fails to make any form of interpersonal attachment and remains in his own world. More usually, however, the failure of attachment in an autistic child results from a biological failure on his part to receive the emotional input from the environment rather than from a deficiency of the input itself (see later). Less overwhelming degrees of disrupted attachment will lead to impairment in cognitive development, socialization and capacity for relationships, and an inability to adjust to stress. This in turn can lead to a form of *functional mental retardation*, or *schizoid* individuals who prefer reduced emotional contact with others. As with other developmental problems, the age at which the deprivation occurred, its duration and the quality of the intervening care are some of the variables that to a large extent determine or lessen the deleterious effects.

Failure of development of basic trust

Basic trust is essential for the process of separation from mother and the development of a secure sense of autonomy. In ideal relationships, a competent assertiveness becomes an accepted integral part of the toddler's character structure. Failure of adequate development of basic trust results in damage to the process of separation–individuation, and the development of the sense of autonomy in normal assertiveness is hindered. Later relationships will also be impaired, closeness and intimacy will be sought after in later life but ultimately phobically avoided when a sizeable investment is demanded (as in a marital relationship), and a degree of paranoia may be evident.

Failure of separation–individuation

Separation–individuation may be interfered with by illness, biological deficits, developmental blocks, lack of basic trust, or basic messages or conditions that preclude further development. Depending on the stage at which individuation is blocked or distorted and on the manner in which it occurs, certain characteristic symptoms or behaviour patterns may emerge. These are grouped in their chronological, developmental order as follows: symbiotic psychosis (see later), passive-dependent, omnipotent, passive-aggressive and aggressive-depressed syndromes. It will be noted that, in general, the earliest blocks represent the most profound disturbance of normal personality development but the least disturbing behaviour, whereas the later syndromes represent the least disturbance of personality development but the most disturbing behaviour.

Passive-dependent behaviour patterns

Between the ages of 12 and 18 months the child who has a 'dominant overprotective' mother who decompensates when thwarted will fail to individuate adequately. He will anticipate a great deal of negative treatment or abuse or feelings of guilt if he fails to meet parental expectations or if he acts more autonomously than the parent can tolerate. The basic message that the child appears to receive is that if he moves away from his mother's immediate jurisdiction, she will not be there when he returns. He therefore feels unacceptable and incompetent as he is, afraid to explore the world on his own and entirely dependent upon his mother's (later generalized to others') goodwill. It is as if the mother's needs may not have been met by her own parents or her husband and her giving to the child is an alternative, but is conditional upon her receiving docile obedience and appreciation in return. Angry explosions can be forthcoming when this is not received. The child is likely therefore to revert to very compliant and subdued behaviour and to be described by others as a 'model' child. The resultant passive-dependent syndrome may not be identified in childhood unless a teacher or someone outside the family labels the excessive compliance and timidity as a problem, or unless a serious separation-anxiety or school phobia presents itself. In older children or adults, however, a covert, underlying resentment about the enforced dependency may emerge directly as a violent explosion or a marital breakdown, or it may simply produce a conflict which is handled by an obsessive-compulsive, a dissociative or a habit disorder, a depression or a psychophysiological problem. These will be described later.

Omnipotent behavioural pattern

The child of the 'indulgent overprotective' parent proceeds beyond the passive-dependent child in separation–individuation, but when he reaches the reality-oriented point of the 'rapprochement crisis' at about 18 months he fails to deal with the fact of his mother's independence adequately and remains blocked at the previous stage where he maintains a delusion of grandeur and omnipotence. This is usually because his mother fails to exert her control effectively, either because her indulgence acts as a defence against her underlying rejection and hostility towards the child and this or other environmental factors render her ineffective, or because she is more dependent upon the child's goodwill towards her than vice versa because of needs of her own that are unmet in other areas. More rarely, the mother may be so overtly terrifying, or the conditions she sets may be so impossible, that the child is simply unable to tolerate the possibility of rapprochement. In any event, the child remains at an entirely narcissistic level, using any manipulative weapon within his arsenal to ensure that his dependency needs are constantly met. There is a marked lack of impulse control, a refusal to accept 'delayed gratification', and overtly aggressive behaviour whenever the child feels that he can get away with this. Control is the key and is maintained at any cost, especially by forcing negative reactions to negative behaviour. If, however, the child meets a superior force, he will temporarily revert to very charming and manipulative behaviour for a while, acting out his frustration in more covert ways such as bullying younger children, setting fires or torturing animals. While these latter are symptoms of the later passive-aggressive syndrome, the omnipotent child is not consistent with these and will revert to more direct methods of control as soon as this option is open to him.

The parents have literally created a 'monster', and when later they try and correct their mistake, they find they cannot control the child without flying into a destructive rage, for which they then feel so guilty that they fall back into their previous pattern of indulgence. It is noteworthy that these children are often the products of unhappy marriages and are indulged by the mother to compensate, but are held in check by the father. They really emerge when the parents finally separate and their delusion of grandeur suddenly becomes true. Sociopathy is a frequent result in later life.

These children are very hard to treat, and residential care is usually necessary in order to gain control over them, the goal of treatment being to push them back into the earlier passive-dependent stage and then bring them appropriately forward through the 'rapprochement crisis'.

Passive-aggressive behaviour patterns

A different pattern develops if the child successfully passes through the 'rapprochement crisis' and is encouraged to separate under certain conditions, but finds these conditions obnoxious in certain ways and is not allowed to protest openly. The conditions may be unclear and therefore impossible (for example, double messages) or clear but unreasonable (for example, you must be perfect; you must be responsible, and so on). Often such children have had a fair amount of positive input and have been encouraged to be independent *outside* the family, but have received a message that they must be entirely subservient *within* the family and never object to parental expectations and demands, no matter how onerous. There is often an ambivalence on the part of the parents towards the child and the expression of the rejecting side of this ambivalence is manifested by the withholding of love and the making of heavy performance demands. The child is also often expected to represent the parents to the world. The child is left with a sense of anger, frustration and resentment against the parent figure or figures for a perceived lack of respect, affection and appreciation, and has enough of a sense of self to fight back, but does not dare to do so openly. At the passive-dependent end of the passive-aggressive syndrome the child is often not consciously aware of his feelings of resentment and anger and his symptoms thus tend to be well beyond his conscious control. Such symptoms would include enuresis, encopresis, and failure to meet parental expectations, especially in school performance. In the middle 'semi-aware' zone occur such symptoms as stealing and lying to cover up. At the more conscious end of the passive-aggressive spectrum are such symptoms as bullying younger children (especially siblings), fire-setting, cruelty to animals, failure to accomplish assigned tasks, and disruptive behaviour in the neighbourhood. In adolescence, drug abuse, promiscuity and truancy would be included.

Each of the above symptoms may have a cause quite outside this syndrome, but when two or more of these symptoms are seen together, as they often are, then this kind of formulation is likely. The hallmark of all these types of behaviour is the ambivalence about the underlying hostility which characterizes them. The latter is evidenced by the fact that precautions about being detected are almost never taken, and when apprehended or accused the child vigorously denies his actions even in the face of massive evidence to the contrary. The behaviour or its inevitable consequences almost always hurt the child as much or more than the parent, but the child seems to fail to learn from this. It is as if the total unconscious goal is *both* to express the anger and to be punished for it simultaneously. Anxiety, fear and guilt are prominent symptoms, but defiance is only shown at the very conscious end of the spectrum.

Therapy is directed at helping both the child and the family to move towards a more healthy and conscious resolution of their anger towards one another. Obviously this is most difficult at the more unconscious end of the spectrum, and enuresis and encopresis will therefore be dealt with later.

Aggressive-depressed behaviour patterns

The aggressive-depressed syndrome results from a child who has successfully negotiated the conditions of the rapprochement phase, but instead of receiving praise and encouragement for this so that he can consolidate a positive self-image and relationship within the family, he finds instead that the old conditions are simply replaced by new and more advanced ones. Thus he is in fact pushed to take on more autonomy than he can handle in his second and third year, and he is being asked to 'grow up' too soon due to unrealistic parental expectations, usually at the expense of ignoring his legitimate dependency needs. The overt expression of his anger and frustration about this is often inadequately handled by one parent, and the other parent often provides an aggressive and violent model, and there may very well be a broken home which has contributed to the child being asked to take on extra responsibility. Parental alcoholism and antisocial behaviour are often extant models. There may be strong family loyalty, but there are usually chaotic controls, and a low level of family cohesiveness. There is a chronic sense of never being 'quite good enough', or able to live up to expectations, and this may be precipitated or contributed to by academic failure secondary to specific learning disabilities or a relatively lower level of intelligence. Such children tend to have a very low sense of self-worth and self-esteem, feeling that their dependency needs and needs for rewards and gratification have not been met 'because they weren't worth it'.

These children have a very high investment in maintaining a pseudo-independence and pseudo-omnipotence in order to cover up their low feelings of self-worth and their unmet dependency needs. They can be very adult-like and charming in their interaction (especially with adults), but they have a low frustration tolerance for criticism or failure, want to win at any cost, and can become very angry and even abusive when they feel put down. They have a high investment in maintaining their independence, and are usually very defiant in the face of any form of discipline, usually stating that 'they weren't hurt', and not infrequently reacting explosively and violently to disciplinary procedures. They become very threatened when anyone attempts to nurture them, and may very well respond provocatively in order to drive the potential 'nurturer' away.

In many ways the aggressive-depressed child presents characteristics similar to the omnipotent child, but there are some essential differences. Control is a central issue for both, but the omnipotent child tries to control others in an effort to get them to meet his dependency needs, whereas the aggressive-depressed tries to maintain control over himself by preventing people from awakening the pain associated with his unmet dependency needs. Both can be very charming, but the omnipotent child becomes aggressive when he feels there is some threat to his constant nurturing, and the aggressive-depressed becomes aggressive when his independence is interfered with and an attempt is made to meet his dependency needs. The omnipotent is essentially narcissistic, and has no tolerance for the dependency needs of others (especially younger children), whereas the aggressive-depressed is more than capable of looking after someone else's dependency needs and in fact thrives on meeting the latter, only becoming threatened and jealous when he sees someone else meeting the dependency needs of a younger child in a way that awakens his own needs. Consequently, the aggressive-depressed tends to be very good with younger children, whereas the omnipotent child either ignores younger children or casually tortures them.

The aggressive-depressed child is often brought to the physician because of defiance and aggression towards other children, the latter usually being the same size or larger than himself (unlike the passive-aggressive or omnipotent child who picks on younger children). More rarely they present in the depressed mode, but they are usually very much in touch with the underlying sadness, loneliness and hurt which they experience and will nearly always be able to identify this for the examiner if asked, which is another distinguishing characteristic. At times they can exhibit pseudo-omnipotent behaviour, protesting that they can do anything and that no one can 'boss them around', but this is clearly a defence against their underlying hurt and depression, and if the challenge is side-stepped and the underlying sadness and depression is identified, the pseudo-omnipotent behaviour will often dissolve into tears.

Treatment of the aggressive-depressed child essentially involves setting limits on the unacceptable expression of the anger, while accepting the anger itself and providing alternative acceptable outlets. Once this is accomplished, the next stage is to side-step and ignore the anger wherever possible and try to elicit the underlying depression. When the latter is identified, some attempt can then be made to help the family to understand and meet the unmet dependency needs, or else arrange for this to be done in the appropriate out-patient or residential setting. In older children, this latter step may prove to be impossible, and one might have to settle for helping the child to channel his aggression into more acceptable activities. In children who do present with depression, mobilizing their anger is the correct route to follow so that they have the energy from this available to them to get their needs met.

Most children who are brought to the physician with an 'emotional disorder' fall into one or the other of the above groupings, the exceptions being those that fall into more specific categories to be outlined in the next section. Although these patterns are described here as resulting from blocks that occur in the initial developmental sequence over the first two years of life, it is important to note that a child goes through the same developmental sequence (although in a much shorter period of time) with respect to each new stressful life event in subsequent years. The tendency within a family is to produce a block at the same place each time the sequence is encountered, but this is not necessarily so and new patterns can emerge and old ones can be altered at any point in the future (especially under a therapeutic process), although with increasing difficulty as the child grows older. Treatment involves supporting the parents and the child in growing from the stage at which he is blocked through succeeding stages to the point where the child can be assertive about his own needs without fear of retribution, while at the same time respecting the needs and rights of others. Thus the passive-dependent child is allowed to be more passive-aggressive; the passive-aggressive child to be more directly assertive; and the aggressive child helped to resolve his depression by allowing his dependency needs to be met and to alter the aggression to assertiveness, all within a framework of feelings of security and self-worth. Needless to say, the parents have had their own reasons for blocking the development at the stage they did, and therefore often require as much or more support during this progression as the children, and family therapy is usually needed. It is particularly important to warn the parents and treatment staff that new patterns of disruptive behaviour will emerge in accordance with these steps as treatment progresses. Failure to do this will lead the trials of passive-aggressive or aggressive responses by a previously totally submissive, passive-dependent child to be viewed as a regression and responded to with harsh and punitive controls, which would be both completely inappropriate and would negate any positive effects that treatment might have been having.

The next section will deal with specific symptoms and syndromes in child psychiatry, many of which will be seen to relate back to the more general patterns just outlined.

SPECIFIC SYMPTOMS AND SYNDROMES*

Syndromes and other types of diagnostic labelling in child

---

* The authors have drawn heavily on two general texts of child psychiatry for this section: M. A. Stewart and A. Gath, *Psychological Disorders of Children*, Williams & Wilkins, 1978 and P. D. Steinhauer and Q. Rae-Grant, *Psychological Problems of the Child and His Family*, Macmillan, 1977.

psychiatry tend to have arisen from the application of a name to a collection of symptoms which have appeared concurrently. On occasion such a pattern of symptoms implies a single aetiology. More frequently, however, the pattern of symptoms is simply an identifiable stage-appropriate reaction to stresses of many different origins, and no aetiological significance whatsoever is implied by the diagnostic label. The classification that appears below, therefore, is of the very roughest, implies no single aetiology (although the commonest likely aetiologies are outlined) and is for convenience only. Even where a single initial aetiology is suggested, subsequent elaboration from other areas will be the rule, for example, the secondary loss of self-esteem and confidence in a child with a learning disability of biological origin.

Disorders of mixed aetiology

Learning disorders

A child presenting to a practitioner with a learning problem at school has initially a very wide differential diagnosis. The diagnostic task is to weigh up the part played by each of the following: general health problems which may affect the functioning of the child, quality of input (teacher and classroom distractions), receptivity of pupil (emotional and motivational factors), organic capacity for input (vision and hearing), general processing ability (intelligence and attention span), specific processing and retention ability (see below), organic capacity for output (speech and fine motor), emotional and motivational capacity for output (performance anxiety, etc.) and quality of output measures (examinations). Each of these has to be considered carefully and accepted or rejected as a possible contributing cause.

Most of the above will produce *generalized* learning problems in all areas and subjects. However, some children with apparently normal health, intact neurological capacity, adequate intelligence and apparently adequate emotional adjustment will nonetheless show learning problems, usually limited to a very narrow range of activity (for example, to read, carry a tune, do mathematics and so on). Since the disability is *specific*, it has earned the title of *specific learning disability*. The aetiology varies, but is usually considered to be of biological origin, sometimes a particular genetic defect (often with a positive family history), sometimes a 'maturational delay' (which will improve spontaneously in time), and sometimes the result of a very specific acquired organic insult (such as perinatal anoxia or lead poisoning). In any event, these children all need special remedial assistance and an early diagnosis to prevent secondary emotional problems. Four common specific learning disabilities are considered below.

Speech and language disorders.   Speech disorders are characterized by abnormalities in flow (stuttering) and/or in articulation (dysarthria). Language disorders may be related to delayed development (autism, mental retardation, deafness, brain damage), a lack of appropriate and adequate stimulation or modelling (elective mutism) or unknown causes.

Although stuttering is seen in a small percentage of normal children, most of these children will stutter for only a few months to two or three years. Persistent stuttering with early onset affects about 1 per cent of children. In this group correlates of low intelligence and poor articulation have been found. On the whole, however, this symptom has not been shown to be correlated with other psychiatric disorders. It does appear to be familial. For the most part, stutterers during adolescence find methods of coping such that their self-esteem is not unduly affected.

Approximately 4 per cent of children have significant articulation difficulties at age 5. By age 7, slightly less than 2 per cent have such poorly formed speech that most of their words are unintelligible. Poor school achievement is an associated factor in about one-third of these. About twice as many boys as girls are affected. Clinically, the main difficulty is in the sounding of consonants, particularly at the beginning and end of words. This may or may not be associated with general clumsiness. Despite school difficulties, most of these children are of normal intelligence. Although at times the aetiology may be obvious (for example, hearing loss, cerebral palsy or cleft palate), for the most part it is unknown.

Language disorder may be considered in any child who has no words by age 2 or phrases by age 4. Although the most common cause is mental retardation, this delay may also be due to deafness, cerebral palsy, autism and those causes of unknown origin which are labelled developmental dysphasia. Most of the latter group exhibit difficulties in the expression of language. Receptive defects are more rare, probably less than one child in ten thousand being affected. These children, like the children with specific language disorders, often have difficulty learning to read. They should always be referred to a speech therapist and it may be expected that about two-thirds of those with expressive disorders will improve while in the majority of those with receptive disorders improvement will be slow with marked residual defects remaining.

In examining a child for mild forms of speech and language disorder, it is useful for the practitioner to give the child a series of directions, for example, 'Pick up the pencil and put it into the glass jar, close the door and then give me that picture of the car'. Simple tests such as asking the child to name objects in the room or repeat a story can be useful. More complex tests such as asking the child to repeat a series of numbers (to test auditory sequences and short-term memory) or to give the order of small figures on the table after they have been removed (visual sequences) may be used in children over 4 who are cooperative and attentive. With the slightly older child, one may ask for fine discrimination in sounds by asking him to differentiate between spoken words such as 'mop' and 'map' or 'fat' and 'rat'. In addition, one would, of course, carry out a full and detailed physical examination of the mouth, pharynx and ears, and test for both hearing and visual acuity.

Specific reading disabilities. Specific reading disability is defined as a reading level that is two years below the level expected of a child of his or her mental age. The prevalence of this disorder varies from 4 per cent in rural districts to approximately 10 per cent in urban areas. This should be clearly distinguished from much higher prevalence figures of 8 to 9 per cent given for 'reading retardation' which includes children whose poor reading is due to lack of stimulation in their environment and whose backwardness would also be seen in a lowering of their overall IQ scores. The boy-to-girl ratio is approximately 5:1 in specific reading disorders, while the prevalence of reading retardation is only slightly higher in boys than girls. In specific reading disorders children may reverse the letters 'p' and 'd' or 'b' and 'd' or whole words such as 'was' to 'saw' and they may have difficulty in giving the proper sounds for letters of the alphabet. Although they can often appreciate the length of words, they have difficulty with the phonetics and cannot break a word into syllables and then put it together and sound it out. There is a definite relationship between delayed language and reading (and spelling) disability but there does not appear to be an association with ambidexterity, although other soft neurological signs have been found to be significantly more common in these children. Some children have difficulty in perceiving and remembering the sounds of letters and syllables but they can read whole words that they have memorized while others, a smaller group, can sound out the parts of words but have difficulty with visual recognition of the whole word.

Follow-up studies indicate that with specific assistance and a supportive environment, most of these children will compensate for their handicap. More than half of them have been shown to suffer in addition symptoms of hyperactivity, distractibility, poor attention span and impulsivity. This group does not fare as well. Unfortunately, it is now becoming clear that the prognosis for improved reading by children with specific reading disability is worse than for children who have generalized learning problems because of somewhat lower intelligence. Specific reading disability does tend to run in families. In all cases, in addition to a careful physical and neurological examination, appropriate psychological and speech pathology testing should be carried out. This may include determination of the IQ to look for differences in the scores for language, abstract reasoning and visual memory; testing the level of academic skills; and specific tests for reading skills to look for recognition, comprehension and phonetic abilities, the ability to copy visual patterns (visual perception) and to detect differences between similarly sounding words, such as 'mop' and 'map' (auditory discrimination), ability to reproduce visual patterns from memory (perception and memory) and the ability to do more complex processing of visual and auditory stimuli including the remembering of sequences. These processes are all assessed in various standardized tests of psycholinguistic abilities. Even the majority of severely disabled children will reach a 12-year-old level of reading if given sufficient professional help and a supportive and understanding environment; this level of reading suffices for most needs in the adult world. It is of interest that, in general, children with visual-motor (written) dysfunction usually become better readers through orally directed teaching than those children who have audio-vocal (spoken) defects who must be taught entirely through visual means. The latter seem to remain preoccupied with decoding words and thus lose the general meaning of what they are reading.

Specific mathematical disabilities. Mathematical disabilities are less frequent but are more commonly seen in girls than boys. This defect is associated with specific defects in spatial localization, short-term auditory memory, right–left discrimination and digit retention, and these children also exhibit multiple reversals in their spelling.

Specific writing disabilities. Specific difficulties in printing and writing are associated with general fine motor awkwardness. A higher percentage of ambidextrous or left-handed individuals occurs in the families. There may be confused laterality and these children may do poorly in sports and have major difficulty when confronted by particularly compulsive primary school teachers. These difficulties are not so often recognized and can lead to secondary emotional problems which may be more serious in their consequences than the primary disorder.

The hyperactive child syndrome

The so-called 'hyperactive child syndrome' is, in fact, the final common pathway of a number of possible aetiologies, the four most common of which are outlined below. The principal signs common to all are: short attention span, impulsivity, distractibility, excessive non-goal oriented motor activity and irritability.

The 'misfit' child. The activity level of the 'misfit' child actually falls within the normal range, but is seen as 'out of step' by parents, siblings or teachers, especially where he is at the high end of the normal range and the parent is intolerant of this degree of activity. There is no necessary history of trauma, family history or associated signs of other disabilities. The child may have good coordination, and although he may appear distractible, he can concentrate when his interest is held on something (for example, television). On the whole, the child would tend to be action-oriented, and may be more non-verbal than his peers. One parent may have a similar history. Secondary emotional and family problems may develop. Treatment involves family counselling and occasionally short-term use of a minor tranquillizer for one or other parent. Activity groups and provision of appropriate outlets for energy (such as sports and exercises) may be helpful.

Learned hyperactivity. Children with learned hyperactivity are normal, but their parents have a high threshold and respond only to excessive and disruptive activity, for example, overly permissive or depressed mothers. The characteristics are similar to those for the 'misfit' child. The diagnosis is often picked up in the family interview by observation, and the treatment of choice is behaviour modification applied by the parents.

Emotional hyperactivity. The emotionally hyperactive child is essentially using his hyperactivity as a defence against his anxiety or anger aroused by problems in his family or living situation. Often defiance, anger or depression 'leak' through and an openly aggressive or destructive history is obtained. These symptoms may also be associated with a typical passive-aggressive syndrome and there is often a vicious circle set up with another family member. This type of hyperactive child tends to be very impulsive, but can concentrate when anxiety or tension is reduced. There will be no evidence of the signs or symptoms associated with minimal brain dysfunction other than learning disorders which are non-specific and secondary to emotional problems. The history usually post-dates the first year of life, and is clearly secondary to emotional trauma, birth of a sibling or other such events. Since the symptom is very useful to the child as a defence mechanism, he usually reacts negatively to attempts to control his behaviour through behaviour modification or drugs. Use of these treatments may, however, unmask a latent depression. The treatment is three-fold. First, to break the vicious circle as quickly as possible, behaviour modification and drugs are used. Anxiolytic drugs (for example, chlordiazepoxide, thioridazine et cetera), are considered the drugs of choice although methylphenidate has been found to be effective in some of these children. Second, concomitant reparative therapy for the primary emotional disorder should be instituted. Third, activities provided by community resources which assist in building the child's self-esteem should be utilized wherever possible.

Organic hyperactivity. Organic hyperactivity is properly an 'attention deficit disorder' and these children usually have other associated signs and symptoms of a broader syndrome known as 'minimal brain dysfunction' (see below). These children also have a higher frequency of minor physical anomalies. The history usually dates from birth and the child is frequently grateful for any assistance, especially the use of drugs, that can be given to him. He has great difficulty concentrating even at times of low anxiety and high interest, and is virtually at the mercy of his disorder. Medication in the form of stimulants (such as amphetamines or methylphenidate) is the primary treatment. It should be coupled with family and individual counselling for secondary emotional problems and remedial measures if possible for the associated symptoms and signs of minimal brain dysfunction. The stimulant drugs increase the child's attention span, decrease distractibility and impulsivity and secondarily reduce the overall level of activity. The usual starting dose of methylphenidate is 0.3 mg per kg of body weight. Children have quite variable responses to different dosages of this medication and a higher dose may be necessary. Methylphenidate should be given one half hour before a meal and its action will characteristically last for approximately four hours. Timing of the dose is important since very difficult behaviour can emerge as the drug wears off. If no changes are seen in the target symptoms during that period of time, methylphenidate is not the drug of choice. This drug, like diazepam in adult psychiatry, has been grossly overused by physicians without adequate testing of its effectiveness in the particular patient. Unlike the group with emotional hyperactivity, this group will often improve with age, although symptoms can be elicited even in adulthood. Periodic trials without medication should be attempted, and because methylphenidate has a retarding effect on growth, 'drug holidays' should be provided to allow the child's growth to catch up to his peers. It is of some importance to note that although the overall prevalence of this subtype is about 6 per cent of school-age children, studies have shown that only approximately 2 per cent are correctly diagnosed and placed on methylphenidate. There are two points that should be made concerning this. The first is that a reasonable percentage of children who could respond to the drug are being handled by more conservative measures. The second is that quite a number of children are being placed on this medication incorrectly. As in all other areas of medicine, accurate diagnosis is essential.

Childhood schizophrenia

True childhood schizophrenia is not usually seen before the age of eight and the symptoms are much as for the adult form. However, it is a rare condition and psychotic symptoms in childhood should raise a high suspicion of organic disorder, especially in children describing hallucinations. The incidence of schizophrenia rises rapidly during adolescence, but during this period of development many of the normal variants of adolescence can make diagnosis difficult. Most children developing schizophrenic symptoms do so gradually and in most the premorbid personality is described as shy, withdrawn or timid. It should be emphasized, however, that most shy introverted children do *not* develop schizophrenia. There is a family history of schizophrenia in approximately 12 per cent of the biological parents.

For the most part schizophrenia is a more difficult syndrome to treat in childhood as the major tranquillizers often produce an unacceptable level of side-effects without sufficient amelioration of symptoms. They are, nonetheless, worth a trial in conjunction with other forms of treatment. Long-term supportive psychotherapy is essential. The prognosis is poor, though better than that for autism.

Presumed biological disorders

Autism

Autism is a syndrome that occurs in about 4 children in every 10 000. Three-quarters of these cases become apparent in the first two years of life while the remaining one-quarter appear to have a period of normal development followed by an apparently precipitous onset of symptoms in the third year of life. Autism is characterized by disturbances in the following areas:

1. Perception (hypo- and hyper-responsiveness to stimuli)
2. Developmental rate (variable and uneven)
3. Ability to relate (people as objects, inappropriate use of objects, poor eye contact)
4. Speech and language (delayed, use of third person)
5. Mobility (especially stereotyped behaviour, rocking, twirling, toe-walking, hand-clapping, etc.)

The principal block in the autistic child is in psychosocial development (which some feel is, in turn, related to the perceptual disturbance) and this has in turn led to considerable controversy as to the syndrome's origins. Currently, it is accepted that the majority of children exhibiting autistic symptoms have organic pathology. Neither the location nor the aetiology is known although recent work has suggested first that there may be an enlargement of the left lateral ventricle (particularly the left temporal horn). Some also believe that a small minority may result from rearing in extremely depriving environments. This group, though small, is theoretically important.

The differential diagnosis includes childhood schizophrenia, mental retardation, major sensory deficits, receptive dysphasia, maternal deprivation and other organic brain syndromes. There are some researchers who believe that all childhood psychoses are part of a spectrum which includes both autism and childhood schizophrenia. The best evidence to date, however, indicates that autism differs from childhood schizophrenia by virtue of its earlier age of onset, the absence of family history, the more 'organic' flavour of the symptoms and the inexorable course. The difference is important, because autism seems to respond best to a combination of behaviour therapy and special education, whereas psychotropic medication, psychotherapy and milieu therapy all have a role in childhood schizophrenia.

One of the most difficult early differential diagnoses to make is mental retardation. Certainly, two-thirds of autistic children perform throughout life at a retarded level, and thus the two syndromes can coexist. Autistic children, however, often have uneven levels of cognitive development, and sometimes normal or even exceptional 'islands' appear where, for instance, entire musical scores can be memorized at one hearing. The chief difference, however, lies in the many other symptoms the autistic child shows, especially the impaired capacity for relationships.

In the differential diagnosis from receptive dysphasia, although both groups have a history of less babbling than normal, and both on testing show a receptive disorder with the autistics having only slightly lower scores in comprehension, there are marked differences in behaviour. Autistic children show less eye contact, are less able to adapt to new situations and exhibit more stereotyped movements such as body rocking, whirling and hand clapping. They also have a history of not playing with other children, unlike the dysphasic group. The autistic child often treats other persons as if they were objects. Although both the receptive dysphasic child and the autistic child have delayed speech, the dysphasic has difficulties centered around articulation and will communicate by gestures in order to relate in a socially meaningful way to others. The autistic child, on the other hand, tends not to use language for purposes of normal social communication. Echolalia, perseveration on idiosyncratic topics and the use of the third person in place of the first person are common.

The prognosis varies with the severity but, in general, by the age of 5 if language has not developed beyond the occasional use of single words, toys are not being used appropriately and the IQ is less than 60 the prognosis is very poor and the child usually is ultimately sent to an institution for the mentally retarded. Children with IQs close to normal and who have some language may develop, on the other hand; they may complete secondary school education and, in rare instances, even continue to tertiary level. Most, even despite apparent academic success, remain loners who exhibit schizoid and neurotic symptoms. Less than 5 per cent achieve a reasonably good adjustment, being able to function relatively normally socially and academically, although they are always labelled as odd or different by their peers. Another group of about 20 to 30 per cent will have a fair outcome and will attend normal or special classes in ordinary schools, while the remainder will require special training and programmes and must depend on their families or institutions.

Mental retardation

The most global developmental delay is, of course, mental subnormality or retardation. In many areas the management of this condition has been removed from the medical to the educational sphere. However, it is still the physician who must make the initial diagnosis and this in itself is an extremely difficult and important task. Mental subnormality is dealt with in Chapter 15.

Minimal brain dysfunction

The frequent association of several possibly organic signs and symptoms with behavioural problems has led a number of people to postulate that there may be a common underlying aetiology of mild neurological impairment in some children. The occurrence of these signs and symptoms together is often associated with a history compatible with mild neurological impairment, for example, perinatal distress, encephalitis, convulsions, trauma and so on. By definition, there are never any gross signs of neurological impairment. This condition is only inferred and has never been demonstrated pathologically, and some deny its existence at all. More than 101 different possible symptoms and characteristics are subsumed under this title. The ten most frequent are:

1. Hyperactivity
2. Perceptual-motor impairment
3. Emotional lability
4. General coordination deficits
5. Disorders of attention (short attention span, distractibility, perseveration)
6. Impulsivity
7. Disorders of memory and thinking
8. Specific learning disabilities
9. Mild disorders of speech and hearing
10. Equivocal 'soft' neurological signs and EEG irregularities

None of these symptoms occurring alone is sufficient to justify a diagnosis of 'minimal brain dysfunction', but two or more occurring together would be sufficient to raise the index of suspicion. For instance, a history of perinatal anoxia combined with hyperactivity, short attention span, delayed speech, and the presence of difficulties with temporal and spatial relations causing a specific disability in reading would be very strong presumptive evidence for the existence of this syndrome.

Investigation for minimal brain dysfunction requires a careful neurological examination looking particularly for such 'soft' signs as mild incoordination, mirror movements or synkinesia, finger agnosia, dysgraphia, and small differences in lateral dominance and lateral discrimination.

Emotional difficulties arise in these children because they are often blamed for things which they cannot help. As with simple specific learning disabilities, treatment is symptomatic including physiotherapy and occupational therapy for fine motor incoordination, remedial education for specific learning disabilities, and medication for hyperkinesis.

Since 'minimal brain dysfunction' can embrace other disorders such as specific learning disabilities or hyperactivity, these terms are frequently confused and used interchangeably both with one another and with a wide variety of other terms. It should be noted that none of these are specific disease entities. They are syndromes which represent the final common pathways of a variety of different possible aetiologies, some of which overlap. 'Minimal brain dysfunction' is the most widely embracing of these syndromes and does imply a hypothetical organic aetiology.

Dementia

Dementia and delirium in adults are discussed and defined in Chapters 8 and 13. The chronic progressive conditions are caused by such entities as neuronal storage diseases, Wilson's disease, Huntington's or Sydenham's chorea, congenital syphilis and tumours and they are often difficult to diagnose in their early stages.

A progressive dementia will begin initially with a halt in intellectual and social development followed by a loss of skills in these areas. The condition becomes obvious as hygiene slips, socially inappropriate behaviour appears and the child's behaviour becomes erratic, unpredictable and out of character (either too aggressive or too withdrawn and apathetic, or both). Neurological signs may appear as late as a year or more after the behavioural signs.

Since the first signs may be antisocial or bizarre behaviour, mood changes, aggressiveness or a steady drop in school performance, the diagnosis may be missed. It is useful to note that virtually the only other psychiatric cause for *declining* performance in school (including intellectual ability and language skills) is depression and its symptoms should be relatively simple to recognize. So too, if psychotic symptoms are present it is useful to remember that autism beginning after age 3 is rare and childhood schizophrenia beginning earlier than age 8 is also unusual.

Delirium

Confusional states are usually easily diagnosed and the signs of the causative condition such as mumps, chickenpox, other infections, the encephalopathies (for example, associated with severe burns), hypoglycaemia, head injuries or drug intoxications are more readily apparent.

Treatment is for both the causative condition and for the symptoms. In the acute conditions only a very limited number of nurses should be assigned to the patient. Other persons well known to the child should be present whenever possible. These simple precautions tend to lessen some of the deleterious effects of confusion. The room should be lit night and day and measures taken to reduce anxiety and assist in orientation.

Presumed psychosocial disorders

Symbiotic psychosis

Symbiotic psychosis is a very rare condition that represents a block in normal psychosocial development. In this instance development is normal for the first year of life, but in the second year when normal children begin to separate from the mother and form a concept of themselves as distinct and separate entities, a block in development produces the symptoms of symbiotic psychosis. Regression occurs both in speech and behaviour with excessive and almost frantic clinging, touching, smelling, licking, feeling and stereotyped behaviour. This must be distinguished from neurotic regression which may, for example, follow the birth of a sibling. The clinging, attention-seeking behaviour is understandable in the latter instance as competition for mother's time, the adjustment to new schedules in the family, and jealousy of the attention everyone is paying to the newcomer. The behaviour and over-attachment in symbiotic psychosis, on the other hand, seem largely purposeless and simple thoughtful attention-giving responses to the infant are not sufficient to reassure him and decrease his abnormal behaviour. The quality of the clinging is also different with the word 'frantic' being, perhaps, the best description.

In the differential diagnosis one might also think of organic pathology in which case neurological and cognitive abnormalities would be apparent.

The prognosis for symbiotic psychosis is poor and those who do improve show residual defects. Some people, therefore, consider it to be a variant of autism, although others relate it to maternal psychopathology.

Passive-dependent behaviour patterns

Besides the general symptoms of anxiety, over-dependence,

fearfulness and social withdrawal, other syndromes such as school phobia, generalized anxiety and phobias, and conversion hysteria may eventually result if a block persists at this developmental level. Although not dealt with here, depression in a later marital relationship is also common.

School phobia (school refusal). School attendance problems can be broken into three sub-groups: truancy, school avoidance and school refusal.

Truancy is essentially an antisocial delinquent act occurring most frequently in males over the age of 12 from the lower socio-economic classes and is often associated with other forms of antisocial rebellious behaviour such as stealing. Truants are usually poor students and experience apathy or antipathy rather than anxiety in association with school.

School avoidance is usually a short-term phenomenon related to a clearly identifiable problem associated with the school or peers such as an examination or an embarrassing or rejecting experience. There is usually anxiety associated with school avoidance, but it is of an 'understandable' nature related to something specific and is self-limiting. A combination of pressure and support usually produce capitulation on the part of the child with respect to school attendance.

School refusal occurs with the same frequency in boys and girls, is commoner in bright children of middle to upper socio-economic families and has no association with other antisocial behaviour. The anxiety is high and may reach the point of producing physiological symptoms (such as vomiting) when the school is approached. It exceeds normal understanding, and despite all support and reassurance there is no 'capitulation point'. There are three sub-categories of school refusal: separation anxiety, school phobia, and generalized withdrawal; these will be briefly described.

Separation anxiety. Separation anxiety usually occurs in children less than 8 years of age who are generally described as good pupils and good, quiet children both at home and at school. The onset may be sudden, and may exist from first school attendance or may be related to some other event which has fed into the separation anxiety, such as the illness of a parent. The anxiety is high, and may well be present in other separation experiences as well as those at school.

There is often a dominant, overprotective mother and an uninvolved, passive or absent father, with the child substituting for the father in the mother's life. Initial treatment involves getting the child back to school on an urgent basis to prevent consolidation of the problem, and subsequent counselling. The mother often has as much anxiety as the child about his leaving home and may need support from the doctor, the father, other relatives and the community in letting the child go. Some re-alignment of the family dynamics is usually desirable.

School phobia proper usually occurs in a child over the age of 8 who displays controlling and 'omnipotent' features at home, but is anxious, lonely and inadequate with peers at school. The dynamics usually involve a 'weak' indulgent overprotective mother with an involved but passive father who colludes with the pathology. Anger is usually not dealt with well in the home, and the child's behaviour there preoccupies the family and takes the pressure off covert marital problems. The result seems to be that the child becomes overvalued at home where he occupies a strong and dominating position, but fails to be accorded such a position of power at school, thereby generating much anxiety in association with the latter. There seems to be little 'separation anxiety' per se, but the child simply refuses to participate in *any* activity (including school) where he cannot occupy an equivalent position to that extant in the home. These children are really quite seriously crippled in dealing with the real world and the treatment is complex. Family therapy is usually necessary, but apart from this the child needs individual work to help him deal with what has become a pathological coping style. He also needs many carefully managed experiences to prove to himself both that he is 'safe' even when not in a position of control, and that there are other ways to gain rewards and a sense of self-esteem in the world. Peer groups are often particularly useful in the therapy of these children, although they have to be forced to attend and a period of residential treatment might be required.

Generalized withdrawal is another pattern of school refusal which has to be watched very carefully. In this variety, the withdrawal is from all areas of life, and the child is often found spending a great deal of time alone in his room. These children become preoccupied with themselves in numerous ways and are often described as 'strange' in some of their behaviours and patterns of interacting. Such a pattern usually marks a serious disorder such as depression or an early schizophrenia and the sooner these children are identified and a specialist consulted the better.

General anxiety and phobias. General anxiety and phobias represent another possible outcome of a block at an early stage of psychosocial development. Phobias may serve as a means by which the child in a passive and dependent stage of development handles fears and anxieties about a separation from the mother by displacing them onto a fear of something that can be avoided. This, in broad general terms, converts a general sense of constant disequilibrium and the assumption that the world is not a safe place into a fear of something that can be specifically avoided and thus controlled. Though maladaptive it is, given the seeming alternative of living with generalized anxiety, a relatively less noxious alternative to the individual involved. Some theorists of the analytical school emphasize a conflict internal to the child in which the emotions the child feels too guilty or fearful to accept are displaced and projected onto an outside situation. This is a useful additional concept and undoubtedly operates in a number of instances, as does the simple learning theory explanation of negative association. Whatever the cause, the choice of feared objects appears to be based on circumstances and learning, but once learned it seems to remain whether or not the individual grows past his original fears to a more mature stage of psychosocial adaptation. In such cases, as well as in cases where the phobia was due purely to a single traumatic incident, behaviour therapy including progressive desensitization or, alternatively, 'flooding' may suffice to ameliorate the symptom. In the toddler this diagnosis is seldom made due to the fact that specific fears of witches, monsters, the dark and so on are normal in this phase of development. In the school-age child, however, most of these fears should have disappeared.

General anxiety, on the other hand, may present with somatic symptoms such as precordial pain, palpitation and difficulty in breathing, sometimes nausea and abdominal pain, although 'hyperactivity' or withdrawal are other common manifestations in childhood.

Conversion hysteria and dissociative states (Chapter 5). Conversion hysteria may also be a means by which the child resolves a conflict that seems unresolvable and, as a secondary gain, manages to solidify his dependent position in the family. Within a family the symptom may serve to focus the family's attention away from internal and potentially disruptive conflicts that could cause a breakup of the family unit. It is a difficult and potentially dangerous diagnosis to make with persistent symptoms unless special care is taken to exclude organic disease.

Passive-dependent–passive-agressive behaviour patterns

Certain syndromes exist that represent difficulties at both the passive-dependent and the passive-aggressive stages of development. They include, for example, dissociative states, obsessive compulsive disorders, anorexia nervosa, psychophysiological reactions and habit disorders.

Obsessive compulsive disorders. Obsessive compulsive disorders (Chapter 5) are normal in 4- and 5-year olds where rituals such as not stepping on the cracks in the pavement seem to be part of growing up. These 'normal' rituals, however, are not followed by intense anxiety if interrupted and do not interfere with schooling or peer relations. Adult obsessional illness is usually heralded by an episode in childhood or in early adult life; such an episode may result from the child suppressing anger at the parents (often for too high expectations).

Anorexia nervosa. Anorexia nervosa is an illness characterized by refusal to eat, a decline to less than 80 per cent of normal body weight, denial of illness, a distortion of body image with a sense of being too fat despite extreme emaciation, amenorrhoea (if menses had begun), lanugo (downy hair over normally hairless parts of the body), overactivity and no known physical or other psychiatric disorder (for example, depression or schizophrenia) that could account for the symptomatology. The central feature is a fear of weight gain, which may or may not be admitted. The prevalence is approximately five cases per one thousand school children, with more than 5 girls being affected for every boy seen. This disorder occurs most often in young teenage girls and is often found to be associated with fears of separation and with attaining an independent adult status. The girl has often been somewhat overweight previously. Around the central theme may be found fears of her new sexuality with the beginning of breast formation, menses and peer group interest in boys. There may even be fear of impregnation, particularly in girls who have had a total lack of sex education. In addition, like most disturbances of a hostile-dependent nature, it is characterized by clinging, demanding behaviour alternating with anger and 'acting-out' directed primarily at the mother. The latter, for her part, is often found to be having difficulty adjusting to the development of her daughter and impending separation. Without treatment the prognosis is bad, with figures of 5 to 15 per cent mortality. With prompt active treatment the prognosis for the immediate physical emergency is good although many of these children will have persistent eating problems.

Immediate treatment usually consists of hospitalization and a careful behaviour modification programme. Permission for visiting by parents and permission to partake in physical activity may be used as rewards for weight gain. It is important that all the rewards be contingent upon weight gain and that careful nursing observation be constantly maintained for many of these young girls will attempt almost anything from vomiting to hiding food to filling up with water before weighings to defeat the programme. The physician should always negotiate with the patient, not with the parents, concerning the weight gain programme. Rarely, tube feeding may have to be instituted as a life-saving measure. Long-term treatment consists of family therapy and often in addition, individual therapy with the young adolescent, attending to her problems concerning growth, development, and separation and individuation.

The need for further treatment may recur from time to time over many years, usually in connection with life crises which in some way symbolize the separation from a secure and somewhat dependent position.

Obesity.   Obesity, although resulting from many other causes such as family eating patterns and genetic predisposition, may also have its basis in a block at the passive-dependent to passive-aggressive phase. It may be a substitute for emotional needs in children who have a sense of deprivation and depression, and in situations of stress it may serve to lower anxiety in these persons. It becomes a problem for the child as athletics and, later, adolescent heterosexual relationships become important and the original poor self-image obtains increasing negative feedback from the environment, resulting in more overeating.

Treatment must be psychological to assist the child in building a more positive self-image, behavioural in changing both the family's and the child's poor eating patterns, and supportive in assisting the child to learn behaviours that will be conducive to eliciting more adequate levels of peer support.

Psychophysiological disorders.   Psychophysiological disorders include breath-holding spells, hyperventilation attacks and certain aspects of bronchial asthma, abdominal pain and functional constipation.

In each of these disorders, the child's level of psychosocial development and the related block make him liable to react to stress with anxiety which activates the autonomic nervous system causing an alteration in functioning in an organ or organ system. This, if maintained, may perhaps cause secondary physical change or will exacerbate an organic disturbance.

In the very young child, breath-holding spells may also be considered in this group of disorders. Breath-holding is a relatively common disorder before age 4, characterized by holding of the breath followed by cyanosis and unconsciousness. It is self-limiting and is used by many children to control the environment. It has been noted that this symptom runs in families.

Habit disorders.   Tics, nail-biting and finger-sucking are of little concern in children below the age of 6 but become problems if they persist. Tics such as grimacing, blinking or shrugging are defined as purposeless, quick, sudden and frequently repeated involuntary movements of circumscribed groups of muscles. They affect about 1 per cent of children with the ratio of boys to girls being approximately 3:1. They usually subside by the time the child is 14. Tics which start between the ages of 6 and 8 and involve the face only have the best prognosis. Tics are frequently familial and these children often have associated anxiety and depression. The rare syndrome of Gilles de la Tourette appears to be primarily an organic condition with secondary psychological complications. It is characterized by multiple tics and barking-like noises sometimes accompanied by coprolalia (swearing). It begins around 8 years of age and may have severe consequences for the child's self-esteem. Haloperidol is the treatment of choice although some adult patients are now being reported in the literature as saying that the cure is worse than the disease in view of the drug's side-effects. Pimozide is being considered as a less noxious alternative.

Nail-biting affects about half the child population between 5 and 17 years of age, somewhat less than 20 per cent biting all nails severely and persistently. It is symptomatic of anxiety. Thumb-sucking and finger-sucking are also common, but in younger children.

In all of the above it is the severity and the persistence of the symptoms that dictates one's approach. If intervention seems appropriate then it is the total person in terms of his or her state of personality development that is the focus of the intervention, and not merely the symptom itself, and such techniques as behaviour modification, hypnosis and medication may be used.

Passive–aggressive behaviour patterns

Enuresis. Enuresis may be purely physiological in origin. Indeed, between the ages of 4 and 9, 12 per cent of boys and 7 per cent of girls will still have primary nocturnal enuresis. In 3 per cent of these, daytime wetting will also occur. By age 14 the prevalence decreases to about 3 per cent of boys and 1.7 per cent of girls. Approximately 1 per cent remain enuretic into adult life. Secondary enuresis, that is, wetting beginning after a period of being dry, is more often of psychological origin. Enuresis has been correlated with many factors including a positive family history, twins, lower intelligence, shorter height, delinquency, early marriage and even numbers of siblings involved in crime. Correlations exist with lower socio-economic class and with speech and learning difficulties. Treatment should begin with supportive psychotherapy for the parents, that is, reassurance and suggestions about home management. This combined with restricted fluids in the evenings, waking the child in the middle of the night to urinate, and the establishment of a reward system (star chart) for dry nights will suffice for a large percentage of cases. If this has not helped over a period of a couple of months and the child is over 6 years of age, a bell and pad system—for conditioning—may be used. A bell rings when the first drops of urine wet the pad and complete an electrical connection. The danger with this apparatus is that the child may receive a slight burn if the bell does not function. Being dry is important to the self-esteem of the child and a trial with this apparatus may therefore be well worth the risks involved, but only with the child's agreement.

Alternatively, a three-month trial of imipramine 25–75 mg depending on the weight of the child may be given at 8 o'clock each evening.

The child should be responsible for cleaning the sheets, changing the bed, taking medication where this is the treatment of choice, and for preparing the alarm system where this is being used.

It is now generally found that antidepressant drugs reduce the frequency of bed-wetting but do not cure it. One-third of the children are cured by the conservative approach above.

Ninety per cent of children are dry after six months of conditioning with one-third of them relapsing between 6 and 12 months after the treatment has been completed. In these latter cases, family therapy is imperative.

Encopresis. Encopresis is a condition characterized by the persistent passing of stools into the clothing after the age of 3. The prevalence rates for corresponding ages are about one-third those listed for enuresis, for example, a rate at 8 years of age of slightly more than 2 per cent of boys and slightly less than 1 per cent of girls.

By the age of 11 these rates have been halved. Most of these children will pass their stools in the late afternoon particularly when under stress and will state that they were not aware that they needed to pass a stool. Many of them also exhibit abdominal pain and/or faecal impaction. About one-third are also enuretic. The family history is positive in about 15 per cent. Family psychopathology is often present and usually centres around issues of power and rebellion. Initial treatment may have to be directed at the medical problem when there is associated constipation and impaction. The differential diagnosis must include aganglionic megacolon (Hirschsprung's disease). Where there is an impacted rectum the use of stool softeners, enemas, or even dis-impaction may be necessary though these procedures and manipulative investigations should be kept to a minimum whenever possible to minimize the degree to which the child's already frightening ideas about his or her bowel functioning may be accentuated. Nevertheless, some specialists recommend that, after emptying the rectum by using enemas and suppositories, one should give light mineral oil once or twice a day for the next few months to prevent constipation from setting up another vicious circle.

Psychological treatment of the condition is much the same as for enuresis and involves an expectation that the child takes care of cleaning himself so that secondary gains are minimized. The child should sit on the toilet for two 10-minute regular periods per day with a star chart for younger children and a reward system for positive outcome each half day, and, later, each day. The more passive child who does not seem to care about soiling will have to be referred to a specialist for help. Only slightly less than 10 per cent of the children will not improve with this intensive treatment. This group often displays serious psychological problems with other associated symptoms such as hyperactivity, non-compliance and learning difficulties. Again, treatment is that of the underlying problems of both the child and the family.

Aggressive–depressed behaviour patterns

Depression. As previously noted, the aggressive-depressed child will rarely present in the depressive mode. Even in those presenting in the aggressive mode, however, the careful clinician will be able to elicit symptoms of sadness, helplessness, hopelessness and low self-esteem, and often vegetative signs such as loss of sleep, poor appetite and various physical symptoms. Recent withdrawal from friends and irritability are also signs. In many instances one observes boredom, somatic symptoms and changes such as fatigue and poor school performance. These signs will often emerge more clearly as the aggression is brought under control, and it is vital to treat this as well in order to prevent recidivism. Such treatment should be mainly directed to the unmet dependency needs and should be largely supportive, giving the older child a chance to talk freely about his difficulties and encouraging and facilitating activities which help to build up his self-esteem. These may range from music lessons leading to participation in a band or rock group for a musically talented youngster to enrolment in an outward-bound school for the athletically inclined. Suggestions must be feasible, practical, and well within the ability of the youngster so that positive reinforcement is virtually assured from the outset. Family follow-up is essential.

Bipolar depression with definitive cycles of mania and depression is very rare in childhood although there have been a few well-documented cases. Treatment with antidepressant medication is useful in some cases of severe depression in adolescence. But its use for depression in younger children is not, as yet, well documented. On the other hand, hyperactivity associated with underlying depression has been well treated with imipramine in latency age children. A specialist should be consulted in these cases.

Suicide. Suicide before the age of 14 is rarely reported and an accurate incidence is therefore impossible to ascertain. However, in North America, it is the second most common form of death between the ages of 15 and 25. In younger children, when reported, it appears most often to be associated with a disciplinary crisis or an attempt to 'rejoin' a dead relative. It would appear that the child does not really comprehend the full seriousness and finality of the act and in some cases it may be seen as a means to punish the parents. In older children and adolescents, however, there are usually definitive signs of disequilibrium and depression including deterioration in school work, decreased contact with peers, marked irritability, low frustration tolerance and other signs such as those listed under depressive equivalents above. A marked change in an adolescent's behaviour, for example, is a critical sign that should alert the physician to the possibility that something other than 'normal adolescent change' is taking place. It is crucial that the physician put aside time to listen in a relaxed attentive fashion to all of the child's complaints and that he obtains a thorough history through contact with the family, school and all other significant figures. Regular counselling sessions are essential and the adolescent should be encouraged to call on an emergency basis if needed. As with all other assessments, attention must be paid to those factors that caused or contributed to the onset of the child's problems, the factors which precipitate his coming to professional attention and those factors that sustain the condition. The family must be involved on an intensive basis.

ADOLESCENCE

The process of development of the normal personality is of major importance up to the age of three but never really stops and it repeats itself cyclically in various ways throughout childhood with a major resurgence at the time of adolescence. Adolescence is best described as a period of intense conflict, where the individual is caught between wanting to remain a protected child on the one hand, and become a free and independent adult on the other. The major four conflicts of adolescence centre around:

1. Dependence–independence
2. Sex: sexuality versus non-sexuality and intimacy versus isolationism
3. Occupation and education: productivity versus self-indulgence and inactivity
4. Values: altruistic values versus egocentricity

The adolescent is vulnerable to symptoms and breakdown due to the strength of the biological drives that come to the fore in this period and the intensity with which he or she attacks each of the areas of conflict mentioned above. Any of the patterns and syndromes mentioned previously may make its appearance under these conditions despite the fact that no symptoms were overtly obvious or sufficient to demand attention in the pre-adolescent years. Also, the presenting behaviours (for example, promiscuity and drug-taking) may differ because of age and different drives and social pressures. The core of pathology and intrapersonal dynamics, however, will be the same as that which was described earlier and the general principles for treatment remain the same.

As is typical of most people in crisis, adolescents frequently try to deal with their conflicts by suppressing one side entirely and embracing the other in the extreme. This frequently results in parents moving to the opposite extreme, and both sides become entrenched in their positions. The art of treating an adolescent, then, lies in gently supporting *both* polarities and helping him to effect a compromise between them. Thus an adolescent in a struggle with authority should be given both due respect for his personhood (supporting independence) and firm guidelines (supporting dependence) simultaneously. One-sided solutions store up trouble for the future. Most often a combination of approaches—individual, marital and family—is found to be best, the pattern depending on the type of problem and the age of the child. Older adolescents are most often better treated as young adults, especially when they are well on their way to leading separate lives from their family. There is no place for rigid authoritarianism, yet indecisiveness or attempts to copy the dress and speech of an adolescent can be just as detrimental to the treatment process. The physician must be a predictable, consistent and secure model. He must be secure and confident both in his job and in his life as a whole, while at the same time attempting to maintain reasonable flexibility and understanding. He must always state clearly and honestly what he believes to be correct but should also acknowledge other routes for accomplishing the attainment of the same basic values. He should help the adolescent to feel responsible and to find his own unique way of becoming his own person. For the most part the physician should be reluctant to accept secrets and must retain the option to disclose whatever he judges to be in the best interests of all concerned. The adolescent should not be expected to meet the same expectations one might place on an adult, but neither should he be in the subordinate position of a child with respect to the doctor. The adolescent is very much in the process of 'becoming' and all of his struggles and conflicts are centered on this task. In the process, the physician is an assistant, perhaps a catalyst, and possibly a model.

Alcohol and drug abuse

One of the most frustrating problems for the family physician is dealing with adolescents who are abusing alcohol and illicit drugs. To experiment with drugs on one or two occasions is very different from belonging to a group where their use is an integral part of the subculture, and they are taken to dull emotional pain or as an act of rebellion against parents. It is important that in addition to a full psychiatric history and family history, the physician obtain all of the relevant details of drug use such as: time, place, in which company, with what effect, type, frequency, dosage and source of drugs used. He should ascertain how the drug-taking began, what now sustains it and what alternatives the patient sees as being available.

The effects of drug abuse can be far-reaching and include the precipitation of psychosis, panic or accidental death with hallucinogens, addiction with heroin and alcohol, violence with barbiturates, alcohol and amphetamine, and a syndrome of gross passivity with long-term use of marijuana and hashish. The treatment is for the acute or chronic physical condition, with hospitalization where necessary, followed by attention to the underlying psychological and social difficulties. With serious cases, specialist help will be necessary and consultation should be sought.

CRISIS SITUATIONS

Theory

A crisis is a disruption of homeostasis and adaptation caused by a threat to the individual against which his usual problem-solving mechanisms do not work. Whether adult or child, the human being is bewildered. Perception is clouded and narrowed and thought is less grounded in reality. The older child becomes preoccupied both with the present situation and with memories of past crises that filled him with similar anxiety, fear and guilt. The reaction to this flood of emotion is seen in the onset of symptoms, coping manoeuvres or both. The child differs from the adult in that he is less developed and has less problem-solving abilities, less experience and therefore less in the way of personal resources with which to handle the crisis. The child is also a dependent organism, and life crises for the child are of a different quality and depend less on factors outside the family than on the threat of removal or disruption of the bonds on which he depends. It is for this reason that the most potent crises for the child are not financial catastrophes, fires, floods or wars, but rather such things as marital breakdown, removal from the home, hospitalization of himself or mother, death of a parent figure, or his own terminal illness and possible separation from his parents by death. The key or threat that runs through all of the foregoing is separation from the parent figure.

Treatment of adolescents in crisis involves a clear delineation of the precipitating event and why he or she was unable to cope with it using past coping mechanisms. The physician must then explain in a clear and succinct fashion his understanding of why the adolescent broke down in this way at this point in time. The aim is to help the adolescent to look consciously at alternative means for coping and to encourage him to try out new methods in everyday life. With the child, however, the process is, if anything, more complex for it is the parents who need to be helped to assist the child through their demonstration of other ways of handling the situation in question. With young children, two situations are of paramount importance, first, hospitalization and second, death and dying.

Hospitalization and illness

Illness in a child will tend to accentuate any problems that already exist. The child who is blocked at a passive-dependent stage of psychosocial development and is shy may become extremely self-conscious, withdrawn and depressed; the child who is in the aggressive-depressed stage and is resentful of authority figures may act out against the physician and nurses. As described earlier, separating from the parent figure(s) is particularly serious between the ages of 6 months and 4 years and causes a characteristic series of events. At first the child will *protest* angrily and demand to go home or to have his parents. This is followed by a stage of *despair* where the child gives up and withdraws. Following this the child may begin to eat regularly and take part in activities but he will not attach to anyone and if the parents should visit, he may remain aloof and *detached*. All stages can cause the parents either to feel guilty that when they visit they seem to make the child worse, or angry at being rejected by the child. Either reaction may be followed by a decrease in visits and thus a vicious circle begins. The third stage, that of detachment, is particularly ominous for, if prolonged, it can have serious consequences in terms of the child's later ability to form close, meaningful relationships.

It is extremely important for the parents to be aware of these feelings that the child experiences in hospital, and even more important for them to realize that their inevitable result on returning home is the expression of considerable separation anxiety. This latter may manifest itself as a temporary regression, reversion to baby-talk, loss of toilet-training, interference with previously established eating and sleeping patterns, and especially increased clinging, temper tantrums and protest at separation from parents on occasions which were previously well tolerated. If the parents respond supportively and reassuringly, these symptoms will disappear, often within a couple of days and certainly within three weeks. If the parents misinterpret these symptoms as 'naughtiness', however, they might well react punitively, thereby increasing the feelings of rejection and separation anxiety and thus keeping the symptoms going for months or years.

The best treatment with the very young child is to admit the mother to the hospital as well. Indeed, this has been shown in surgical cases not only to avoid the deleterious effects of hospitalization, but also to lower significantly the post-operative complication rate. If this is not feasible visiting by the parents should be frequent, regular and predictable. The child should bring to hospital some of his own toys and favourite doll and be cared for by a limited number of staff to whom he can become emotionally attached. This in turn is not without its problems, for the over-attachment of nursing staff may lead to a loss of objectivity and consequent emotional difficulty for them as the disease and treatment progress. They may even become competitive with the parents and unconsciously discourage visiting. Regular staff meetings in which the emotional impact of dealing with seriously ill children is openly discussed and worked through are a necessity for optimal nursing and medical conditions in the large paediatric or general hospital.

The child must also be prepared for all procedures. Many are painful and some, such as those to do with ears and eyes, deprive the child of part of his perceptual world. All procedures are frightening and all are made worse by fears of the unknown. Pain may be viewed by the young child as a punishment and all children fear deformity and being different (this peaks in the early adolescent years).

Severe illness such as leukaemia may cause blocks along any of the developmental lines and, in a vulnerable child, may cause regression. Characteristically, the parents will exhibit guilt, anger and resentment and will, in their feelings of helplessness, mourn the loss of the child 'who might have been'. Rejection or over-protection may be the parents' behavioural response. The parents must be helped to support appropriate expectations and to ensure that peer relations are encouraged and that the child maintains his or her academic standing. The physician must help the family including the other children to express feelings and thus defuse resentment, anger and other effects, as well as helping them to understand the several meanings (psychological, social and financial) which the illness has for the parents and other siblings. He must also very carefully elucidate with the parents all of the strengths or assets that both the child and the family have and how these can be maximised to the benefit of the patient.

In summary, the physician should be just as alert for new

behaviours which are out of keeping with the child's previous behaviour and which signal definite psychological pathology, as he is for physical complications of the primary physical disease process. The two are inseparable in the sense that deterioration in either sphere will have serious and detrimental repercussions in the other.

Death and dying

Perhaps one of the most difficult problems for any of us is the management of the dying child and his or her family. The child through the pre-school years does not really comprehend the finality of death and his greatest fears are of separation. Between 4 and 8 years of age, fears of mutilation become more important and it is only at or around the age of 8 that the full meaning of death is understood. The pre-school child may feel responsible and may in turn feel that he might be able to do some magical thing that would cause the dead person to wake up or to come back. The prospect of death in the adolescent, on the other hand, most often arouses anger and frustration and an undirected resentment, 'why me ... look what I might have been', and so on. The family will undergo marked stress, often with feelings both of resentment against fate and against the dying child, and guilt that they have not done or are not doing enough. Siblings may feel left out and the family ranks may close. The physician walks a difficult path between being honest and realistic, and yet encouraging the family through his actions and treatments to continue with some hope. The stages the individual goes through can be described as *denial*, followed quickly by *anger* and *protest* ('Why me?' or 'Why my child?') followed by *bargaining* ('If I'm good then .... '). Next follow *despair*, helplessness and *depression* over what might have been in the past, and what might be in the future. *Reconciliation and acceptance* is the last stage, involving coming to terms with the reality in an appropriate way. This last stage may, of course, never be reached by the patient but if it is not reached by the family the consequences for their lives, in particular for the siblings, may be quite severe. One should recognize that the entire medical team will go through all of these stages and the manner in which they are resolved can either help the child and his family and other patients on the ward or it can be to the detriment of all concerned with, at its worst, the child being ignored and anger and resentment being discharged onto the child's family and one's colleagues. Support and acceptance of the stage reached by any involved person is the best way of helping him or her go through this grieving process.

Child abuse

Child abuse is also a crisis, though of a different nature. The incidence is reported as more than 5 cases per 10 000 population and the real incidence is probably a great deal higher. It may be physical, sexual or psychological. The distribution is roughly 50 per cent below, and 50 per cent above, 6 years of age, with boys outnumbering girls until age 12 when the reverse becomes true. Predisposing factors include prematurity, inappropriately high expectations, parents who were themselves abused as children, and parents who have had children in part to fulfil their unmet needs (for example, to be loved and to be needed).

A child who fails to attach appropriately to its mother, fails to form basic trust and develops and remains fixed in one of the general pathological patterns of behaviour previously described will evoke considerable frustration and anger in parents. Physical abuse may be the result. As an adult, both this individual's personal sense of emotional emptiness and his anger at the world may force the continuance of this early pathological behavioural pattern. This, plus his or her family history of 'permission' for violence learnt from his abusing parent may (depending on circumstances) lead to physical abuse of his or her own child. It is also now recognized that the child often invites abuse by virtue of its temperamental characteristics or by virtue of a misfit between its temperament and that of the mother.

A high level of suspicion must be maintained if any of the following factors is present: the history of injury keeps changing or is different from one informant to another, or does not correspond with the injuries sustained; the parent is hostile to enquiry, delays in bringing the child in, seems detached or states that she has difficulty with her impulses to hit the child; the parent frequently moves her place of residence, has little opportunity for recourse or help from others for relief. One should also have a high index of suspicion if the child shows evidence of neglect, is unusually fearful, is hypersensitive to staff, has a history or shows evidence of multiple previous injuries, denies previous known abuse, seems emotionally detached and depressed and is viewed as 'bad' by the parents.

In most jurisdictions the physician must report such cases to the appropriate authorities immediately but, apart from this legal act, the physician must make every attempt to explore the situation in an observant but understanding fashion, attempting to appreciate the stress the parent has been going under from his or her own point of view.

Treatment is likely to be a specialist matter except in very mild cases. Treatment is first and foremost for the parents, and recent techniques in parent-effectiveness training may be of use. Parents should be taught other methods for handling their children. Often education in such activities of daily living as preparation of a balanced diet, shopping and budgeting may be of immense benefit. Above all, the parents should be given nurturing parenting themselves, which they can then pass onto their children. If the child is left at home or returns to the home, someone must be available to the parents twenty-four hours a day. Before one can safely consider that some progress is being made, the parents should be seen to be developing a better self-image, more interests outside the home and a positive image of their child. With younger children, the mother is usually the abuser and psychotherapeutic work should initially focus on the mother–child interaction and explore the precise circumstances of each event in sufficient detail to be able to elucidate the common precipitants or triggers. At the consultation, some of these mothers may exhibit model behaviour with their child even to the extent of being too calm with what might temperamentally be an extremely difficult child, and they may give a history of a build-up of tension as each event was handled carefully until they suddenly exploded. In such cases the physician should, if necessary, help the mother to see this progression. She should then be encouraged to formulate means for effective intervention such as: implementing constructive controls at the first sign of escalating trouble, calling for assistance, or obtaining day-care to allow herself some time off. Although child abuse evokes an angry reaction in most of us, it does not occur 'out of the blue'. There are very clear causes—either historical, psychological or environmental—in the child, the mother or the family system and it is the physician's job to delineate clearly these causes and see that appropriate management is carried out. Treatment is almost invariably long-term. The prognosis is often serious and is predictably worst when drugs, alcohol, and a history of violence and marital and vocational instability are found. In some of these families the child may have to be permanently removed from the home by the appropriate government authorities.

PHYSICAL DEVELOPMENTAL MILESTONES*

This list of milestones has been chosen to avoid the need for special material. The ages suggested are approximate and any single failure should not be considered significant.

1 Month	Watches mother's face when she is talking to him
	Will regard ring on a string 1 metre away
	Quiet when a bell is rung
6 Weeks	Smiles at mother
	Eyes follow moving person
2 Months	Smiles at others, vocalizes
3 Months	Will hold rattle for a minute or more
	Watches own hands
	Turns head to sound
16 Weeks	Held in sitting position—head held up constantly
	Looks around actively
	Hands come together as he plays

*Prepared by Dr R. A. Bugler.

5 Months	Able to grasp objects Crumples paper Takes objects to mouth
6 Months	Holds bottle, grasps feet Tries to recover a toy Imitates some noises
7 Months	Keeps lips closed if he doesn't want any more food Responds to name Vocalizes syllables, Ba Ba
8 Months	Sits for a few seconds unsupported
9 Months	May move by rolling Pulls self to stand Can pick up a piece of string
1 Year	Walks with both hands held Rolls ball back to one Plays peep bo Understands one word
15 Months	Creeps upstairs Walks without support Imitates mother in sweeping
18 Months	Four or five words more than Da Da or Ma Ma Uses a spoon and gets some food in mouth Walks three steps or more unaided Will point to mouth, hand, toes if asked to
24 Months	Knows some common objects, cup, door, pussy Imitates action. Waves, clasps hands or nods head Will fold a piece of paper if shown
30 Months	Holds pencil in hand instead of fist Knows his own sex Helps to put things away
3 Years	Can stand on one foot for seconds Can help to set the table Joins in play Can do some dressing of himself May count up to 10, knows one colour

3½ Years   Puts two halves of picture together
             Will fold a paper twice
             Understands concept of two

 4 Years   Goes down stairs one foot per step
             Can button clothes
             Attends to own toilet needs

 5 Years   Copies a triangle
             Gives age
             Compares two weights

 6 Years   Copies diamond shape
             Names four coins
             Knows some opposites—boy, girl

 7 Years   Will repeat three numbers backward
             Able to read simple sentences
             Subtraction in units

12

Emotional and Sexual Disorders in Marriage

One attraction of marriage is that we share a private world. What our friends see is of small significance compared to what takes place after they have left. If that private world should become poisoned, unpleasant or painful it is difficult to know what to do. The kindly suggestions of a third party are of no help. Lasting solutions to emotional and sexual problems would appear to be those which are discovered in the private world by the couple who inhabit it.

The inviolability of this private world is probably important to the development of the marriage, and this partly explains the reluctance of many doctors to intrude. If we attempt to enter, we are deterred by the display of violent and uncontrolled feelings. Although it is widely appreciated that marital disorders are important causes of psychiatric illness in all members of the family, their treatment is uninviting. Marital problems are perhaps the most unwelcome of all psychiatric consultations. Yet they add new dimensions to psychiatric work. Joint consultations, like family therapy, can operate on the basis of different assumptions from individual psychotherapy. The effort is challenging and some of it can be undertaken by general practitioners. The principles are the same as those discussed for family therapy (p. 142).

ASSESSMENT OF MARITAL PROBLEMS

There are many ways in which marital problems may be presented. There are some cases of agoraphobia in which the wife seems to be saying that she feels herself to be a prisoner in her marriage. Depression which is relieved by the absence of the spouse may imply that the marriage is the cause. In other cases, one partner openly brings the problem to the doctor. This can be done in two ways. It often takes the form of an accusation ('My husband is making me ill, Doctor, can't you stop him ...'), and whether or not the accusation is justified it is usually safe to assume that the *complainant* is emotionally disturbed. The normal spouse of a disturbed person will bring the partner's disturbance to the doctor (I'm so worried about my husband, Doctor, he does the most dreadful things'). Quite frequently the couple will come together with their problem, and this perhaps is the best way of all.

The consultation may start, therefore, with a joint interview. If not, it can be argued that one should be requested. When conducting these interviews it is important not to attempt to take a history but to encourage the partners to uncover their problem in the presence of the doctor. The main interventions which are needed are those which attempt to clarify what is being said ('You seem to be saying that your wife does not appreciate what you do for her') and those which counter attempts by one partner to block further discussion. It is very important that both partners succeed in a candid exposition of their point of view, and whenever possible one partner must not be allowed to kill the discussion through silence. In this context, silence means withholding what ought to be expressed, and this is anti-therapeutic. Tears must not be allowed to stop the interview, and a paper handkerchief may be offered instead of sympathy. A related type of intervention which some consider very valuable is to draw the attention of the participants to their particular recurring patterns of interaction.

A joint interview will quickly establish a number of facts. Complaints about the partner's behaviour are often transformed into requests for help. For example, the woman who formerly complained of her husband's excessive sexual demands will recognize that she is frigid and perhaps seek treatment for it. There is no substitute for the observations made at a joint interview; you do not need to be told who is the attacking partner—it takes place in front of you. This is the nearest that one will ever get to the private world of the marriage. From this vantage point one can often make a good guess (not always accurate) regarding the need for individual treatment. In some joint interviews the partners respond to each other and one can feel an emotional shift during the interview. In other consultations one or both partners show themselves to be inflexible, for example, by insisting that the doctor should label normal behaviour of the partner as pathological. This may show that joint interviews are unlikely to succeed on their own and that individual treatment may be needed if the marriage is to be helped at all. Alternatively the physician may sum up the situation by drawing attention to the points of conflict, and remarking upon the consequences of the ways in which each partner is treating the other one. The therapist then can tell the couple what options they have, for example, for one or both to change in significant respects, to continue as they are or, perhaps (if this has been raised and with due caution), for them to separate. Strong intervention of this last type requires both experience and good judgement. The effects may not be immediately apparent—indeed some worsening may appear—but follow-up often yields a favourable outcome. We have seen patients conclude they will separate, despite our careful efforts at reconciliation, and yet they have reappeared happy and still united after a few weeks; and we have struggled to avert a separation out of fear that the more dependent partner would not survive, only to find that both partners were enormously better after parting.

Some marital and family therapists never see one member of a couple or family alone. Most are more pragmatic and arrange individual interviews in accordance with the circumstances, but not without careful consideration. For family practitioners and psychiatrists or others in training, it is usually highly desirable to supplement the joint interview with an individual examination. The aims of this interview are twofold: firstly, to take a full history of the individual and of his part in the marriage; secondly, to decide whether there is any psychiatric disorder in need of treatment. Often the separate interview produces information which has to be kept from the partner. This includes extra-marital liaisons and also loss of love and interest for the partner and the marriage. Intriguing though such information may be, it is frequently better not to know it, so as to be able to deal with both partners without the handicap of secrets shared with one partner only. Information given in confidence inevitably has to be kept confidential.

It sometimes happens that the other partner (often the husband) is never seen. He may stay away because of a complete lack of interest in helping the marriage; more often because he suspects that the spouse has enrolled the doctor as an ally and he fears that a consultation will turn into a reiteration of her complaints. He may feel guilty about his behaviour and expect to be criticized. He may be anxious that the doctor might question his normality. Some feel betrayed if there is a possibility that their secret weaknesses may have been disclosed to a third party. Finally, there is the possibility that the patient is keeping doctor and spouse apart. In all these cases it is worth while to write to the missing partner (with the patient's permission) tactfully inviting him to attend and reassuring him that his point of view will be taken seriously.

AFFECTION AND SEX

One of the important things about the relations between man and woman is that the connection between sexual activity and personal feeling is inconstant. We like to think that in the 'normal', 'mature' individual, sexual intercourse will only take place in permanent relationships. In fact, this is not always true. The sexual drive has its own autonomy, and cannot always be conveniently disciplined by the expectations of society and the personal relationships of the individual. It also has its own disorder. Sexual failure may, therefore, be a consequence of a disturbance in the emotional relationship or due to the intrinsic psychological problems of the individual.

The effect of neurosis

A failure of understanding can lead to unfair accusations from wives who believe that their impotent husbands no longer love them or indeed love someone else. While this may be true, it is more likely to be the result of a neurotic disturbance which has been precipitated by recent significant events in the patients' life history. Other sexual difficulties, such as premature ejaculation and other neurotic symptoms, may be present. These are patients in whom impotence is a symptom of a neurosis.

The discussion in earlier chapters on the aetiology and psychopathology of neurosis applies equally here, but attention must be drawn to the choice of impotence as the main neurotic symptom. Most neurotic patients experience some diminution in sexual capacity, but impotence is only the presenting symptom in a minority. It may arise either because conflicts over sexuality play a predominant part in the structure of the neurosis or else because the marital relationship has been caught up in the neurosis, and the impotence is a way of acting out these conflicts towards the wife. Naturally, these two explanations may both apply in varying proportions in any particular case. It is necessary, therefore, to take a very careful history of the sexual education of the patient, paying as much attention to what was not said as to overt prohibitions. A home in which sexual taboos were never mentioned implies that sexuality is indecent and 'wrong'. Having been warned of the 'dangers' of masturbation, and the sinfulness of premarital heterosexual experiences, even petting, it is easy to understand how the unfortunate man is incapable of changing his sexual attitudes on his wedding night.

On the other hand, if the wife refuses to be seen, the possibility is raised that it may be her attitudes which are playing a large part in causing her husband's impotence. Sometimes wives refuse to attend not because they fear they have something to hide but simply because they are too prudish to discuss sexual problems with the doctor. As always, when a relative refuses to attend, this is a very significant finding. A man who is unsure of his potency will find it very difficult to summon up enough self-confidence in front of a wife who is prudish and shamefaced about sex, perhaps believing that sex is wrong or dirty. Ill-controlled aggression will also wreak havoc with the sex relationship. Any sensitive man may find it hard to be potent with a nagging woman, and some women possess an especial knack of puncturing the self-confidence of the male. If such a marriage breaks up, the man may find that he is fully potent with a woman who has an easy accepting attitude towards sex. Conversely, the husband may use his impotence to hit back at his wife. One of our patients was a man who was unable to be aggressive towards his wife. Although a successful executive who could be aggressive in business affairs when required, he was meek, withdrawn and impotent at home. His wife complained bitterly of his lack of feeling towards her. He was encouraged to deal with her in a more normal way, and although this led to occasional rows (which were previously unknown), the marital relationship improved remarkably and his potency returned.

The same comments can also be made about the women who fail to respond sexually. Failure in making love shows itself in more ways than difficulty in intercourse. Such women dislike the playful kisses and caresses which most women welcome from their husbands even when coitus is not contemplated. They will accept sexual demands only under certain conditions, for example, in bed, in the dark, alone in the house. They will refuse sexual advances in unconventional circumstances. Apart from their sexual life, frigid women tend to be irritable and ungracious towards their husbands and neglect the minor courtesies of married life. These associated symptoms mark off clearly the frigid woman from the type of woman who welcomes sexual intercourse and enjoys it without actually attaining a recognizable climax.

In considering the psychological background to frigidity, the same general pattern which was discussed in relation to impotence applies equally here. Many frigid women are more guilty about sex than they realize, largely due to their mother's reactions to their sexual experiments in childhood. 'I could see from the look on mother's face that she was shocked,' said one of our patients when describing how she was caught masturbating by her mother. As with men, a frank discussion of sexual matters with someone in authority (the doctor) goes a long way in helping the patient to unlearn her prudish attitudes. Many of these women would do well to ponder the words of Montaigne:[59] 'The daughter-in-law of Pythagoras said that a woman who goes to bed with a man ought to lay aside her modesty with her skirt, and put it on again with her petticoat.'

In many women frigidity is but one symptom of the disturbed relationship with their husbands. One patient discusing her refusal to have an orgasm said with a flash of insight: 'Why should I give it to him on a platter!' The same patient, during her psychotherapy, became more easily aroused by her husband after a row in which her aggressive feelings had been abreacted and no longer remained to disturb her sexual response.

Women who complain of frigidity present different types of psychological problems. Although homosexuality is not very common among frigid women, many women are worried by occasional homosexual feelings and an occasional lesbian experience, without this being a bar to normal heterosexual adjustment. Occasionally, an unsuspected lesbian discovers the meaning of her frigidity by finding herself sexually aroused by a nude pin-up discovered accidentally in her husband's belongings. More common are the markedly immature girls who are quite unprepared for the emotional demands of marriage. Their sexual difficulties range from a frank refusal of coitus to the passive resistance of a completely anaesthetic frigidity. These marriages tend to break up in a characteristic fashion: the girl flies home to mother and will not live with her husband. Another group of women are uneasy in the feminine role. One of our patients attended the consultation without her wedding ring (at that time, and usually still a significant omission). She explained that her childhood had been made unhappy by her father, who appeared to despise girls. She had a great desire to be better than the opposite sex and obtained great satisfaction in attaining higher marks than the boys in her class. She obtained a degree and worked as a physicist. She became fond of a very intelligent, kindly but ineffectual scientist who pressed her to marry him. In a fit of pique she agreed. This marriage was not very successful.

Sexual activity was usually confined to mutual masturbation. She had an affair with another man 'to show her independence'. She was a very efficient woman and was continually upbraiding her husband for his ineffectiveness about the house. 'If he puts up a shelf, it falls down,' she said. According to her he could not even light the stove properly. Her criticisms of him led to violent scenes in which her husband would lose his temper when she had goaded him sufficiently. These scenes distressed and exhausted her greatly and were the reason for her seeking treatment. She had some awareness that she was in part responsible for these difficulties, but insisted also that her husband should have treatment. After some months of psychotherapy normal intercourse had been resumed and her life at home was much more peaceful. She broke off treatment by declaring that if she continued in psychotherapy any longer she would be turned into an average woman and would start wanting to have a baby and this was no part of her plan for life.

This patient was fairly representative of this group of women. They are very critical of living in a man's world, to which they present an attitude of envy, competitiveness and aggression: 'Anything you can do I can do better'. In other ways they are intensely feminine women, often well groomed and attractive above the average. Classical psychoanalytical theory held that the basic conflict is their difficulty in accepting the fact that their body is inferior to the male in lacking a penis ('penis envy'). Certainly their competitive attitude towards men suggests that a deeply held inferiority feeling may well be the driving force, assuaged only by material proofs of their superiority.

The trend of this discussion so far must not be taken to imply that any woman who aspires to a successful career is impelled by envy of men; far from it. What is distinctive about these women is the way they organize their emotional security. In our culture, the majority of women find their emotional security in the love of their husbands. However successful they may be in their career or profession their primary security lies in their husband's faithfulness. It might be argued that this attitude has a sound biological basis in the woman's recurring periods of helplessness at the time of labour, but cultural and social traditions are probably more important. For many men emotional security lies not only in the affection of their wives (however highly they may value it) but also in their confidence of their own ability to organize a favourable adjustment to their environment. The women under discussion tend to organize a system of security for themselves after the masculine pattern, and many feminists are to be found among them. They are liable to acute anxiety if they fear they can no longer control their environment (to be at the mercy of a man) and this naturally leads to sexual difficulties. Some attempt an uneasy compromise by insisting on being literally on top of the man during sexual intercourse.

Finally, there are the frigid women with an obsessional temperament who regard men as 'unclean'. This attitude may be shown quite obviously in remarks such as that men do not take enough baths, are untidy, and the like. Often enough there is the implicit idea that men need more baths than women. This attitude may spread to clothes, so that frigid women of this type have a great reluctance to handle and wash their husband's soiled garments. It can be shown that this aversion is linked with frigidity rather than the general aversion to dirt which so many obsessionals describe by the fact that such women have much less difficulty in dealing with soiled nappies. Naturally, these difficulties greatly interfere with coitus (which is often a messy experience for many non-obsessional women) and may even prohibit sexual relations. Even touching or being touched by a man can be an unpleasant experience. It is perhaps not irrelevant that in colloquial speech, 'touching' can have a sexual connotation, and in these women even shaking hands can carry disturbing sexual overtones. Associated with this revulsion from physical contact there is always to be found an anxious hostility to the opposite sex which they take little trouble to conceal. What is more deeply hidden is their ardent desire for a sexual relationship in which their passionate feelings would have no constraint. As is so often the case in psychological disorder, an attitude of excessive control and restraint serves to guard the person from the 'dangers' of an uninhibited outflow of feeling.

There are two further general points to be noted in the

histories of these frigid women. First, frigidity often appears after childbirth, as indeed is also the case with other neurotic symptoms. There are probably a number of reasons for this, including fatigue from meeting the needs of young babies and toddlers but the effect of the emotional demands of motherhood on a neurotic personality are likely to be the most important if the difficulty persists despite the availability of adequate contraception. Fear of another pregnancy may also play a part. Second, frigid women are prone to commit adultery. The rationalization they offer for this behaviour is usually that they are seeking sexual satisfaction, but this is unlikely to be a complete explanation. Some women conduct these affairs to bring humiliation and pain to their husbands. In such cases one suspects that sexual tension may not be as important a motive as aggression against the husband which leads both to frigidity and adultery. In some women these extramarital liaisons represent an acting-out of childhood fantasies of which the patient may not be aware. With a repressive upbringing, sex is forbidden in the home (and this is carried over into the marital home) but is practised, albeit guiltily, outside the home. A clandestine affair fulfils these conditions very well, in a similar fashion to the case of promiscuity discussed in Chapter 5.

Although there are many differences in psychosexual development between men and women, it will be clear from this brief discussion that there are two basic psychological factors which are of importance in cases of sexual disorder. The first is a failure to be fully aware of the extent and depth of sexual feelings. Upbringing must play a part in this failure which is brought about by the mechanism of repression. The second disturbing factor is an unacknowledged hostility to the partner. This hostility can arise for different reasons. If it cannot be fully discharged in a row it interferes with the capacity to respond sexually; or, it may be expressed by rowing about sex.

Rows about sex

Sex is the cause of many arguments. 'My husband is over-sexed' is still a frequent complaint. At the outset it must be noted that there is a big variation in the frequency of sexual intercourse. According to the findings of Kinsey and others, married couples in the twenties may have frequency of coitus of up to twenty times per week, although three is a more average figure. The average frequency gradually declines to once a week in the fifties, but there are many exceptions to this figure. Naturally, people vary in the sexual as in other appetites, and it may be that the libido in some couples is ill-matched. In a normal marital relationship, satisfactory compromises are usually attained. When there is a complaint of excessive libido on the part of the other partner, there is usually the implication that 'unfair' demands are being made. The complaint is made with an edge of hostility and rejection: in other words, the complainant is showing some of the signs of frigidity (or impotence). Few normal women complain of excessive libido on the part of their husbands, although they may privately wish for a little more sleep. In other instances, the normal spouse does not press his or her sexual demands on an unwilling partner. To do thus, to the point of arousing complaint, suggests that he or she is making use of the libido aggressively to discomfort the other. A complaint of excessive libido in the other partner, therefore, always implies a more widespread disturbance in the emotional relationship of the marriage, and it is this which should be the object of treatment.

Pathological increase of sexual desire does occur in some mental illnesses. It is very common in hypomania when, associated with the impairment of judgement which occurs in this condition, it can lead to sexually extravagant and promiscuous behaviour much to the distress of the family and of the patient after recovery. This fact alone may make mental hospital treatment necessary. Much the same can happen in schizophrenia, except that the deterioration of behaviour which occurs in this condition may lead to even more bizarre deviations from normal conduct. A respectable wife became a prostitute at the start of her schizophrenic illness. Brain damage can also lead to similarly disinhibited behaviour. Occasionally, depression can lead to a temporary increase (or perversion) of libido, although the reverse is more often true. In all these conditions the hypersexuality is always accompanied by other signs of the psychosis, and the correct evaluation is seldom difficult.

Mention has already been made of sexual misbehaviour in the neuroses. The ambivalent attitude of the hysteric towards sex may lead her to an imprudent encouragement of a willing male whom she has no intention of satisfying sexually. This can lead to a very difficult situation. While it would be a mistake to brand all extramarital liaisons as neurotic, this is unfortunately true for many. Compulsive sexuality is described, in which coitus brings no satisfaction but is nevertheless repetitively sought, but this is rare. In women this is known as nymphomania.

Techniques in lovemaking

Another commonly occurring question is: 'Is it normal?', referring to unacceptable aspects of lovemaking. The problem raised by this question is not the normality or otherwise of the sexual activity, but the fact that one partner is attempting to force an unacceptable activity on the other. The complaints of one partner may also be the first moves of an attempt to break the sexual connection altogether. Types of sexual activity vary greatly in different marriages, and in a normal marital adjustment there is an agreement as to what can be done for the mutual satisfaction of both partners. It is the marital relationship as a whole, not a particular facet of sexual behaviour which demands scrutiny.

Nevertheless, perhaps due to ignorance or a repressive upbringing, there are occasional examples of couples who derive pleasure from certain types of lovemaking and yet are troubled by doubts as to whether or not it is 'normal'. Normal can have two meanings in this context: biological and statistical. As regards the first definition, it can be said that all love play is normal biologically provided it results in coitus, although there are occasional exceptions here if circumstances prevent full intercourse. However, a persisting preference for mutual masturbation is certainly unbiological and indicates the presence of some psychosexual disorder.

The statistical definition of normality is bounded by culture and class. Homosexual preferences once regarded in both

Britain and North America as abnormal, are currently not considered so by American psychiatrists. What is taken for granted in one society is regarded as positively perverse in another. Difficulties sometimes arise when the marriage part- ners come from different social classes and cultures, some- times indeed when the physician belongs to a different sub- culture from his patients. In our opinion, therefore, it is wise not to pronounce judgement on any variety of sexual activity provided it is acceptable to both partners and is not obviously unbiological in its aim. The position to be adopted in coitus, the admissibility or otherwise of oral-genital contact, the infliction of pain through biting, even the question of whether the body should be naked or not, in darkness or in daylight are only a few of the topics on the propriety of which many people hold decided views, although in other sections of society (as Kinsey has shown) the very same activities are regarded as commonplace. We suspect that some practices are singled out ('love bites' are a good example) because they appear to have a social class association: nice people don't do things like that.

JEALOUSY

Of all the emotions which can disturb a marriage, jealousy is probably the most destructive, partly because there can be no adequate defence against a jealous suspicion. Even if the grounds for a particular accusation can be shown to be false, the innocent victim is uneasily aware that the next attack will be equally unpredictable and unavoidable. It is extremely difficult to decide at what point jealousy is to be called morbid. Indeed the word itself suggests an overvaluation of circumstances. A man who produces concrete evidence in court of his wife's unfaithfulness is hardly described as jea- lous. The propensity to develop this reaction is greatly influ- enced by tradition and culture. In groups such as the Inuit (Eskimo), who used to practise sexual hospitality, jealousy is relatively rare and, therefore, is more likely to be regarded as morbid when it arises. In other cultures the experience is so universal that only the most irrational forms would be regarded as abnormal. In our own culture, lack of any jealous reaction during courtship is sometimes taken as evidence of lack of love.

Many writers, in discussing this topic, relate jealousy to a sense of property. Jealousy is therefore a normal reaction when it is suspected that those rights are being infringed by a third party. Clinical experience suggests that this is not the most important element in the jealousy which disturbs marriages in our society. Most jealous accusations are not only in the form 'What has he done to you' but assert 'I suspect you love him more than me'. Fear of loss of love, therefore, would seem to be the basis of many jealousy reactions. In this, as with many emotional problems, the nursery appears to provide the paradigm for the adult reaction. Jealousy of siblings for their mother's attention and love amounts to a demand, which may be insatiable, for greater show of affection. The child behaves as if the supply of love is strictly limited, like food in a famine, and the kisses which his siblings receive reduce the number left for him. Clearly, it is the insecure child who is most insistent on these material proofs of affection. A child who knows that he can call on more than sufficient reserves of affection is less disturbed when his siblings claim their share.

Seen in this perspective, jealousy must be understood as a neurotic phenomenon, in that it is the non-adaptive persistence into the adult world of a pattern of demands and anxieties which normally belong to childhood. We are excluding from this discussion the justified suspicions of a deceived spouse; indeed, it is surprising how unsuspecting are people in this situation! A patient who was referred on account of her unreasonable suspicions about her husband's faithfulness confessed with bitter tears that she believed that her mother had never loved her. She had no confidence that she could even merit faithful love. A discussion with a Marriage Guidance Counsellor of her anxieties about her mother's love led to a disappearance of the morbid jealousy.

A different basis for jealousy is the presence of a wish for greater sexual freedom. The jealous accusations of the alcoholic give a hint to the promiscuity in which he might indulge if it were not for his impotence. One of our patients accused her husband of homosexual practices and cited as evidence pornographic photographs of undeniably heterosexual nature which she found in his pocket. There was some reason to believe that the husband had an extramarital affair, but none that he was homosexual. This case illustrates the way in which these accusations are determined by a projection of (unconscious) wishes and fantasies with a complete disregard of the facts available. Another patient spent many hours in examining the hairs which she found on her husband's jacket, trying to determine if they belonged to her. At the conclusion of her psychotherapy she told us that these accusations arose out of her own sexual frustrations. Although unaware of it at first, she came to realize that she wanted to have lovers and envied men their supposedly greater sexual freedom. Her jealous attacks gave some outlet not only to her frustration but to the libidinal dreams hidden beneath it.

Arguments about jealousy can be divided into three groups. In the first place one partner maintains his right to enjoy extramarital friendship. Superficially this would seem to be an argument over the rules of marriage. In fact it amounts to open defiance of the partner. One couple remarked sadly, 'We show our love by hurting each other'. In the second group are the marriages in which the accusations are denied but nevertheless the accused partner manages to leave 'clues' behind which do not fail to imply his infidelity. It is believed by many therapists that in such marriages the partners are colluding unconsciously in acting out a situation of conflict which has a hidden meaning for both of them. In the third group the jealousy reaction represents a morbid development in one partner only, sometimes psychotic in nature (p. 262).

It will be seen, therefore, that emotional and sexual difficulties are inextricably intertwined. Failure in making love means a failure in loving. Often enough the sexual difficulty is a symptom of a more general disturbance in the relationship. Sometimes it arises out of a specific sexual inhibition in one or both partners. There are some people who seem to be incapable of sustaining a full relationship with anyone of the opposite sex. There are men, for example, whose impotence is total and permanent. Usually they marry later in life without the usual history of girl friends and heterosexual contacts in early adult life. As one gets to know such men better it becomes evident that their sexual incapacity is only one symptom of an impotent way of life. They lack the normal thrusting aggressiveness which one would expect in men with their intellectual capabilities, and usually their careers are undistinguished. Meek, respectable and friendly, they are well liked but carry little weight with their peers. Sometimes they marry aggressive wives towards whom they have a dependent relationship. It is sometimes said of such men that they are latent homosexuals. Although this may be true, their histories very rarely give evidence of occasional escapades of homosexual behaviour, and it must be remembered that there are many men who are capable of active sexual relationship with both men and women. To our mind it seems more likely that they have suffered a repression of their sexuality which impoverishes all aspects of their life, not only their marital relations. The prognosis for this group is very poor.

It would seem, therefore, that there are some problems in marriage which can only be helped if the therapist is able to share the private world of the partners but in other problems he has to be able to deal with the inner difficulties of one partner; often he has to do both. Sometimes matters prove to be less simple. The 'helpful' partner can have had some pathological needs which were satisfied by the other's idiosyncrasies. Altering the latter because they have become too obtrusive may require re-adjustments in the former. For example, a man who used to play the role of tender husband to a sick wife will have to accept that he cannot continue to be both father and mother in the household when she recovers.

EVALUATION OF MARITAL AND SEXUAL PROBLEMS

In this confusing situation it is more important to understand the presenting clinical situation than to attempt to arrive at a diagnosis in depth after the first interview. This is partly because few couples disclose the whole of their problem at the initial interview, but a more important reason is that if the doctor has correctly evaluated the fundamental disorder he still has to deal first with the presenting problem if he is to get full cooperation. However, lengthy initial joint interviews of 1½ to 2 hours can result in a reasonably full appraisal of the problem, as well as, sometimes, good therapeutic results. *Presenting problem* refers to three clinical situations.

1. *Conflict in relationships.* This is a situation of non-cooperation between the partners. Marriage may be regarded as a problem-solving institution, and some marriages fail in this respect. As noted in the previous section, this failure may be the declared reason for the consultation; in other cases the conflict takes the form of blaming the partner. This situation must be dealt with first because if the partners cannot help each other the doctor is unlikely to succeed on his own. He too can expect non-cooperation. Restoration of a cooperative atmosphere may solve all the problems of the couple; alternatively one of the other two basic clinical situations may now be disclosed.

2. *Emotional disturbance in one partner.* Some patients have insight that the cause of the trouble lies in themselves, for example, in an ungovernable temper or in an attitude of revulsion towards sexual activity. The other partner is perceived as helpful and supporting, and there is no tension in a joint interview. Some cases present in this way, in others this insight develops in the course of dealing with one of the other basic situations.

3. *Sexual failure without overt emotional disturbance.* In these cases the couple perceive the problem primarily as a failure of bodily function. They protest that they have a good relationship in all other ways and that individually they have no problems regarding sex. They are often wrong in these protestations, and dealing with this situation often leads eventually to the emergence of one of the other two situations.

Each of these three situations requires its own therapy. The skill lies first in recognizing which situation is confronting the doctor and employing the appropriate therapy and second in recognizing when the situation has changed, requiring a different therapeutic approach.

Conflict in marriage

'What nice trees you have', the wife's affected brittle voice did not conceal her hostility as she stepped into the consulting room. Many couples warn the doctor of their conflict before he has even had time to greet them and in others it comes to light during the interview.

Conventions

The first task is to redefine the conflict in a way which allows helpful discussion. As in other games, the participants of a marriage have to play by the same rules. In disturbed marriages the couple often refer to different conventions without realizing it. Sometimes this occurs because of a disparity in social and cultural background, and it helps to make this difference explicit. Although two families belong to the same culture, each family chooses to employ only certain of the values, attitudes and possessions which are available. Most young people are surprised to find that families which they had considered to be like their own in fact have made very different choices, and they may not discover this until after marriage. Some brides, for example, are hurt when they discover that the husband is unwilling to disclose how much he earns. The tension is naturally greater if one chooses to marry someone from a different culture.

Elizabeth Bott[8] pointed out that marriages differ widely in the manner in which the partners work together. Some families have strict conventions as to what is women's work and what is men's work, while in other families the couple share the tasks. Her evidence suggests that couples who continue to live in the same locality in which they grew up tend to lead a separate social existence after marriage, a man with his friends and a woman with her relations as they did before they were married. These are the families in which the roles of husband and wife are kept most distinct. Couples who have moved away from the areas in which they grew up tend to lead a joint social life, going out together and entertaining friends. In these families tasks are more likely to be shared. Difficulties arise when one of the partners continues to live near his family (for example, by working in the family business) and the wife comes from afar. In this situation the wife will demand more sharing of leisure time activities and household tasks than the husband expects. Lack of awareness of these basic social patterns leads to bewilderment and conflict.

Another obstacle to adjustment which is more clearly seen

is in those cases in which the married partners are of opposite extremes of temperament, for example, hysterical and obsessional, and there is a complete lack of understanding regarding the limitations and potentialities of the partner's personality. What is taken for granted by one is regarded as criminal negligence by the other. This naturally leads to frustration, irritability and anger.

Hostility

Often a simple explanatory approach does not work or else the issues are too trivial, perhaps cannot even be remembered. At this stage it is best that the doctor remains silent and listens carefully. Without prompting some couples will develop a blistering attack on each other. The most fruitful interviews are often the ones in which the worst things are said. Open defiance, 'I'll sleep with whom I like'; rejection, 'I'm leaving you now'; and hate may be very freely expressed. Any attempts on the part of the doctor to offer a helpful interpretation are brushed aside. Indeed the doctor's main difficulty is in sitting still and restraining himself from putting a stop to it. H. V. Dicks made a wise comment:

> I have difficulty still with such painful situations, and have to summon all my recollected experience to withstand the wish to cut them short or to pour oil and sweet reason on these hurtful contretemps.[18]

Strangely enough these terrible scenes are often followed by a reconciliation. It is hard to believe that warmth and love lie hidden in the vicious rows, but that is the ambivalent truth of the marriage bond. It is as if the presence of the doctor sanctions the release of the frightening emotions. When they have been expelled in safety the couple are then free to love each other.

It would seem as if no relationship is free from this ambivalence. Lorenz[42] has shown in his ethological studies that the formation of intense bonds between mating pairs occurs only in animals with strong drives of territorial aggression. Man is one such animal. He suggests that bond formation is necessary to protect the mate from being attacked or expelled. Perhaps many of the conflicts in marriage should be understood as attempts to assert rights over abstract 'territories' such as use of time or money. If these natural feelings of anger and resentment are left unexpressed they poison the atmosphere so that even simple issues develop into rows. This is the drawback to a simple therapy of explanations: until the disturbing feelings are thoroughly ventilated no reconciliation is possible.

The issue here is not whether one should be able to control one's temper. It is certainly important to be able to do so and sometimes very necessary. The important issue is firstly that people should be clearly aware when they are angry, and secondly if the anger does not dissipate quickly it is usually less harmful to have a row than to sulk for days. It may not be generally appreciated that there are people who are frightened of getting angry. For some there are strong moral prohibitions, for others there are fears of reprisal such as being attacked in return or being abandoned. The feeling of being angry may be so disturbing that the patient is not actually aware of being angry; or, if he is aware, he is completely unable to show the other person how deeply he feels. For such couples, the consulting room becomes a safe arena in which battle can be joined and relief gained from pent-up feelings.

Losing one's temper is not always therapeutic. In some quarrels one person loses his temper not in order to assert his rights but in order to squash the display of anger in the other person. This leads to mutual enragement, with exhausting and unresolved quarrelling. This is especially liable to happen if one person is depressed. Depressed people are not only irritable but also sensitive to and intolerant of anger in other people as well. Antidepressant treatment has a specific part to play in the resolution of this type of conflict if only because it effectively increases the patient's tolerance of hostility.

It is often surprising how quickly this method of treatment can work. In many cases only a few interviews will suffice although they may have to be repeated after a little time.

Motives and purposes

There are other cases in which the couple are hurt and bewildered by their conflict. Quarrels may be unresolved because the true issues are never brought out.

It is important to look below the surface when attempting to understand a marital complaint. Disputes about money, for example, are rarely solved by the advice of an accountant. The important motivation is more clearly shown by the effects of the behaviour on the partner. Reckless overspending of the housekeeping money and stringent attempts to control expenditure are both ways in which the domestic finances can be used as a weapon against the other partner. Indeed almost any facet of behaviour can be turned to this end provided that it is sufficiently objectionable to the victim. Sexual maladjustment is often the keenest weapon in the marriage combat, and this type of analysis can also be applied to extramarital liaisons. Although in some cases great care is exercised to conceal the sexual activity so that the liaison can continue as long as possible, in other cases the faithless spouse either takes no trouble to hide his irregular behaviour or even flaunts it in front of his partner by a so-called confession and creates great distress and unhappiness. Sexual satisfaction is clearly low in the hierarchy of motivations of such behaviour.

The following case illustrates the way in which the real problem of a marriage can become obscured.

One couple came for treatment because of the husband's inability to manage his debts. Although earning a good salary, he would contract petty debts which he would forget to pay. He was especially forgetful about H.P. payments, so that on occasions the television would be removed by the debt collector. These unnecessary humiliations made his wife furious. She was a school teacher, and on one occasion in the class one of her pupils asked her for five shillings which the pupil's mother had lent the husband. He worked in an accounts department and never made a mistake in handling his employer's money; but all attempts to help him budget the family money failed completely.

In joint interviews it was revealed that formerly he had been a sergeant in the army. While at an overseas posting he became aware that his wife was having an affair with a soldier in his office. He did not dare tackle the soldier for fear of looking a fool in the sergeant's mess and he lacked the courage to have it out with his wife. The situation was never resolved. On returning to the U.K. he left the army and took a civilian job, and the difficulties began.

It was suggested to the couple that the husband's behaviour was unconsciously a method of paying his wife back for all the humiliation she had inflicted on him when in the army. They were encouraged to discuss the affair, and with prompting the husband gradually became able to express the resentment he had felt.

On follow-up some months later the wife reported that the financial troubles had never recurred and that her husband was liable to lose his temper if offended. She realized that their 'normal' rows were a safeguard against the recurrence of her husband's previous hurtful behaviour. The doctor met them accidentally in the street several years later. They were both very happy and the husband had now trained as a teacher.

Other couples complain of a dearth of emotional life in the marriage. Lovemaking becomes boring, the wife finds herself increasingly disenchanted with the chores of home care, the husband sees himself as valued only for his pay packet; in the end the couple become estranged. One accuses the other of silence or of retreating to work or the pub.

A clergyman's wife was referred on account of depression. She had been adequately treated with antidepressants and at the time of examination was free of signs of an endogenous depression. She was still miserable and complained of her husband's silence.

In joint interviews they explained their situation. When first married they both held the highest ideals of the behaviour expected of a clergyman and his wife. No discourteous word passed their lips. The husband was a reserved man who found great difficulty in revealing his inner feelings. As time went on the wife became increasingly distressed at her inability to preserve the inner calm which she felt was expected. Her husband's silence (meal times often passed without a word being spoken) made it impossible for her to express her dissatisfaction.

Superficially, the joint interviews were unremarkable. Quietly, the wife spoke of her difficulties and with hesitation the husband disclosed the difficulties he felt in expressing himself. Both found the interviews painful but rewarding. They broke off treatment with the wife still needing to take antidepressants; they had abandoned sexual relationships many years previously and had not resumed when last seen.

Although difficulties in communication are often the result of undeclared resentment, more often they are due to the reluctance of one of the partners to show his feelings. This often occurs in sensitive people who are easily hurt. They build up the habit of silence partly for fear that they may lay themselves open to ridicule (one man traced back his reserve to the shame he felt at public school at being a bedwetter) and partly because they fear that an open expression of feeling may hurt others as much as it would hurt themselves.

The outcome

When the presenting problem of the marriage is conflict, failure to communicate and cooperate, it is essential that the couple be seen together. They both have a half share in the problem which only comes to flower when they are together. It is also extremely important not to miss the signs of a depressive illness. Little progress can be made in treatment until the depressive symptoms are controlled by medication, and this applies equally to cases in which the cause of the depression is unconnected with the marriage and to those in which the depression is a response to the emotional conflict in the marriage.

In the absence of depressive illness, lack of progress in joint interviews may indicate that one or both of the partners have neurotic problems in their personality and require individual treatment. Indeed one function of joint interviews is to define the indication for individual treatment and to help the partner concerned to accept the fact that he needs it. There are, therefore, five outcomes of the clinical situation of a conflictful and uncooperative marriage.

1. Resolution of the problem by means of antidepressant therapy.
2. Resolution of the problem by means of joint therapy.
3. Demand for individual treatment for one or both of the partners.
4. No change, perhaps with acceptance of the situation.
5. Separation.

In the event of the third outcome, it may be objected that joint interviews are a waste of time. If the doctor can assess the need at the initial interview, why not recommend individual treatment straight away? Unfortunately when first seen many patients often insist that their symptoms are the result of the bad behaviour of the other, which is no basis for individual treatment.

Separation leading to divorce is a rare outcome of joint interviews because couples intending to part are more likely to go to a solicitor than a doctor. Occasionally, two people are held together by a sense of guilt or false loyalty and when this becomes clear they are able to reach a decision. It would be superficial to call this outcome failure, because it frees both partners from a situation which has prevented their development as individuals. In the end, people are more important than marriages. The effect on children is discussed in the previous chapter, but often such decisions are delayed until the children are older.

Emotional disturbance in one partner

The essence of this situation is that the patient is aware of a disturbed emotional attitude to some aspect of the marriage and that any marital distress that occurs is solely the result of his or her own problem. There is, therefore, agreement between the spouses as to who is in trouble and that the trouble is psychological. It is this which distinguishes it from the other two basic clinical situations.

Here the doctor is on more familiar ground and the general principles of treatment apply to marital problems as much as to any other. Of first importance is the treatment of psychotic conditions, which may present as morbid jealousy. Some patients spend hours searching the clothing of their wives for spots and stains which they aver are from the semen of their rival. The utter unreality of their statements leads to the opinion that they are in fact deluded. The presence of other symptoms, such as passivity feelings, in some cases points to a firm diagnosis of paranoid schizophrenia. In some ways these are the easiest cases to manage, because many will respond to appropriate treatment. Many cases are, however, not so easy to evaluate. They present their jealous suspicions with delusional force, and yet outside the topic of marriage they show no sign of psychosis and do not as a rule respond to treatment directed at the supposedly underlying mental illness. One of our patients was convinced that her husband intended to murder her, and yet could give no reason for this belief. These delusions were unshaken by ECT or phenothiazine tranquillizers, but to our surprise she left hospital to rejoin her husband! In our experience these marriages are always disturbed even before the advent of frank delusions. Some patients who have always had suspicious natures seem to be liable to develop delusions of jealousy as a reaction to intolerable emotional strain. These cases must be distinguished from delusions of jealousy which occur in paranoid schizophrenia and are associated with other characteristic signs of that condition. Such patients may have had a satisfactory marital adjustment before the advent of the illness, and the delusions of jealousy can be expected to clear up if the basic illness responds to treatment. When jealousy is the reaction of a suspicious personality to a disturbed marriage the prognosis is much less certain. It is surprising how little attention has been paid to these distressing and not uncommon conditions, and it may be that the distinction between these two types of jealousy is not as fundamental as clinical impressions suggest. Certainly some therapists consider that there are often, or even always, aspects of the mutual relationship which sustain the psychosis and which require attention whenever one partner has chronic emotional disturbance. We do not wholly accept this view but the possible contribution of the 'healthy' partner should always be considered.

Depressive illness may also present as morbid jealousy. Many depressed patients feel unworthy and this attitude leads them easily to believe that their marriage partner would prefer another. Retrospective jealousy is a difficult variant of this theme which occurs when one partner learns of sexual misbehaviour before marriage. Sometimes antidepressant therapy will clear both the depression and the jealousy but often the relief is partial. The jealous person suffers intensely in the thought that there is a flaw in the person whom previously he idealized.

There are two other symptoms which need careful consideration in respect of the diagnosis of depression. The first is irritability and aggressive behaviour. One patient sought help because he was afraid he might harm his wife and child, yet at interview it was obvious that there was a warm and loving relationship between them. Bad temper had been a feature of his personality throughout his adult life and had also led to difficulties outside the marriage. He improved greatly on nortriptyline.

Loss of interest has previously been noted as a cardinal symptom of depression; sometimes this takes the form of loss of libido. A mild puerperal depression is, therefore, often the cause of lack of interest in sex following a confinement. Careful examination will usually reveal other depressive symptoms such as intellectual retardation.

Many of these difficulties are made worse by alcoholism, and some patients are aggressive only when drunk. When sober they seek help for the sake of their spouse. The premenstrual syndrome may also lead to recurrent episodes of marital disturbance.

Inhibitions

In the majority of cases however it will be clear that the patient has an emotional problem and is looking for someone with whom a helpful discussion can take place, which accords with the definition of psychotherapy given in Chapter 9. There are no special technical features to be discussed: they are the same sort of human beings whose needs were considered in the chapter on treatment. What they have in common is the need to be able to love and be loved more freely. Two types of problem recur frequently.

Many of these patients recreate in their own marriage the problems which they had with their parents. One woman, for example, was chilly and rejecting to her husband as her mother had been to her when she was a little child. She lavished on her own small daughter the love which she had needed herself when she was at her daughter's age. The situation resolved as she became aware of it. The wife and son of another patient experienced the same cold and critical treatment which the patient had received from his father. Relief came only when he was able to identify with warm and accepting father-figures. Other patients cannot shake off a deep bond with a parent which interferes with the development of adult relationships. One man dated his troubles to a particularly vivid dream at the age of twelve in which he had intercourse with his mother. His marriage had broken up because of his lack of emotional commitment and later he became impotent. In all these cases a childhood relation with a parent was disrupting their adult love relationship.

A different type of problem was shown by a young woman who experienced a great aversion to sexual intercourse soon after she began an oral contraceptive. She loved her husband deeply and felt the lack of sexual outlets. During psychotherapy she became aware of aggressive and vicious trends in her nature. At one point she described her revulsion to sexual intercourse in words which suggested that she felt as if she was about to be raped. She then realized that she feared that her husband would attack her with the same viciousness which she experienced in her fantasies of battering babies. She had projected on to her husband the aggression which she had disowned in herself. Another woman patient had enjoyed being seduced by her father. As she grew up she attempted to deny her sexuality by an extreme modesty which persisted to disturb the sexual relations in her marriage. In these cases trouble arose in the sexual relationship because the patients were unable to accept a part of their nature.

In the individual treatment of cases such as these, the disturbance in sexual relationships is only a facet of their impaired ability to love. By resolving their anxieties, psychotherapy can assist them to be more self-giving in all aspects of their loving relationships. One couple complained that intercourse was 'no more than two people having a simultaneous orgasm'. Paradoxical though it may seem, the couple were fully justified in their complaint. The wife was inhibited and ungiving in all aspects of her loving and came for help when she feared that her husband could stand it no longer. An orgasm without meaning is worthless.

This clinical situation is often the presenting problem. Occasionally it is disclosed when conflict in a marriage has been resolved. Often it is revealed during the course of treatment in the third type of situation in which individual anxieties are first denied.

The resolution of this situation usually reveals no further problems. Occasionally the other partner will seek help.

Sexual failure

In the third clinical situation the couple present their complaint primarily as one of bodily failure, disclaiming any

psychological or relationship problem. It is necessary, therefore, to describe the more frequent sexual complaints and
because overt emotional disturbance is absent the possibility
of an organic cause must also be borne in mind.

Impotence

By impotence is meant the failure to gain, or maintain, an
erection. Difficulties in erection are very common with the
newly married and on the honeymoon. Any situation in
which sexual desire is heightened excessively can cause impotence in the male. According to Strauss,[72] it was not uncommon in soldiers returning home after a long spell of
overseas service. Impotence may be relative, in that intercourse is perfectly satisfactory with the loved mistress, but
not with a nagging wife. Excessive fatigue, or awkward
circumstances, may also be the cause of temporary impotence in an otherwise healthy man. Although impotence
brought about by the above situations may be the first sign
of a psychological disorder, it is important to stress that
this is not necessarily so; many normal men will experience
impotence under these conditions, and, in the absence of
psychopathology, it will respond readily to reassurance and
counselling.

Age is commonly believed to have an important effect on
the sexual activity of men. Kinsey showed that the amount
of sexual activity varied immensely with age as far as men
were concerned, there being a steady decline in activity from
early adult life to old age. More recent work[66] suggests that
in fact what happens is that the frequency of sexual intercourse declines to three or four times a month in the sixth
decade. From that time on the level of sexual activity does
not change until interrupted by a serious illness in one of
the spouses, after which it is not resumed. If the couple are
fortunate in being free from serious illness coitus may be
continued beyond the eighth decade. The steady decline in
activity which Kinsey demonstrated was apparently due to
the accumulating risk of serious illness in old age. There is
nothing abnormal or unusual, therefore, in sexual relationships being preserved in aged couples. Naturally, this depends
on the vigour and sexual interest of the individual, and those

who have never gained much satisfaction from sexual activity find the wife's menopause a convenient pretext to abandon it altogether. A common pattern of impotence of which age is the cause is the remarriage of a widower. Although potent with his first wife, there may be a gap of a few years in which there is no sexual activity following the end of his first marriage. Efforts to reestablish sexual intercourse with his second marriage several years later may meet with failure. Once the regular practice of sexual activity ceases in middle life, it may be impossible to resume.

The importance of androgen deficiency is hard to assess. Cooper[16] showed that impotent men could be divided into two groups: those with a low sex drive (few ejaculations) and an early insidious onset had lower levels of urinary testosterone than impotent males with a high sex drive. There is some evidence that low testosterone levels may be the consequence of infrequent orgasm, and not the cause. Administration of sublingual testosterone rarely improves the condition. It is worth trying in men over forty years of age, provided there is no evidence of prostatic malignancy, but it must be conceded that when it does appear to be beneficial this may be a placebo response. Long-acting preparations of testosterone enanthate are available for intramuscular injection.

Physical illness does not often present as impotence. Diabetes mellitus and neurological conditions affecting the spinal cord, such as multiple sclerosis, are the most important causes. Occasionally, impotence can be a symptom of temporal lobe epilepsy. Impotence is, however, a side effect of a number of drugs. It is commonly associated with hypotensive agents and has been described as a side effect of poldine. Antidepressants have a paradoxical relationship to impotence. In some cases, especially in middle-aged men, impotence can be the presenting symptom of a depressive illness. The physician must not be misled by the explanation that the depression is due to the impotence: the reverse is the case, and the characteristic signs and symptoms of depression will be elicited on enquiry. Antidepressant treatment will usually bring about the resolution of the condition. In other cases in which the sexual function is unimpaired by the depressive illness, impotence can be a side effect of the tricyclic antidepressants.

It is not clear why this should be so. It is known that the tri-cyclic drugs have an effect on the bladder sphincter because they are helpful in nocturnal enuresis. Occasionally anti-depressants improve premature ejaculation. In both cases the results seem likely to be due to an anti-cholinergic effect on parasympathetic function. In some instances the reduction of potency may have to be accepted as the price to be paid for the relief of depression.

Prostatectomy does not cause impotence, but the destruction of the internal sphincter causes the semen to leak into the bladder so that the patient lacks the sensation of ejaculation: usually he is sterile. Arthritis may make coitus so painful that it has to be abandoned. Impotence may result unless the couple can be counselled into accepting a way of gaining sexual satisfaction compatible with the physical disability.

Premature ejaculation

By premature ejaculation is meant that state of affairs when the man ejaculates either before or soon after penetration. Occasionally, the semen may be ejected in a dribbling fashion and not in spurts. Some men appear to believe that they should be able to control their ejaculation almost at will, and although this may be true for a small minority, it is an unrealistic ambition for the majority of males in our culture; in Kinsey's survey 75 per cent of men ejaculated within two minutes of penetration. It is nevertheless realistic to plan treatment to enable the man to postpone ejaculation long enough for his partner also to reach orgasm.

Clinical experience shows that premature ejaculation is closely tied to impotence. Many patients go through a phase of premature ejaculation before impotence supervenes, and on recovery premature ejaculation may appear again before normal sexual habits are regained. All that has been said about impotence applies, therefore, to premature ejaculation.

This account of both impotence and premature ejaculation is not complete without a discussion on secondary anxiety. For most men, successful sexual practice is essential for the well-being of their ego, and any disorder of this function arouses the greatest feelings of anxiety and inferiority. Having failed once, for whatever reason, the man approaches the next occasion for sexual intercourse in a state of great tension: he feels he must succeed this time, for the sake of both his wife and his vanity, he fears that he is bound to fail and the whole experience is approached as if it were an ordeal in which his manhood will be put to the test. As anxiety and tension are the greatest enemies of potency, he is naturally more bound to fail next time, and so the anxiety grows. As he learns to dislike and fear sexual experience, so he puts off the occasions, and the longer interval between intercourse tends to make worse these disorders and especially premature ejaculation.

Failure of ejaculation

Failure of ejaculation is a rare disorder in which erection is satisfactory but ejaculation does not take place. This disorder accounted for only 3 per cent of men attending a special clinic for sexual difficulties.

Frigidity

The term *frigidity* is usually meant to cover lack of orgasm in women. Although this is true it does perhaps misplace the emphasis. There are many women with contented married and sexual lives who rarely, if ever, experience orgasm. When a woman complains of frigidity (either on her own initiative or prompted by her husband) what she is really complaining of often turns out to be a desire to avoid sexual intercourse. This can vary from an absolute refusal of intercourse with vaginismus to the passive resistance of the woman who is completely cold and unresponsive.

Before accepting a complaint of frigidity as valid a careful enquiry should be made. First, one must be sure that penetration in fact occurs. Next, one must be satisfied that the woman is aware of the two different types of orgasm which occur. The patient's confusion on this point can be pardoned as the textbooks are so often contradictory. In our view it must be accepted that many women achieve orgasm only through clitoral stimulation, some achieve orgasm from penetration and a few rarely achieve orgasm at all, although they find intercourse pleasurable and welcome it. Some women seek advice because they realize that their friends have different sexual experiences from themselves or are vainly trying to achieve an orgasm by a method of love-making which does not stimulate the area which is erotogenic for them. Provided that intercourse is a pleasurable experience and is recognized as an essential part of their marriage, we reassure such women. The woman who enjoys love-making but does not reach a climax is, we feel, less in need of treatment than the woman who attains an orgasm but attaches no importance to it, who is 'not bothered' if she goes for a long time without intercourse, or who restricts her sexual activities with rules and prohibitions——only in bed, no lights, and the like.

Psychoanalytic theory used to suggest that women who are unable to reach a vaginal orgasm are psychosexually immature. It is undoubtedly true that in the course of successful psychotherapy the woman's capacity for orgasm can increase considerably. On the other hand, there are so many women with neurosis who are capable of vaginal orgasm, and so many without obvious neurotic character traits who lack that capability that it seems to be unwise to equate psychosexual maturity with the capacity to experience vaginal orgasm. The biological status of the female orgasm is doubtful, to say the least. It is obvious from a biological point of view that coitus must be pleasurable to ensure that conception occurs but otherwise the orgasm appears to be irrelevant. It seems to us that the need to release sexual tension by means of an orgasm is less important in the female than in the male. The need to be loved and the desire to become pregnant (of which the woman is often not fully aware) may in many cases be of greater importance, sometimes with inconvenient results for her social life.

A further difficulty lies in the nature of the female orgasm. Often it is not a critical experience, as in the man, but consists of several peaks. Many observant women are unsure whether they achieve orgasm. Some women (Kinsey reports 15 per cent) report multiple orgasms during a single act of coitus.

On the other hand, one should be suspicious of the complaint that lack of sexual responsiveness in the woman is due to inadequate lovemaking on the part of her partner. One of our patients in psychotherapy reported that when she was in the right mood, she experienced a climax as soon as penetration occurred. When she was depressed, coitus could be prolonged indefinitely without any response on her part. Undoubtedly there are some husbands who are inept at sexual intercourse, but this complaint can also be a cover for the wife's frigidity.

In the same way, failure to achieve a satisfactory sexual adjustment may be due to ignorance, but it is more likely to be the result of a disturbed attitude to sexuality in both partners which forbids the experimentation which occurs in a normal marriage. Preoccupation with sexual technique may serve as a diversion from difficulties in the emotional relationship in the marriage.

To close these general remarks it is perhaps unnecessary to point out the truth of Bergler's observations that in order to achieve an orgasm most women need to love their partner tenderly. If this is not the case it is not abnormal for the woman to fail in her sexual responses although in these circumstances women differ greatly in the way in which they respond.

We would suggest that the term *frigidity* refers to three distinct but related complaints.

In the first place we are in accord with the view of Masters and Johnson[45] that the best indication of sexual arousal in women is vaginal lubrication. Failure to lubricate must indicate failure of sexual arousal. This may be associated with a complete lack of sexual sensations when the genitals are touched.

Second, some women complain of pain during sexual contact. This may be experienced on simply touching the genitals (when it is often caused by a lack of lubrication), at penetration, or only with deep penetration. This is called *dyspareunia.* Local conditions in the vagina or, in the case of deep dyspareunia, endometriosis, must be excluded by a physical examination.

Third, there is the element of refusal. This is often associated with panic and sometimes only occurs when the act is half completed. The vaginal secretions dry up and all pleasurable sensation is lost. Some patients become so anxious at the point of intercourse that their husbands desist and never actually achieve penetration. The most extreme form of refusal is *vaginismus*. Attempts at penetration on the part of the male precipitate widespread muscular spasms in the woman, chiefly in the adductor muscles of the thighs and the extensors of the spine. Apart from the adduction of the legs, sufficient extension of the spine will render penetration impossible.

Refusal of coitus differs from other types of frigidity in that it may bring about certain social consequences. If the marriage is unconsummated, the husband may apply for a nullity suit; in any case the woman will be childless. Other types of frigidity do not interfere with the carrying out of the sexual act, although they may limit sexual pleasure. In this respect the woman with vaginismus has a greater incentive to recover (and this also applies to the impotent man) than a woman who has one of the other types of frigidity.

Apart from local and pelvic lesions, it must be remembered that depressed women lose interest in many aspects of life especially their sexual relationship. The oral contraceptive has been shown to have a similar effect. Antidepressant treatment although restoring libido occasionally appears to reduce the woman's capacity for orgasm. The significance of this is not understood.

Contraception

Because the couple present their problem as a simple failure of bodily function, it is always necessary to exclude a physical cause for the complaint. The next point of importance is adequate and acceptable contraception. Fear of pregnancy is a fundamental cause of sexual failure in both men and women. In many cases the onset of the problem follows an unwanted pregnancy or a pregnancy scare. Even when no clear history is obtained, it is surprising how a marriage will improve when this fear has been dealt with. Some women, to their surprise, will obtain an orgasm for the first time in their lives.

Satisfactory contraception must also be safe. If no more children are wanted, it must be absolutely safe. Sheaths are often an added difficulty to a couple who have sexual problems, although occasionally helpful to men with premature ejaculation. This is also true for the cap, except that some doctors advise the cap for young women who are frightened of their bodies. The regular insertion of the cap helps them to accept the physical reality of the genital tract. Vasectomy may be useful in older couples. The incidence of psychological complications seems to be very small; impotence following an unwanted pregnancy can even be cured by this operation.

Another essential prerequisite for satisfaction in coitus is a warm secure location. It is surprising how frequently couples are inhibited by a cold bedroom, a small child who shares the room or even thin walls and a squeaky mattress! It is also important that time is put aside for lovemaking and that it is not relegated to the end of the day when both are fatigued.

These common-sense considerations must be dealt with first. This will be enough to help some couples to overcome their difficulties. In others it becomes obvious that the failure to solve the practical problems covers up other problems. The refusal of a woman to allow her child to sleep in another room can then be seen for what it is: a safeguard against excessive sexual arousal. One patient persistently failed to attend a contraceptive clinic. She then developed the habit of falling asleep downstairs rather than in the conjugal bed. When the doctor interviewed the husband he disclosed that unknown to his wife, he was a homosexual and did not want a revival of their sexual relationship. Attempting to deal with the practical problems is a potent instrument for uncovering the truth about the sexual relationship.

Learning to enjoy loving

When both medical and practical considerations have been reviewed, there will still remain a number of patients who firmly assert that they have no other problem except the physical one. They may be right, because for some sensitive individuals failure in lovemaking is so embarrassing that the next occasion is approached with an apprehension which becomes a self-fulfilling prophecy, and this applies to both men and women.

In this situation (it is worthwhile to explain this mechanism in a joint interview) the practitioner is advised to use a form of retraining adapted from Masters and Johnson.[45] This will either be successful or else it will uncover anxieties or conflicts which can then be dealt with as in the first two clinical situations.

The first step is to learn *pleasuring*, to use Masters and Johnson's term. Instead of ordinary lovemaking the couple are instructed to learn how to caress each other's body, but they must avoid specifically sexual areas. This involves them lying close without their clothes and with the light on, to discuss exactly what type of caress the partner prefers. This intimate sexual information, which is unique for each individual, is much more important than the general advice to be found in manuals of sexual technique. The couple return to the doctor after two or three weeks, when they are invited to discuss what problems have arisen. It may be that they found that they were more prudish that they realized or perhaps they found difficulty in talking about how they felt. Occasionally, unexpected problems arise, as in the case of the curate who experienced any type of caress as an unpleasant tickle. In discussion it emerged that he struggled against the temptation to be a big baby which was powerfully aroused in the situation of lovemaking. His wife suggested that it was not wrong to relax and enjoy being a baby, provided that he was an adult outside the bedroom. He accepted this and made good progress.

The importance of this approach is that right from the start the couple are taking an attitude of joint responsibility towards their sexual problem. They discuss it step by step. It is also extremely important to ensure that they keep to the prescribed limits of lovemaking for each stage. If difficulties arise then it becomes easier to define exactly what goes wrong.

If all goes well the couple are then allowed a greater range of sexual activity, but attempts at penetration are banned. If the problem is primarily with the man's erections, the wife must experiment with different ways of caressing the penis to find the way of touching which her partner finds most sexually exciting. Masters and Johnson advise that the wife should sit up with her back to the headboard of the bed, her husband lying between her legs with his head away from her. In this position he can relax and allow his wife's caresses to arouse him, knowing that his erections will not be put to the test of penetration. Dry mucous membranes can be painful to the touch, so the couple are advised to use a lubricating jelly. This enhances the sensation in the penis. Masters and Johnson observe but cannot explain that couples who refuse to use a lubricating jelly never succeed in overcoming their problem, and this has been our experience also.

If premature ejaculation is the problem, the wife must know how to control this by the 'squeeze' technique. The ejaculatory reflex has two stages. In the first stage both the internal and external sphincters are contracted and the semen gathers in the prostatic urethra. In the second phase the external sphincter relaxes and the semen is ejected. Once the first stage of the reflex has started it cannot then be stopped. The man, therefore, has to warn his partner that the urge to ejaculate is growing nearer, and before the first stage of the reflex is reached she must grasp the penis with two fingers on the dorsal surface, one on either side of the coronal ridge, and her thumb on the central surface at the attachment of the frenulum. She must squeeze hard; an erect penis can take a great deal of pressure without it being painful. The urge to ejaculate will die away. Some of the erection will be lost, and caressing the penis can begin again. In this way the woman can learn how to control her partner's erection and ejaculation. His problem becomes their joint responsibility. In this way confidence is built up in both partners.

If it is the woman who is slow to arouse, Masters and Johnson suggest that the man sits with his back to the headboard of the bed, with his wife sitting between his outspread legs. Her back rests against him, with her head on his shoulder. Using a lubricant jelly, the man explores the most sensitive areas of sexual arousal in his wife's genitals. Masters and Johnson call this the 'non-demand' position, because the wife can relax knowing that nothing further is expected of her. Some couples find it helpful to have a bath together when learning how best to stimulate each other.

This stage of lovemaking must be continued until the wife

is confident of her husband's erection and ejaculation. In the case of failure of ejaculation the wife must persevere until she is able to bring about an ejaculation. When the wife is slow to arouse the husband must persevere until the wife begins to lubricate, which is a sign that she is now ready for penetration.

This stage is the most crucial in the treatment. Sexual anxieties which were denied at first may become apparent by now and will need to be dealt with. At this stage the need for psychotherapy may well become evident, not to the doctor who will have suspected it for some time but to the patient. In this way the foundation is laid for successful treatment.

Many couples will arrive easily at this stage, but the first attempts at penetration need to be carefully prepared. The couple must be strongly warned against the conventional position for coitus. Instead, Masters and Johnson advocate a position in which the man lies on his back with his wife kneeling over him, her knees about in line with his nipples. In this position she can handle his penis and only insert it when she feels she is ready and when she knows that the erection is satisfactory. This position is important for the frigid woman because she can control coital movement. In the conventional position she is pinned under the man and her coital movements are driven by his rhythm. This is one of the causes of anxiety which dries up the vaginal secretion. In any case it is probably wise for the woman to use some lubricating jelly before penetration is attempted. For the man with sexual difficulties this position is also helpful, because the wife has the responsibility of maintaining his erection and introducing the penis into her vagina. In the conventional position many men fumble at this point and lose their erection. For men with difficulty in obtaining an ejaculation the wife should bring him to the point of ejaculation before inserting the penis.

Once intercourse has been satisfactorily achieved in this position then the couple are free to experiment with other positions. Masters and Johnson note that the majority of their patients eventually preferred the left lateral position because that gives both partners equal control over coital activity.

This approach to sexual difficulties is important because it emphasizes the need of the couple to discuss together what they are doing. Nobody is on trial: the sexual response of each is the responsibility of both. This approach also illustrates a fundamental point in psychotherapy. The art of psychotherapy often consists in helping the patient to come face to face with his anxiety. This cannot always be achieved in sexual anxieties through discussions only. A careful approach to sexual activity, akin to the desensitization procedures for phobia, will succeed either in overcoming the anxiety or focusing it to a point at which the patient becomes aware of it and needs to talk about it.

The success of this treatment varies. If there are no serious underlying problems, five or six consultations will bring about a dramatic improvement. When underlying problems are brought to the surface, some patients will break off treatment while others will enter successfully into psychotherapy. Even in those who are forced to discontinue, there is perhaps an advantage gained in frankness, in that both patient and doctor have some insight into the real nature of the problem.

Non-consummation needs to be dealt with rather differently. The therapy of this condition has been reported by Friedman.[24] This requires a woman doctor who first examines the woman vaginally. This requires a subtle mixture of tact and firmness. While the examination is being carried out the patient will often disclose anxious fantasies about her body. Many of these women prefer not to acknowledge the existence of their genital tract (for example, they will not use tampons) and the doctor's examination affirms that it exists. Immediately afterwards the woman is instructed to insert her own finger inside her vagina, confirming to herself that it is there. It is suggested to her that she practises dilatation of the vagina with her fingers, perhaps in the bath where she has comfort and privacy. Fingers are a more natural and acceptable instrument than glass dilators. When she realizes that her vagina will accept two or three fingers, then she must invite her husband to try with his fingers. When she is comfortable with this, penetration soon follows.

In this approach to marital and sexual difficulties investigation and treatment are not separate processes. Successful treatment of the presenting problem challenges and uncovers further problems which will require a different therapeutic approach. In any situation presenting as conflict, no matter what is at issue, the difficulties must be dealt with by joint interviews with both partners. The ability to work together and with the doctor must be the first aim. When this has been achieved individual problems can then be defined and the need for individual treatment can be accepted. If the complaint is one of simple failure of bodily function and providing that organic causes can be excluded, retraining the couple to rediscover sexual pleasure will either succeed or uncover problems in the relationship or in the individual. The clinical skill required is that of recognizing quickly enough which of the three situations is being presented to the doctor. Many of the failures of treatment arise from the doctor's failure to recognize what the presenting situation has been and hence he continues to employ an inappropriate therapeutic approach.

THE UNACCOMPANIED PATIENT

So far the discussion has assumed that both husband and wife come for treatment. There are cases when only one spouse will attend. This may not matter if the patient seeks help for a problem inside himself without in any way implicating his partner. Occasionally, there are problems such as promiscuity in which it is vital that the spouse is kept in ignorance of the real nature of the patient's difficulties. All too often, however, the spouse is missing because he is not prepared to face an interview. Even in these cases sympathetic listening will often help the patient to live with his situation. A specially difficult problem is when one partner has lost his love for the other. This is shown usually in a profound lack of interest in the spouse, the marriage, in efforts to help the marriage (they find it hard to find time to come for an interview), in the sex relationship, but rarely in overt hostility. Extramarital liaisons are common but by no means the rule. When taxed with their loss of love they frequently find less difficulty in admitting it than their partner has in accepting this new situation. One often receives the impression that these marriages have been quietly crumbling away, with little or no transaction of feeling between the unperceiving partners until some chance event makes it clear to one partner that the marriage has died. Marriages may continue like this for some time for the sake of the children or for reasons of respectability, but the unloved partner finds the position most painful and needs a good deal of support.

Some patients make use of the doctor's understanding to work out a different approach to their problems. One married woman discovered she had never loved her husband only when she fell in love for the first time with another man. She was determined to save her marriage for the sake of her children. She approached the Marriage Guidance Council, and the patience shown by the counsellor enabled her to work out a different emotional basis for the marriage. Accepting the fact that she no longer loved her husband, the wife discovered a hidden reserve of affection and pity for him which enabled her to carry on. The client was very grateful for the help she had received; in fact all the counsellor had done was to listen with understanding and tolerance.

13
Old Age

Old age predisposes people towards psychiatric illness. First, the special biological and psychological effects of ageing increase the vulnerability of the individual to physical and mental illnesses, and, second, social isolation and emotional stresses often become both more common and less easily dealt with as we age.

Biological and psychological changes in old age

It is customary to take the age of sixty-five years as the dividing line between middle age and old age. We do so here as a matter of practical convenience, but with the proviso that before this age the major alterations of temperament and the marked changes in physique which are attributable to old age must be considered abnormal whereas after this age they gradually begin to appear in a substantial proportion of people. We hope thus to have achieved a reasonable compromise between the views of Miss Daisy Ashford (aet. nine years) who in her book, *The Young Visiters*[1] described Mr. Salteena as 'an elderly man of 42', and those sprightly octogenarians who consider men of sixty-five to be juveniles. At any rate it is after the age of sixty-five that those routine physical and psychological changes appear which we regard as characteristic of old people. These changes in their mild form are an increasing slowing of metabolism, bodily activity and thought, a gradual loss of physical strength, changes such as loss of elasticity in the tissues, a narrowing of interests, a tendency to emotional rigidity and self-centredness, a gradual impairment of memory, an exacerbation of pre-existing neurotic trends and a not unnatural preoccupation with means of warding off the effects of increasing physical decrepitude. There is, too, a diminution of the senses which predisposes to accidents and minor physical disabilities. All these effects, and especially the psychological ones, predispose the individual to eccentric standpoints which may cause social friction and from these lesser effects greater ones may grow in any particular case, for example, the emotional rigidity may lead to bad-tempered crotchetiness which becomes so bad that the family will no longer keep the old person in its midst, the preexisting neurotic patterns may develop into undue persistent anxiety or irritable hypochondriasis or paranoid querulousness; memory and attention may fail sufficiently for the old woman to be dangerous if left solely in charge of gas cookers or fires. In these ways the common biological and psychological changes of old age may lead to social difficulties.

Organic causes of mental illness in old age

In old age the vulnerability to mental illness is enhanced *pari passu* with the vulnerability to physical illness. The doctor regularly has more work to do when the patient passes the age of sixty-five. Partly, this happens because some degenerative cerebral or arterial changes bring mental changes in their train.

We have already touched on this in Chapter 8 in the discussion on dementia. In Chapter 18 we mention the emergency situation which can arise when a severe delirium (confusional state) develops, and it is pointed out there that such deliria occur more readily in those in whom some degree of dementia is present already. About 5 per cent of the population over 65 in Great Britain and North America have a moderate or severe dementia and another 5 per cent have a mild but definite degree of dementia. In its less urgent form dementia still often presents as a social deviation, sometimes a severe one. In the milder forms of dementia the individual may be forgetful, untidy, prone to wander and get lost and inclined to neglect personal hygiene. In the more severe forms these characteristics are all exacerbated with, for example, loss of recognition of near relatives, helplessness in feeding and walking, incontinence, the development of delusions and hallucinations and abnormal mood states such as agitation, depression and fatuous euphoria. Fifteen to thirty per cent of patients presenting to hospital with a provisional diagnosis of dementia have treatable conditions. The position in this respect in general practice is unknown but may well be more favourable. Thus potential causes of dementia must be thoroughly sought out with all available harmless techniques. The varied treatable organic diagnoses are discussed in Chapter 8. Particular mention needs to be made of depression which can be mistaken for dementia. Mild changes with ageing should also be discriminated from dementia; a little slurring and increased rigidity, more problems than in the past with memory, or a tendency to live in the past by no means necessarily amount to a significant dementing change.

After the above possibilities have been excluded, two main types of process can be regarded as causing progressive dementia. The commoner (affecting about 60 per cent of chronic cases) is the *Alzheimer* type of *dementia* (called early onset dementia if pre-senile, late onset dementia if arising after the age of 65). It is associated with characteristic neuropathological changes, especially plaques and neurofibrillary tangles and granulo-vacuolar degeneration, which are most pronounced in the temporal lobes. Survival from the date of onset ranges from months to over 10 years. Slow virus infections due to neurotropic viruses cause at least a few of these cases, often with neurological signs such as spasticity and extrapyramidal rigidity (Jakob-Creutzfeldt disease).

The second type of chronic dementia, *multi-infarct disease* (formerly atherosclerotic dementia) is responsible for about 20 to 30 per cent of cases. It may be marked by episodes of deterioration with partial recovery, by major or minor strokes, by the occasional presence of physical signs of vascular lesions and by the occurrence of emotional lability (that is, sudden and unjustified variation from one mood

extreme, such as elation, to another, such as depression).
Multi-infarct dementia also has a somewhat better prognosis
than Alzheimer's disease but the distinction between them
often cannot be made with any reasonable degree of certainty. In particular, multi-infarct dementia is not reliably
correlated with changes in the extracerebral vessels apart
from those such as the internal carotid which supply the
brain.

We emphasized earlier in Chapter 8 that dementia no
longer implies an irreversible process. It is worth repeating
that a few dementias are remediable and that a few apparent
dementias are the result of depression which is also remediable. These cases represent some 15 per cent of those presenting in one series of both younger and older patients with
dementia.[44] In addition a higher proportion, perhaps some
25 per cent, may be suffering from conditions which it is
possible to arrest. Whatever the exact figures there is at least
an important minority for whom a diagnosis of dementia
implies a responsibility on the doctor to take further action
in regard to investigation and treatment.

Emotional stresses in old age

The loss of worth-while occupation, bereavement and social
isolation are probably, in addition to severe physical illness,
the worst stresses which most people are called upon to face
during their lives. All these calamities happen most commonly in later life when the organism is biologically failing
and is least fitted to resist and survive. It, therefore, often
happens that old people have to contend from a position of
weakness with difficulties which would be a strain to anyone.
In consequence, it is not surprising that, besides presenting
the doctor with more psychiatric work than any other age
group, the old frequently suffer too from the most intractable conditions. Nevertheless, there remain many instances
where the prognosis may be as good, or almost as good, as in
younger life and the practitioner can find that the old who
present as misfits or worse may yet show remarkable powers
of recovery. Attention to the many remediable factors which
predispose to illness in old age and sometimes treatment of

the basic illness itself (where, for instance, it is a depressive disorder) will often serve to transform the individual and his situation. Neurotic disorder also occurs in old age, not only in terms of longstanding symptoms but also as new psychological symptoms when circumstances induce them. For example, a man of 70 developed hysterical weakness when he had to retire from work and spend more time than he liked with his dominating wife. After very thorough neurological and psychiatric investigation, this particular problem was eased by marital therapy and joint interviews. Bergmann[7] has confirmed that some 11 per cent of elderly people over 65 and living in the community have neurotic disorder manifesting itself after the age of 60 years. He found that social factors contributed somewhat to neurotic illness, thus isolation and bereavement in such patients were relatively common compared with normal controls. However, a predisposed personality or major physical illness were more important in promoting neurotic responses in the elderly. This again emphasizes the need for thorough and effective treatment of physical conditions in elderly patients.

Psychiatric management

Despite the gloomy view which is often taken, many of the psychiatric disorders of old age respond well to treatment. They include neurotic reactions, depressions and some of the deliria and even dementias, and in these cases the management will be in accordance with the usual principles. The remaining conditions are mostly the so far irreversible degenerative disorders and their management merits some further attention.

Dementia implies a lessening of awareness, rigidity, failure to cope with new situations, impairment of memory and disorientation. It is, therefore, important that where such patients are concerned (and this applies equally to home and hospital) they must be cared for in a stable and unchanging environment. Indeed, removal to a hospital or nursing home, however necessary such a change may be, will sometimes prove to be beyond the patient's power of adjustment and lead to a rapid deterioration. Change of nursing attendants can be almost as upsetting. Nursing care needs to be of the highest: incontinence can often be prevented by regular use of the commode. Diarrhoea can be a distressing symptom for the elderly patient. When this is not the result of faecal impaction, lack of vitamin B due to an inadequate diet can sometimes be the cause.

Agitation and restlessness are often a major difficulty, particularly at night when they are associated with insomnia. Current evidence recognizes what general knowledge has always known, namely that old people sleep as much as younger ones but in a different pattern. They take midday naps and they fall asleep earlier or wake later. It is perhaps wrong to attempt to alter this pattern too much. If nocturnal sleep is badly disturbed, however, some simple irritants should first be considered. A cold bedroom, an uncomfortable bed which has, like the patient, deteriorated over the years, a full bladder, a loaded rectum can all cause sleeplessness. When such ordinary causes have been dealt with hypnotics may then be used. Barbiturates should no longer be employed because in addition to their other disadvantages they provoke confusion in the old; and chloral (or dichloral phenazone) should be avoided if possible because of the interaction with other medication. It is best to use nitrazepam or perhaps flurazepam supplemented if necessary with small doses of a sedative antidepressant like trimipramine if the patient is depressed, or a phenothiazine like chlorpromazine if the patient is mildly confused.

It is also important to try and provide good awareness of their surroundings for any patients with a tendency to confusion. This is particularly relevant at night so that a night light may be the best prophylactic against restlessness and hallucinations on nocturnal waking. We have even known auditory hallucinations at night to be eliminated in the case of a very deaf man when a colleague advised him to wear his hearing aid during sleep. The minimal increase in sensory input which this provided prevented his previously regular hallucinations on waking.

By day it is equally important to provide the patient with familiar, readily recognizable surroundings. This reduces the liability to confusion and consequent restlessness. Sometimes the nursing attendants—whether family or professional—fail to understand the extent of the psychological impairment in these patients. Getting lost is the natural consequence of disorientation and failure to dress oneself is more likely to be due to a dressing apraxia than naughtiness. Being uncooperative may be due to a sensory aphasia, or a motor apraxia. When the nurse realizes the extent of her patient's limitations the crises tend to arise less often.

More severe and intractable restlessness and confusion can usually be controlled by small doses of phenothiazines, carefully adjusted to cause the minimum of side effects. By day the less sedative ones such as trifluoperazine will be preferred, and by night the more sedative as just indicated. In general all psychotropic medication (and much other medication also) should be given in lower doses than to younger adults because it is excreted or metabolized less efficiently in the elderly.

After all this it must be said that there is as yet no potent treatment for multi-infarct disease or for Alzheimer's disease. In the former, anticoagulant treatment has not been well demonstrated to be effective and the claims for vasodilators await confirmation. Hydergine alkaloids have a statistically significant effect in improving some elderly depressed or confused patients but the locus of the effect is uncertain and also its degree is modest. Success in the management of multi-infarct disease and Alzheimer's disease rests on attention to detail.

How long the patient can remain out of hospital depends upon the resources of his home environment and the extent to which this is supported by local medical and social services. In recent years, there has been an increasing development of community services aimed at maintaining the old in their homes or in suitable accommodation other than long-stay institutions. This work depends primarily upon the help of the family doctor aided by hospital staff and by social workers. A full geriatric and psychogeriatric service includes effective short-stay inpatient assessment and treatment units, day hospitals, home visits by social workers and nurses, a meals-on-wheels service, chiropody, social clubs and even 'granny-minding' arrangements which help to maintain a normal psychological adjustment in familiar surroundings with established acquaintances. With these techniques many district services have succeeded in caring for the elderly without chronic institutional admission.

It is worth emphasizing that behind all such successful community care there must also be adequate hospital and local authority accommodation. Community services fall into disrepute if they are relied upon to meet the needs of those who are too ill for them. 'Short-stay' units can only function properly if they are not blocked by long-stay patients. Such blocking occurs readily if there is in fact nowhere for the small proportion of grossly confused or difficult old people to go. This happens if there is not enough of any or all of the three most relevant types of residential care: geriatric, psychogeriatric and local authority. In such circumstances—and they still exist in many parts of Great Britain—an exceptionally difficult burden is carried by the family and the family doctor.

14

Loss of Memory

A complaint of loss of memory is sometimes made by the patient and sometimes by his relatives. We discuss it next because we think that the inattentiveness and forgetfulness which trouble old people are probably the most common forms of amnesia for which the advice of the general practitioner will be sought. We devote a separate chapter to it because the topic readily counterpoints a number of different physical and psychological mechanisms.

In the case of loss of memory in old persons the forgetfulness will generally seem to be for the habits and experiences of recent years; by contrast, it is usually held that information from childhood is retained to a surprising degree. Investigations of memory for remote events indicate that these standard views are not wholly correct. In fact if memory for recent events is impaired, so too is memory for remote ones, and to the same extent. The man in the United States who in 1977 has forgotten that Gerald Ford was the last President, will also have forgotten that Franklin D. Roosevelt was President at the time of Pearl Harbour. He will, however, remember both those personal and those public events which have been repeatedly rehearsed in his memory in the years since they occurred. He will thus recall his own birthday and, perhaps, the school to which he went together with the name of the current President.

An interesting pattern of memory loss is observable after

head injury. Depending on the severity of the injury there is, in states of concussion, a loss of memory for events immediately prior to the accident. This loss decreases as the patient recovers but may never be wholly restored, particularly as regards the last few seconds before the accident. The return of memory after ECT (EST) shows a similar pattern. In these cases it would seem as if scenes and information registered just prior to the traumatic event may not have had sufficient time to become established in the memory—perhaps because the cerebral cortex continues to process such material for some time after it is first observed. The disturbance for the period just after acute trauma to the brain tends to be different in that, when the patient recovers consciousness, in addition to a worsening of his ability to retain the facts registered by his perceptual apparatus there is also likely to be an impairment of his level of awareness. The result of this is that the amnesia for periods following head injury tends to be more patchy and longer lasting than that for the time before the head injury. It is marked by the recall only of the more outstanding events which took place during the period of partial return to consciousness.

In old age when the organization of the cerebral cortex begins to be impaired by degenerative disease it would seem as if the pattern of breakdown in one respect is the same as that for retrograde amnesia produced by head injury. The better-established memories are retained, the others lost. That process, which is seen in relatively pure form with retrograde amnesia, is modified in old age, however, by the diminished alertness and failing ability to register material which the dementing subject shows. A patchy impairment of memory for current experiences will, therefore, be noted as well. In this respect the changes found in old age are comparable to those which appear in anterograde (post-traumatic) amnesia for the period following loss of consciousness, when too the registration of new material is impaired.

In all patients with loss of memory in old age it is important to remember the differential diagnosis of depression. Loss of memory is one prominent aspect of dementia, and the possibility that a depression or a remediable cause of dementia may be promoting the loss of memory must be considered and carefully investigated if necessary. We discuss this aspect of the investigation of dementia in Chapter 8.

Current scientific studies of memory particularly emphasize the distinction between the period of short-term memory lasting not more than thirty seconds after an event, and long-term memory which covers all memories relating to elapsed periods of time greater than thirty seconds. This is in sharp contrast with the traditional clinical view in which immediate memory (of about half to one minute), recent memory (applying to events of hours, days and even weeks past) and remote memory (applying to months and years gone by) were distinguished from each other. The current distinction is, however, the only one which is scientifically validated. It proves particularly useful in studies of the remarkable *Korsakow's syndrome*, sometimes called the dysmnesic state. In its pure state this is a rare clinical condition which has as its hallmark an almost total failure of recent memory. More often there are also other disturbances of memory and intellectual function as in confusional states and dementias. Patients afflicted with the pure syndrome fail to recall simple material which may have been presented to them only a few seconds previously; this predisposes them to produce detailed but imaginary stories of their doings or those of the people they meet, a practice known as confabulation. This means that the patient builds up false statements of events which are outside the span of his memory so that he will tell the doctor who has seen him daily in hospital for three weeks that they met that morning in the local working men's club or that the nurse is a shop assistant who served him at the grocer's yesterday. Such developments, while making his ideas seem extremely comic to the observer can leave other mental functions, such as speech, learning and judgement relatively unaffected. It is this which distinguishes the pure Korsakow syndrome from dementia, with which similar memory disturbances can also be associated. In the latter condition there is a global impairment of all mental functions. The Korsakow syndrome can be a sequel of any delirious state, from whatever cause. When it follows a simple delirious state the prognosis is usually good. When it follows an alcoholic delirium (delirium tremens) recovery is much less likely. However, about 20 per cent of patients with an alcoholic Korsakow's psychosis recover fully and a further 20 per cent improve substantially. Korsakow's psychosis can also occur as a result of a subdural haematoma, tumour or almost any organic condition and especially those which disturb brain function in the region of the mammillary bodies or the fornix system.

The type of loss of memory which presents most difficulty in the differential diagnosis is none of the foregoing, however. It is the amnesia which may occur for a circumscribed period in patients who may show no other sign of loss of memory or impairment of cognitive function. This is the conventional 'blackout' or fugue state. The practitioner will properly refer this for specialist investigation. Its possible causes include epilepsy, hysteria, depressive reactions, schizophrenia, toxic deliria, hypoglycaemia and simulation.

In the case of depressive reactions and confusional states there will usually be ample evidence of the presence of these illnesses which may have given rise to a tendency to wander and ignore current happenings during the period of wandering. There may also be partial recollection for the period of the disturbance. Their recognition is not difficult. In the case of epilepsy, hysteria and simulation there will usually be complete loss of memory claimed for the period in question. Where this happens because of epilepsy it will be due to an automatism and associated almost invariably with a focal lesion, most often in the temporal lobes. There will be very few cases of epilepsy indeed in which sufficiently thorough investigation fails to establish the presence of an ictal disturbance. If the clinical evidence alone is insufficient, the EEG may well give valuable information. If epilepsy is suspected, however, it is essential to realize that one normal EEG does not rule out the condition and that special EEG techniques may be required to determine the presence or absence of a focal lesion. (These include activation procedures like hyperventilation, photic stimulation and sleep recordings.)

In the case of hysteria or simulation it is necessary to establish a suitable motive, of which the subject may or may not be aware. For hysteria, evidence of an appropriate premorbid personality is also desirable and, for simulation, some overt confirmation of the deception will probably be required. Simulation is, however, a rare phenomenon and in the case of hysteria a tentative exploration of the case by either hypnosis or narcoanalysis* may result in the recovery by the patient of the lost memories.

The above characteristics will also apply to the types of hysterical amnesia which persist up to the time of interview. In these the pattern of events is that the patient is generally found lost without any recollection of his previous life. He may be identified by a card or notebook in his pocket and it generally transpires that he has been missing from his home for a few hours or days, in which time he has been wandering about. As with the epileptic or the other sort of hysteric who has had a circumscribed fugue, the hysteric with a persisting amnesia will be able to deal perfectly well with current data and with any facts presented to him after the time of losing his memory for his previous life. Thus he will offer his name because it was on the card in his pocket or on the envelope of the letter which he was carrying. But he will not remember his wife's name or whether he had children or what was his occupation and so forth. However, if others produce these facts he will accept them and remember them although unable to produce them originally himself as long as the condition lasts. The point to note is that whilst the patient's amnesia serves to cut him off more or less from his past life (in which he is always in some sort of trouble) he usually remains willing to live in the present and therefore does not forego any of the skills, such as the proper handling of current information, appropriate to his current situation. Very occasionally, in grossly unstable personalities, the amnesia may extend to all aspects of the immediate environment. One patient, for example, not only lost her memory but asked in a childlike fashion what the television set was. Other patients may appear to forget simple laws of arithmetic. It seems likely, however, that an element of simulation occurs in such cases, which are then known as the Ganser syndrome.

Very brief attacks of loss of consciousness have to be

---

* This is a technique in which the patient is interviewed in a drowsy state following an intravenous barbiturate injection.

distinguished occasionally from some of the foregoing. They include syncope, various forms of epilepsy and hyperventilation attacks. The history of syncope is characteristic with an initial feeling of faintness and usually evidence of pallor and perhaps sweating. Often faints are promoted by the hypotensive effects of medication. In these cases there is usually a history of fainting on getting up from a sitting or lying position, and a drop in blood pressure can be found on comparing it in the recumbent and standing positions. In patients with epilepsy the introduction of medication often serves to alter the fit but not abolish it completely. This results in modified forms of grand mal and psychomotor epilepsy which, without the previous good evidence of epilepsy, can be confused with hysterical blackouts. Hyperventilation attacks are often also considered to be hysterical and sometimes may be, but more often they are due to anxiety. Sometimes one may demonstrate convincingly to the patient that overbreathing produces his attack and breathing into a paper bag stops it. Stokes-Adams attacks and other circulatory disturbances should also be considered in reviewing the causes of brief blackouts. Cerebrovascular disorder may give rise to one other form of moderately prolonged amnesia, *transient global amnesia*. In these attacks the patient, without other signs, suffers a generalized loss of memory particularly in regard to his surroundings. Angiography may be expected to demonstrate an appropriate lesion related to cerebral atheroma and impairment of the cerebral circulation.

It remains to mention one extreme form of the complaint of impaired memory. Many patients with depression complain bitterly of impaired memory, together with difficulty in concentration. It has long been recognized that, although such symptoms can be caused by an early dementia, they are nearly always caused, in younger patients, by the presence of depression. A failure to maintain drive and difficulty in attending to current events are bound to lead to some temporary forgetfulness. Formal memory tests of such patients almost always show normal results. When the depression recovers, memory is felt to have become normal again also by the patient. We have the impression that the problem is a little more evident clinically nowadays because the use of antidepressant drugs frequently produces a substantial improvement in depression without immediately restoring all their normal drive to patients. Occasionally, indeed, the antidepressant drug is blamed for mild apathy and forgetfulness. The correct response in such cases may not in fact be to reduce the medication as the patient suggests but rather to increase the dose. However antidepressants can also sometimes cause mild memory impairment, so, particularly if the depression appears to be under good control, the alternative policy of reducing the dose may be indicated first. All such decisions as the last depend on careful inquiry and a detailed consideration of the clinical situation.

15
Subnormality

When someone, because of lack of comprehension, fails to master the techniques necessary to maintain his place with others in society we generally tend to think of him as being unintelligent. This estimate is always a comparative one. We look about and see what others can do and then decide whether the person in question is more or less able than others. However, if the individual has not had the same training as those who perform better than he, we may consider him to be potentially more intelligent than he appears. A successful trade union leader or business man who left school early will not be thought to be less intelligent than a college student because the latter has passed some examinations whilst the former has not. Likewise, the congenitally blind or deaf may be found to have the potentiality of learning to read provided that suitable methods are used to teach them and they will not necessarily be considered to lack the power of understanding. However, once allowance has been made for these particular cases and even for more special ones such as specific inability to read (dyslexia), which may exist in someone whose attainments are otherwise at least as good as average, we do tend to regard as unintelligent those who fail to acquire the skills and abilities of the population at large. This, in its most general way, is what is meant by subnormality of intelligence (formerly called mental deficiency and known in North America as mental retardation) and the reader should note that it is essentially a social and statistical concept. The reader should also note that by accepting this approach we, and he, are saved from committing ourselves to a belief in 'intelligence' as some mysterious absolute quality measurable only by strange procedures called intelligence tests. In accordance with informed opinion in modern psychology, we see intelligence as a measure of skills gained by the subject or patient. These skills may or may not be capable of increase, but they are not solely manual ones. The term *skill* as used here covers the ability to manipulate words and figures, to find one's way about in the world and even to judge the nature of social and emotional relationships.

In fact, subnormality of intelligence is itself a social concept which is used for medical and legal purposes. The expression is found in the Mental Health Act (England and Wales) of 1959, replacing the older classification of the Mental Deficiency Acts. In the 1959 Act subnormality is defined as

> a state of arrested or incomplete development of mind (not amounting to severe subnormality) which includes subnormality of intelligence and is of a nature or degree which requires or is susceptible to medical treatment or other special care or training of the patient.

Severe subnormality is likewise defined as a state of arrested or incomplete development of mind. It is, however, 'of such a nature or degree that the patient is incapable of living an independent life or of guarding himself against serious exploitation, or will be so incapable when of an age to do so'.

In North America it is usual to use a slightly different scheme of classification into mild (Wechsler IQ range 69-55), moderate (54-40), severe (39-25, the latter figure being extrapolated) and profound (less than 25). Corresponding degrees of deficit are described; the mildly affected are able to reach 6th school grade with special education by the late teens and may be socially and vocationally adequate but they need guidance under severe stress; the moderately affected can reach the 4th grade, need special education and can do unskilled and semi-skilled work but need more supervision and guidance when under mild stress; the severely affected can contribute partially to self-support but need full supervision.

The reader who reflects on these definitions will be able to make his own gloss as to their meaning and scope. They will imply that the defect is either congenital or else acquired in the developmental period; for practical purposes this is usually infancy but may extend to cover childhood and adolescence; they imply that adults who have obtained skills which they subsequently lose are not included in these definitions; and they imply, finally, that the criteria for classifying a person as subnormal are pragmatic ones, namely whether he can hold his own in society without more help than the average person or whether he will ultimately come to harm by virtue of his lack of intelligence unless provided with special support and care.

Causes of subnormality

The foregoing provides a framework for examining the aetiology of subnormality, which is usually attributed to two major sets of causes. The first set is the influence of heredity, the second that of miscellaneous pathological conditions. In general we expect the children of normal parents to be of normal intelligence and we are not usually surprised when the children of those whom we think unintelligent are also found to be dull. As one might expect from these common-place observations it is probably the case that there is a large hereditary influence upon intelligence, although this view is disputed, and it seems that a proportion of those who are subnormal represent one extreme of the curve of normal distribution of abilities in the population at large. In these cases the subnormality is attributable to poor endowment by a number of genes whose joint effects are responsible for the degree of intelligence which the individual may manifest. In this respect intelligence may be compared with height where the final measure is also related to endowment by a number of genes.

The parallel with height extends to the second major group of causes leading to subnormality. Any process which inhibits growth or damages the skeleton during the growth period may clearly reduce the height reached by the individual to something less than his potential limit. The same is especially true for intelligence. Occasional genetic mishaps, infections

encountered during fetal life and subsequently, toxic processes affecting the organism *in utero*, irradiation, birth
injury or other later head injury and endocrine and metabolic
disorders may all result in damage to the brain which brings
the individual below the level of normality. Amongst genetic
mishaps the acquisition of an extra chromosome in mongol-
ism or in Klinefelter's syndrome may be mentioned as
instances of the special handicap sometimes imposed by
chromosomal abnormalities. With respect to infection, rubella
during the early weeks of pregnancy is particularly noteworthy, as well, of course, as meningitis in infancy and later,
and congenital syphilis. Amongst endocrine and metabolic
conditions, cretinism and phenylketonuria (the latter due, of
course, to a recessive gene) may also be instanced. Finally,
in this list one may note that even in cases where the aetiology of the pathological process is not completely settled,
for example, hydrocephalus or cerebral diplegia, its association with subnormality in a significant proportion of cases
cannot be disputed. It is, therefore, certain that a proportion of cases of subnormality must result from the effect of
organic disease processes upon what would otherwise have
been a normal organism. About 25 per cent of all cases are
estimated to fall in the moderate, severe or profound groups
and nearly all of these patients have known somatic causes
for their condition.

A third contributory factor to the development of subnormality now requires comment. This factor is the effect
of experience at critical times upon the development of
intelligence. We are accustomed to think of intelligence as
the ability, often, to solve problems without previous experience. However, it would seem that this apparently innate
genetic endowment can be improved by suitable experience—
particularly in the early years of life and at any rate before
puberty. We do not refer here to the ability to improve
scores in intelligence tests. By suitable instruction in the
requisite techniques both adults and children may be able
to improve their scores in these tests by some 10 to 20 per
cent. We refer rather to the fact that children who gain only
a limited acquaintance with verbal, spatial, mechanical and
other skills seem to be at a disadvantage in adult life, when
the development of their abilities is considered, compared

with those whose experience has been less restricted. It is as if during childhood the food of intelligence is experience and in those who are not adequately nourished the adult organism's abilities will be stunted.

In much the same way an individual may fail to gain his full potential stature if reared on a diet which whilst not poor enough to cause rickets still is not enough to permit his growth to the maximum possible height. This consideration, whilst of general interest, is of special practical importance with borderline cases of subnormality—especially those which become apparent in childhood. It implies that quite a large number of individuals, particularly those in whom there is no organic damage and for whom the parents have until then failed to provide the best possible environment, may be considerably and permanently helped by suitable training and education. Therefore, even if subnormality is due in most cases and in greater part to organic or hereditary causes which can be altered for the better only occasionally (as in phenylketonuria), there is nevertheless a significant respect in which environmental influences and appropriate teaching or management can be used to improve the prognosis and indeed the 'level of intelligence'. It is, perhaps, instructive to realize this not only for its own sake but also because it gives an example of how unrealistic it is to suppose that the nature-nurture controversy in psychological phenomena can ever be settled by attributing psychological effects wholly to one or other of these causes. In addition, it is instructive to recognize how a seemingly fixed prognosis of unalterable subnormality may also at times be changeable for the better.

It should be mentioned that the 'head-start' programme in the United States aimed at correcting the postulated effects by improving schooling for disadvantaged children. The programme is generally regarded as having failed in its aim. That does not necessarily prove the original hypothesis wrong; perhaps the necessary social and verbal nourishment has to be provided in the earliest years of life for proper intellectual growth to take place. The quality of care, and the presentation of verbal and visual stimuli to the infant, may be critical in the first years and even in the first months after birth. But even in later years, careful training of subnormal children and adults has been shown to yield good results.

The intelligence quotient

It is convenient at this point to discuss what is meant by the intelligence quotient (IQ). Intelligence tests were first developed by Binet working with children and in this work the scores of children of different ages were compared. If a child performed as well as the average for his chronological age he was then said to have a mental age equal to his chronological age. If a child performed as well as the average either of older or of younger children his mental age was accordingly held to be greater or less than his chronological age. It was then considered that the ratio of mental age to chronological age tended to remain constant. It has since been found that is is not so and a ratio of this type, therefore, cannot be used. This ratio did, however, give a fair estimate of the relative abilities of the individuals and the test positions which they would hold in relation to their fellows; when multiplied by 100 it gave a figure which could be used for comparative purposes irrespective of age and which was known as the intelligence quotient. So long as it is seen as a comparative measure and not an absolute quality, this quotient still has its uses even though it tends now to be derived in various tests for adults from the position which the individual's score holds in relation to that of others, rather than from a mental age/chronological age ratio.

The exact figure in an intelligence quotient may never be relied on as evidence of subnormality. It is usual to regard the figure of IQ 70 as being about the borderline between dull normals and subnormals and the figure of 55 as marking the approximate borderline between subnormals and the severely subnormal. Nevertheless there are many people whose test performance is less than 70 who function adequately in the community and who, therefore, cannot be held to be sufficiently socially deviant to be classed as subnormal whilst on the other hand there are numbers of patients in institutions whose test performance is somewhat better than 70 (by various measures) but who are so incapable socially or emotionally that they require hospital or other care. The test of whether an individual is subnormal lies in his social adaptation, and his IQ can often give only a partial guide to the likelihood or otherwise of his living a successful life in the community. For individuals on the borderline of subnormality success depends very greatly upon their emotional stability.

The consequences of subnormality

In the case of severe subnormality of the most extreme sort the individual needs complete nursing care from birth to death. Lesser, and more common, degrees of severe subnormality may necessitate institutional residence or permanent supervision by others for the individual who cannot read or write, handle money or find his way about. The cases which present most problems to the practitioner are those where the subnormality is relatively mild and the individual pursues a tenuous existence in the community. Mere lack of intelligence in itself will not necessarily cause an individual to deviate from social patterns, nor, if it is sufficiently mild, will it alone prevent him from leading a successful and happy life. But in the face of personal crises, economic difficulties or cheap temptations to damaging pleasures it is the very dull or subnormal who most easily give way. Whilst neurotic symptom-formation is the perquisite of everyone the stress of dealing with unfamiliar situations is bound to be greatest for the subnormal and it is therefore the dull who most readily produce gross conversion symptoms. There is even some reason to believe that they are more prone to schizophrenic illnesses too. Likewise, the dull and subnormal constitute an undue proportion of problem families, and other deviant groups such as delinquents and prostitutes. Yet dullness or subnormality is never the sole cause of these social deviations. Qualities of personal drive, temperamental stability and modest contentment can protect the subnormal against the pitfalls we mention, but being dull generally increases the risk of these misfortunes.

Management

In the first months of life subnormal children are often like any others—greedy, wet, dirty and prone to sleep and when not asleep to cry. They are loved also like other babies. Some are recognized to be abnormal at birth— especially those with Down's syndrome—and in the case of others the parents learn with dawning anxiety that their child is not performing or progressing as it should. It has been shown that the older the age of the child the more accurately the parents recognize the degree of backwardness in development which their progeny show.

When parents first learn of their child's handicap or potential handicap they usually and not surprisingly react with ambivalent feelings. There is in many a wish that the child had not been born, as well as, still, tender love for him. Guilt at the first of these feelings, anger, and projection of the unwelcome emotion on to others are common. The same applies to the parents of other children born with physical rather than mental handicap. At one hospital it was shown that the mothers of children with congenital heart disease were almost uniformly critical of the doctors involved in the care of the children. Medical advisers and social workers have, therefore, to walk delicately when they convey information to parents about a child's mental retardation. These problems are found particularly by paediatricians and family doctors. Even when he has made a spot diagnosis of the condition, as with Down's syndrome, or cretinism, the doctor should not introduce his conclusions to the parents at once; it is far better to complete a full examination first and draw the mother's attention to the possibility of some trouble than to announce it bluntly and precipitately. Thus after the first examination, it is often wise to convey the conclusion tentatively and to arrange for a further review, after a few days, preferably with both parents.

Similarly, when dealing with a child in whom the diagnosis is less obvious and the degree of subnormality less severe, the instruction of the parents has to be a gradual process. The physician may quickly recognize that a child of three with arrested hydrocephalus, occasional epileptic fits and backwardness in walking and talking is not going to be of normal intelligence. The parents with their appealing and affectionate child need longer to accommodate themselves to the idea. Once they have recognized the situation there are many possible problems which can arise in relation to the subnormal child and the rest of the family. The parents take up positions on whether they want any more children, who or what is to blame for the state of the affected one, whether they shall seek institutional care for the child so that the mother can return to work, whether grandmother can help, and so on. Many of these problems are the normal ones of ordinary families, but exacerbated by the extra dependence of the subnormal child. It is logical to offer two or three sessions of joint counselling or therapy to many families in this situation or the option of occasional later sessions if desired.

As with normal children management of their problems can be rewarding and the majority of subnormal children find acceptance and love within the circle of their family and its friends. The few who are a very severe nursing problem may spend all their days in institutions but many of them tend still to be visited and cherished by their families. Sometimes indeed they attract a special concern which is detrimental to their siblings. On the other hand some of the most painful cases for parents are those where a previously healthy child sustains a head injury or meningitis which alters him completely. This is perhaps the hardest form of subnormality for parents to see affecting their children.

When school age is reached a variety of provisions becomes available. Training centres with special transport services and appropriate staffing are normally provided for the severely subnormal. The combination of physical and mental handicap is often dealt with in local education authority schools for the former. Other schools provide education for those who are subnormal but educable. Of recent years it has been demonstrated, particularly by Tizard and his colleagues, that even the severely subnormal can learn tasks which have been suitably adapted for them. The training and education of the subnormal is thus not a topic for pessimism.

The management of the adolescent and adult subnormal, like that of psychiatric illness in general, now also tends to be based increasingly on the idea of care in the community. In some respects this has always been more feasible for the subnormal than for the psychotic. The subnormal individual grows up to his place in the community, rather than drops lower down from one he has attained. Both groups were always, and still are, better accepted in rural environments where they are under less pressure and face less hazards than in the urban one. As society steadily becomes more complex, with a greater premium on literacy and social skills, the less intelligent are in difficulties not just because there are fewer routine jobs (that is not wholly correct) but more because they cannot cope with the increase in paper work and general knowledge which is required. Hire purchase, social security benefits, telephoning the gas board from a newly altered phone box, rather than being able to walk round to the office—all these provide difficulties for the less literate, amongst whom the subnormal are always found. To counteract this situation an increased social work service is necessary but is not always available.

It is customary now to talk of all long-stay admissions to general psychiatric and subnormality hospitals as promoting a disadvantageous 'institutionalization'. What is often not recognized is that many such hospitals are well run and provide their residents with a range of appropriate corporate and individual activities which is unlikely to be fully replaced when these hospitals are closed. The hospital craft departments (joinery, upholstery, and the like), services and occupational treatments offered many opportunities to place patients in useful and satisfying activities. Outings, film shows, sports and other recreations were provided to an extent which enabled many to live happily within their limitations. Community care has still to prove that it can do as well as the best efforts of the chronic hospital system.

16
Deviation of Personality and Behaviour

Many psychiatric states lead to social deviations on the part of the patient. In other words they lead him to act in conflict with the general rules, conventions or ideas of moral conduct which are approved by his society. In many of those states it is at once apparent or at once seems likely that the patient is ill, for example, acute schizophrenia, phobic anxiety. In this chapter, we wish to consider, however, a different group of cases—cases where the social deviation is prominent, but the decision that the patient has a psychological abnormality is only made later. As an example of such a sequence of events we would instance alcoholism where the observer may first say 'Disgusting' about a patient's behaviour and subsequently exclaim, on reviewing the train of disaster and the quirks of personality which handicap the individual: 'It's a disease!' Besides delimiting our present subject from more obvious types of illness on the one hand it has to be separated also from conditions which although eccentric or unusual are not necessarily abnormal in any pathological sense. This must lead to a consideration of standards of normality.

Psychiatrists are often accused of seeing the abnormal in the normal. This generally happens, first, because almost all behaviour may be described as tending towards the satisfaction of conflicting emotional needs rather than theoretically rational aims. Second, it happens because most variations from the recognized rules of behaviour represent a more extreme form of tendencies which can be observed in nearly everybody. For this latter reason, however, psychiatrists can generally counter the accusation just mentioned with the equal truism that they also tend to see the normal in the abnormal. Accepting these arguments we can rarely see hard and fast dividing lines between normality and abnormality. If the deviation is sufficiently gross to disturb the individual or his neighbours treatment will be sought. If not, no action will usually need to be taken, the criteria for treatment thus being socially determined. Indeed, if one of the meanings of mental health is understood to be adjustment to society, then plainly our criteria of mental health are profoundly influenced by the ideals and standards of the society in which we live. Further, no action will be taken for those deviations which are recognized but at least not regarded as unhealthy. At least in this society, nuclear disarmers, suffragettes and other political activists have been able to break the law, sometimes with moral credit, without being offered allegedly therapeutic brain-washing.

Other deviants are less fortunate: alcoholics and homosexuals are among those who have to risk the censure and perhaps sanctions of society when their abnormal behaviour is discovered. It may perhaps be worth pointing out that our own judgements concerning praise- and blame-worthiness are determined to a greater extent by our contemporary culture than many of us care to admit.

The recent changes of law concerning homosexuality and abortion illustrate the conflict between alternative systems of contemporary mores, with the eventual victory of what previously had been a minority viewpoint. It will be generally agreed that it is no part of the physician's role to distribute praise or blame towards the behaviour of his patients. When help is sought by a patient (or by a Court with the patient's consent) in the unlearning of an undesirable pattern of behaviour, medical or psychological treatment may be available for some conditions, and in certain cases the patient can be assisted in achieving an adjustment which best satisfies his emotional needs and brings him into least conflict with society. On other occasions, the doctor may be asked his opinion as to whether illness has impaired an offender's responsibility, as defined in law. This definition may well appear to evade many of the subtleties of the relationship between moral responsibility and illness,* but this is the question which is addressed to the doctor. Indeed the doctor's activities in this field are contained by the requirements of the society in which he practises. The same principles which help to account for the behaviour of delinquents are equally applicable to other irrational forms of behaviour which stand uncondemned by society, such as the emotional need for some people that offenders should be punished, but these subjects are commonly unavailable either to research or to therapy. It will be understood, therefore, that the deviations of behaviour referred to the doctor often appear to be selected arbitrarily by custom and tradition rather than on the basis of scientifically established fact. Nevertheless, certain major conditions, situations or characteristics can be recognized as predisposing the individual to social deviations. In particular we would instance psychoses, subnormality of intelligence, old age, psychopathy and extreme degrees of neurosis, as especially tending to cause social deviation.

In some of these conditions, for example, schizophrenia, the behaviour may be so bizarre, violent and irrational that there is no disagreement that the offender is mentally sick. A minor degree of depression, the insidious simple variant of schizophrenia, the compulsive and repetitive life patterns of some neuroses may all give rise to a behaviour which has not been determined either by a rational conscious choice or by normal emotional needs. The aberrant behaviour may result merely in a failure to live as vigorous and effective a life as could be normal for the individual, and the consequent failure to deal with social obligations may not readily

---

* For a discussion of this see Merskey and Clarke.[51]

be recognized as due to a disease process. More tragically, the morbid behaviour may lead to trouble with the authorities

Aberrations due to psychosis or organic disease

Many types of perversion or sexual abnormality may arise during the course of severe psychoses and the homosexual attitudes which may be seen in paranoid states are of particular theoretical interest. All these psychotic conditions, however, are usually so pronounced that there is no difficulty in recognizing the pathological setting of the abnormal sexual behaviour. Sometimes also abnormal sexual behaviour appears in persons who are not obviously psychotic and who have until then led blameless lives. Such behaviour may, then, be the first sign of a dementing process due to organic disease, for example, senile degenerative or atherosclerotic brain disease or even cerebral tumour, notably in the frontal regions. The significant feature here is the contrast with the patient's normal personality and the behaviour to be expected of him on the one hand and his actions and attitudes on the other.

There is lastly a group of cases in which an aberration of behaviour occurs in individuals who have hitherto been lawabiding and respectable, and yet there is no evidence of brain damage. The offences usually comprise exhibitionism and sexual interference with young children; to this group can be added non-sexual delinquency such as shoplifting. These offenders are almost all over fifty years, and there is some indication that they are suffering from mild depressions. It is difficult to make this diagnosis when they are first seen after the offence, because they are naturally agitated at being the cause for scandal. They do, however, improve with antidepressant treatment, and if they are reviewed some months later they will report that they had been suffering from tiredness, lowness of spirits, lack of concentration and sleeplessness for some time before the offence was committed. They often ascribe these symptoms to 'overwork' and, therefore, neglect to seek help. It should not be forgotten that a mood of mild depression will prompt a wide variety of delinquent behaviour from shoplifting to promiscuity in certain individuals who are normally of a character beyond reproach.

PERSONALITY DISORDER

A recent survey of problem families[75] showed that the most important psychological disorder associated with deviant behaviour was a disorder of personality rather than psychosis or neurosis. Most definitions of personality disorder are unsatisfactory. A *Glossary of Mental Disorders*[26] lists ten types, as does Schneider.[69] The new American Psychiatric Association scheme (DSM-III Draft Guidelines) recognizes still others. In effect, most authorities define the disorder by describing abnormal personality traits. The difficulty with this type of definition is that it also seems to apply to one's friends and colleagues who may have well-defined obsessional or hysterical personalities. The natural reluctance to classify them as abnormal is founded on an important insight: what right have we to diagnose as abnormal an individual who lives effectively? This problem is raised acutely in Henderson's[29] concept of the creative psychopath. Men and women of genius may be difficult to live with, eccentric and statistically rare, but it is surely wrong to label them as diseased.

Idiosyncrasies may help us to recognize a person, but they do not define him. A person is defined by his work in the widest sense of the word: what he has achieved, created, understood. At the very least, it is no small achievement to have led an independent existence and brought up a family and many people make more important contributions to life than this. Yet it would be wrong to use achievement as the only measuring stick for personality. Fate may arbitrarily break the work of any man or woman; their aspirations and values ('constructs' to use Kelly's term[35]) tell us more about them.

It is extraordinary how patients will reveal themselves. One man will wish to be judged only by the success which others can see, a woman by her power of attracting men ('I am getting old'). Whether or not we admire their lives, the pattern of aspiration and achievement, what is sought and what is rejected, can be recognized and understood. This is important clinically because the stress which will cause illness is often one which threatens the pattern. The ability to create such a pattern we believe is the hallmark of normal personality function. We would diagnose the presence of personality disorder when this pattern is missing or when the values which inform the life pattern are frankly pathological (as in paranoid personalities) or when the pattern is confused and self-defeating as in some neurotic personality disorder. Abnormal personality traits and isolated episodes of abnormal behaviour do not in themselves justify the diagnosis of personality disorder; the life of the patient must be evaluated as a whole. This implies that the diagnosis cannot be made until the individual is fully mature. It must also be remembered that criminal behaviour is quite likely to be the result of social and cultural pressures. It is only in the recidivists or unsuccessful criminals that a high rate of personality disorder is found.

The *antisocial* and the *inadequate* are two types of personality disorder in which the subjects fail to make anything of their lives. The antisocial personality has also been called the *psychopathic* or *sociopathic*. The characteristic behaviour of individuals with antisocial personality disorder is an apparent inability to care deeply for other people, antisocial characteristics, a refusal to postpone present pleasures for future benefits and an obvious incapacity to learn from past mistakes. Apart from this last characteristic, most of us at some time in our life are liable to act in a mildly antisocial manner, especially with the help of alcohol. It is only when this type of behaviour has been an outstanding characteristic from early years that the diagnosis of psychopathic disorder can be made. Even in such cases, reliable behaviour may be expected for unpredictable but fairly long periods, especially if the patient is in a sheltered environment.

This aggressive type of personality disorder has little tolerance of frustration and is liable to outbursts of rage and temper. A typical history of such a patient is that he is of illegitimate birth or orphaned early or at least comes from a broken home. They are inattentive scholars, frequently playing truant from school and are little influenced by punishment. They often go to approved school, Borstal or prison because of offences such as larceny, housebreaking and stealing and driving away motor cars. They are resentful of discipline and it is particularly characteristic that they do not seem to learn from experiences which would deter the average member of the community from repeating such escapades. They are adventurous and prone to take risks but rarely succeed in the army except in war-time when they may win distinction in action. In civilian life they take numerous jobs and scarcely ever settle to any one trade. They may be variously affable or moody. Sometimes they make easy and friendly contact with all manner of people but then fail to sustain the promise which their attractive behaviour has evoked. Others pick quarrels easily and readily believe themselves badly done by. Sexually, they tend to be promiscuous and their marriages are often short-lived. They come to the doctor's notice most frequently because of suicidal attempts made in periods of intense but short-lived depression. After such attempts they are often surprisingly cheerful and remarkably calm. Women rarely follow this pattern so far as the aggressive features are concerned but may show similar behaviour in the other respects—particularly truanting, petty theft, promiscuity and suicidal behaviour.

So far as their physical characteristics are concerned, antisocial personalities do not differ from the general population except in one respect. Their electroencephalograms show in excess a phenomenon which occurs to a minor extent in normal adults and a major extent in children. This is the occurrence of slow activity, particularly in the temporal regions. Such slow activity occurs normally in children and also in about 5 to 10 per cent of the population at large. It occurs in about 30 per cent of inadequate personalities and in about 60 per cent of aggressive antisocial personalities. Since the behaviour of psychopaths is in many ways like that of children, since they tend to improve as they get older and since there is a certain amount of evidence that their failure to grow up into a normal adult pattern of life is related to childhood misfortunes, it is peculiarly fitting that the single organic abnormality found in them should be an immature pattern of their cerebral electrical potentials.

The childhood misfortune just mentioned is the basis for one theory of the origin of antisocial personality. This theory, advanced in its most cogent form by Bowlby[9], holds that the development of antisocial traits is caused or facilitated by deprivation of loving maternal care at critical periods in the growth of the child and especially before the age of five. The consequence of such deprivation in the first instance is that the child protests with tears and neurotic symptoms, but at a later stage in effect gives up hope of forming lasting human relationships and so develops the forms of aggressive or affable yet ruthless and uncommitted behaviour which are prominent in antisocial personalities. Whilst this theory is certainly not valid for every antisocial personality it does appear a reasonable view to take in a significant number of cases. It fits well with the occurrence of mixed forms, especially those having plentiful neurotic symptoms and is also compatible with the tendency to mature in later life and to have EEGs whose development can be regarded as retarded.

In one other place this alteration with age is further taken into account. The Mental Health Act of 1959 (England and Wales) provides for the detention of antisocial personalities in hospital until the age of twenty-five, without their having broken the law, subject to the usual safeguards of appeals to Mental Health Review Tribunals. In doing this the Act also takes the brave, but for its purposes essential, course of attempting to define psychopathic (antisocial) disorder. This it describes as

> a persistent disorder or disability of mind (whether or not including subnormality of intelligence) which results in abnormally aggressive or seriously irresponsible conduct on the part of the patient, and requires or is susceptible to medical treatment.

The Act qualifies this description and that of all the other mental disorders with which it deals by providing that no one may be dealt with for mental disorders under the Act 'by reason only of promiscuity or other immoral conduct.' The informed consensus appears to be that this section of the Act is reasonable in spirit and useful in practice. Although the wording is inevitably somewhat imprecise, we feel that in routine clinical work the implications of what is meant by psychopathy have become sufficiently standard for its use in the Act to be a success—as so far appears to be the case. We think this also means that the concept of psychopathy is a useful one in the wider framework which we have attempted to establish.

As will be expected from the foregoing description, the management and treatment of such patients is usually unrewarding. If the characteristic antisocial behaviour extends after the age of thirty, little improvement is to be expected. With younger patients, and especially adolescents, a more hopeful prognosis can be entertained. Treatment consists more in guidance and support than in analytical psychotherapy. Much reliance has been placed on training institutions such as approved schools, but recent reports of follow-up studies have been discouraging. Admission to a psychiatric hospital or unit, while giving much needed relief to the family of the antisocial personality, very rarely results in a material improvement of behaviour. The failure of social learning which lies at the heart of the antisocial personality's disability still defies satisfactory treatment.

Some other personality disorders are often referred to as being *inadequate*. It is perhaps worth while to consider the meaning of this term in more detail.

Inadequate can be used in two ways. Absolutely, it describes the situation in which the personality cannot face up to some commitment. Clearly, there are situations in face of which almost anyone is inadequate. Relatively, inadequate implies a standard: the majority of people could be expected to cope with the problem. Neurotic patients are often described as inadequate but in many cases this is plainly an oversimplification. A neurotic personality does not preclude a person from possessing exceptional gifts. From biographies one may be justified in believing that both Charles Darwin and Florence Nightingale suffered from disabling neuroses, but neither could be described as inadequate. Indeed the hallmark of the neurotic personality is that apart from those aspects of life involved in the neurotic conflict they function at a normal level. If inadequate is to have a specific meaning, distinct from neurotic, it must imply that the person has less than average ability to cope with all aspects of life, yet is distinguished from the subnormal patient in possessing intellectual ability within normal limits.

It is this definition of inadequacy which applies to the personalities of some unemployed. A large proportion of them not only fail to secure satisfactory employment but also fail to maintain a family life. Many have no regular sexual outlets at all. They lack recreations and hobbies. On interview they make a characteristic impression.

> The ineffectiveness these patients displayed in all aspects of life was also apparent on interview. They waited upon the words of their interlocutor, and rarely ventured to put forward what they wanted in life or what they would like to do. Although some might fairly be described as retarded in speech, they varied in their verbal facility; but when the interview touched on topics which, it might be supposed, would awaken their self-interest, their talk became vague. Their complaints and dissatisfactions, their present difficulties or previous happiness, their hopes and fears for the future, whatever was in question, would arouse no definite affect of point of view which could be seized upon and discussed. A striking feature was their tolerance of the worst conditions and their seeming inability not only to obtain satisfactions but even to desire them.[74]

Anxiety and hysterical symptoms are very common, and there is usually a history of neurotic symptoms in childhood as well as bed-wetting and temper tantrums.

It may be assumed that this is a constitutional anomaly of personality but there is some evidence that loss of their father during childhood occurs more frequently than might be expected. It might be speculated that lack of a suitable model hinders the masculine identification of the developing boy who later finds difficulty in fulfilling the male role in our society. It is difficult to persuade such men to make a better adjustment to work but some improvement has been reported with inpatient treatment at least with patients under forty.

In women who are inadequate personalities, the syndrome is very like that in men, but they have less opportunity to show their unreliability at work and there is more evidence to their shiftlessness as homemakers, promiscuity and tendency to hysterial symptoms. They have great difficulty in handling money. Serious debt indicates personality disorder in women just as a poor employment record does in men.

In *paranoid* personalities there is no lack of direction in their lives. They are often consumed with bitterness about the unfair treatment they have received. One of the tragic outcomes for men with this personality is that they often provoke the persecution of which they complain. Antagonistic, hostile and ungrateful, they complain about any help they are given. This attitude quickly alienates all who try to assist them. They are prone to develop psychotic episodes, but they differ from those with true paranoid states in that their delusional complaints tend to settle if they are moved to a different environment—until their behaviour creates fresh difficulties.

Schizoid (known in DSM-III as *introverted*) personalities may be recognized by their strategy of retreat. They avoid intimate affective contact with other people. The emotional warmth of a close relationship which is a source of strength to ordinary people is perceived as a threat by those with a schizoid personality. Many normal people possess schizoid traits in their personalities and are able to make a few close relationships, perhaps many, but are very much at a loss outside the secure circle of their home. When the disturbance is sufficiently marked to merit the diagnosis of personality disorder the affected individual is in full retreat from the world. Often unable to work, they are sometimes unable to leave the house. The greatest wish of one patient with this disorder was to become a hermit.

Sometimes schizoid personalities are subject to phobic symptoms in addition. It is important not to confuse symptoms like agoraphobia or schoolphobia with the schizoid personality. It is important also not to use the label *schizoid personality* when the patient actually has a schizophrenic illness. This is sometimes done out of uncertainty but the practice ought to be avoided. The American Psychiatric Association Draft Diagnostic and Statistical Manual-III suggests recognizing introverted and schizotypal personalities. The characteristics of the two types are listed briefly in Appendix 2. The schizoid personality as just described is the introverted personality in the American classification and schizotypal describes a severe personality disturbance with characteristic eccentricities and peculiarities in addition to introversion. The distinction appears to be a helpful one.

The *neurotic* disorders of personality have already been discussed in Chapter 5. A summary is also given in Appendix 2. Obsessional and hysterical traits are present in most people. In extreme cases the needs of a neurotic life style so distort the pattern of the patient's life that it becomes sterile and self-defeating.

Cyclothymic personalities have already been described in Chapter 7. The swings of mood may become so marked and continuous that effective living is impossible.

It will be seen that disorders of personality present a different dimension of disturbance to those of neurosis or psychosis, although it is obvious that they provide a ready soil in which psychiatric illness can develop. They are also often associated with complex disorders of behaviour.

DEVIANT BEHAVIOUR

Sexual perversion

A sexual perversion may be defined as sexual activity which aims at achieving satisfaction without coitus, when the latter is reasonably or properly available. The fundamental characteristic of a perversion is thus that the normal reproductive aim of the sexual activity is lost whilst some alternative such as a homosexual relationship is positively preferred. It follows that it may not be perverse for a man to accept homosexual contacts or to masturbate when he has no access to suitable women, or for a girl to accept petting to orgasm by her fiancé when she feels it would be improper to do more. However, where the practice followed ignores acceptable opportunities for a normal heterosexual relationship and, even in addition, may break the law or firm social rules, it is correctly regarded as a perversion. Members of the American Psychiatric Association approved, by a majority vote, a committee recommendation that they should not consider homosexuality as an illness. The draft DSM-III guidelines exclude affectionate homosexual relationships between consenting adults from the category of personality disorder but include 'egodystonic homosexuality', by which is meant a complaint of persistent insufficient heterosexual interest or a pattern of sustained homosexual arousal which is unwanted and a source of distress to the individual. This uneasy compromise will allow at least some patients to claim medical insurance for treatment. The DSM-III also recognizes other types of homosexuality as a disorder, for example, paedophilia. The American decision to exclude established homosexual preference from the category of disorder has not been followed in Britain where the biological implications of a condition which inhibits procreation probably still carry more weight and where the law and public opinion, although not penalizing relationships between consenting adults, are unwilling to see homosexuality as a normal variant.

The most common sexual deviation is homosexuality and the next most common is exhibitionism; we discuss both of them briefly below. Other deviations such as transvestism, fetishism and scoptophilia are much rarer and many of the considerations which apply to exhibitionism also apply to them. In addition it should be noted that there are many other sexual disorders which are not perversions since their direction is not abnormal and which are not dealt with in this chapter. Examples of such conditions are impotence, ejaculatio praecox and some cases of frigidity which represent a failure to achieve normal sexual activity rather than an alteration in the goal; these are described in Chapter 12.

Homosexuality

An overt preference for physical relationships with members of the same sex constitutes a homosexual deviation. Figures have been given to suggest that one in twenty-five of the total male population are affected in this way. In unmarried men alone the incidence is several times greater and Kinsey estimates it at between 12 to 13 per cent. In unmarried women the incidence is estimated at 4 per cent. In addition 37 per cent of normal heterosexual men are thought to have had homosexual contacts with orgasm at some time in their lives, particularly during adolescence. Even ignoring these transitory relationships an enormous number of people are affected by the established deviation and this is especially true of males. It is commoner than diabetes mellitus and at least four times as common as the schizophrenic illnesses which fill our hospitals.

Although it has taken some time for the probable incidence to be recognized, our knowledge of the figures is still much better than our knowledge of causes. There is some evidence from identical twin studies that constitutional factors are important. Until recently there was no evidence that there were any hormonal differences between homosexuals and others. Now it begins to appear that there may be some differences in the secretion of sex hormones in homosexual compared with heterosexual males. However, it is still too soon to say how important this evidence may be. Some homosexuals do adopt manners, habits and even the clothes of the opposite sex; some of these comprise a special rare subgroup convinced that they really belong to the opposite gender from the one represented by their anatomic sex and external genitals and they may attempt to persuade doctors to carry out plastic operations which would promote their identification with the sex which they wish to become. Yet one of the most consistent findings in cases like Klinefelter's syndrome or Turner's syndrome, where there may be anatomical and hormonal grounds for uncertainty as to the patient's sex, is that in general sufferers from these intersex conditions identify themselves easily with the sex which they believe to be their own whether or not they are correct in their belief on physical grounds. Their psychological history determines their sexual outlook. Females with these conditions think and act as males if they have been treated as males and as females if they have been brought up as females. Likewise, those who are anatomically males behave as males if brought up as boys and as females if brought up as girls. In fact overt homosexuality has no reliable association with any anatomical or endocrine disorder so far described.

Amongst psychological factors that have been claimed to be important in the production of homosexuality is the presence of a strong emotional attachment to the mother. The life of Marcel Proust, a homosexual, exemplifies this, and his dependent attitude to his mother appears clearly in his most famous work, *Remembrance of Things Past*. It also often appears in clinical history-taking that homosexuals have had such a relationship with their mothers and it is certainly possible in theory that such attitudes might prevent a male child from developing a normal heterosexual outlook. A dominant mother who shows perhaps rather special taboos regarding sexual topics is not found only in the life histories of homosexuals; this pattern occurs frequently with adult patients of both sexes who have a history of sexual difficulties of any type. What is perhaps more specific in the history of homosexual men is the fact that their fathers either were missing or were weak individuals or else brutal and antagonistic. In all these instances, there is lack of an acceptable father with whom the growing boy can identify and learn how to be fully masculine. On this basis indeed there have been credible sporadic claims of cures being obtained in overt homosexuals by analytical psychotherapy.

In any discussion on aetiology it must be remembered that homosexual behaviour is widely distributed: it is common enough in all mammals, it has been and is permitted in many human societies, and in a few communities it is even valued more highly than heterosexuality. In our own civilization it is easy to identify a normal phase of partial homosexuality in early adolescence, from which the majority mature into a heterosexual attitude. It would appear, therefore, that homosexuality is one of a number of biologically available sexual outlets. Cultural factors appear to be predominant in determining the extent to which homosexuality is available as a sexual outlet. The fundamental disability, therefore, in a homosexual would seem to be his inability to sustain a heterosexual relationship.

To summarize, therefore, we may say that although homosexual behaviour is normally one of the available sexual outlets, in our culture this is not usually so after adolescence apart from exceptional circumstances. A combination of a certain genetically determined constitution with a special constellation of psychological influences inside the family may be sufficient to prevent heterosexual adjustment and favour an aberrant sexual outlet.

As regards treatment and prognosis, much depends on whether the patient is still in the toils of a delayed adolescence (perhaps with tentative heterosexual experience) or is an established invert. While something may be hoped from psychotherapy in the first case, as regards the established invert there is only a small chance of achieving a sexual reorientation. Indeed, such is the moral abhorrence that some homosexuals experience towards heterosexual intercourse, it is at least doubtful if they seriously wish to change in that direction. Total suppression of sexual drive may be of great value to the panic-stricken homosexual in danger of offending the law, but this at least can only be a temporary measure; it involves the administration of oestrogens (even in certain countries voluntary castration) and care has to be taken not only because of unpleasant feminizing effects but also because it may be welcomed by the patient since it may gratify his phantasies of female identification more than it reduces his libido. Psychiatric help may, however, be of considerable value in supporting the patient through emotional crises, particularly the frustrations in love, to which the unfortunate homosexual is liable. Further, there is a considerable number of people who at some stage have homosexual difficulties which lead on to neurotic difficulties. For example, an anxiety state may be provoked by the exposure of someone with unconscious homosexual drives to the risk of being involved in a practising relationship, or else someone growing through a homosexual phase in adolescence may be alarmed by his feelings. In these cases appropriate psychological and medical support may be of considerable value at the critical time. In particular it will be possible to advise some individuals at least that their troubles may be only temporary or that the extent of their homosexual inclinations need not prevent a satisfactory heterosexual adjustment.

Apart from this, psychotherapy is indicated in individuals who are aware of both homosexual and heterosexual interests and who wish to confirm themselves in a heterosexual pattern. This is a situation in which patients can be helped both by analytic therapy and by positive supportive attitudes. Behaviour therapy too has a role to play in some cases and should be considered favourably as an alternative approach. We are not in general keen on aversive techniques of treatment which can easily satisfy latent masochistic attitudes in patients—and sadistic ones in therapists—but mild aversive measures have achieved some successes and cannot be wholly rejected. Covert desensitization which relies on associating repugnant thoughts and feelings with the behaviour which it is desired to avoid represents a still more benign aversive method. These are not the only methods of behaviour therapy available and positive reinforcing schedules encouraging the practice of heterosexual interests and ideas can be worth trying (see Meyer and Chesser[54]). They require the help of someone versed in the technique.

Exhibitionism

Whereas it is more or less acceptable for women to display in public some parts of their bodies which modesty normally requires to be covered the same is not true for men. Perhaps this is because women do not appear to derive the same satisfaction from displays of the male torso which men get from displays of the female body. Similarly the perversion of exhibitionism is peculiarly male and only men are charged with it. Although not so common as homosexuality its frequency is still very high. As many as 2279 men were convicted in only one year. Since only a proportion of offenders can be caught there must be many more who commit the act or are disposed to do so.

In exhibitionism the individual suddenly displays his genitals to one or more females and sometimes masturbates at the same time. What marks it as a perversion is that with it there is no attempt to achieve intercourse. It is further typical of most offenders that they would be disconcerted if the female approached them and they derive great satisfaction from the horror, shock or frightened response which their action evokes. They are rarely interested in showing their genitals in private to a cooperative woman, but they may persist in committing the same offence in public situations so that ultimately it is inevitable that many of them are caught. Intelligence has almost no bearing on this aspect of their behaviour and although it may perhaps arise more readily in the mentally subnormal there are very many instances where the offence has been committed in this seemingly foolish way by well-educated and otherwise responsible persons. One of our own cases, for instance, repeatedly exposed himself in the neighbourhood of his home and even from his own front window.

Exhibitionists tend to fall into two groups: adolescent and adult. In the adolescent there is very often a clear history of stress, perhaps sexual (such as the marriage of an elder sister) but more often occupational. These boys are often in jobs for which they are unsuited either on account of temperament or capability. The prognosis for this group tends to be good provided that their problems are given attention and that they receive the necessary support and guidance at this difficult time. The problem with adults is more difficult. Frequently, the offence is committed repeatedly and punishment appears to have little effect. On examination they appear depressed and deeply troubled apart from this sexual disorder. Nevertheless, even in these cases success may attend the efforts of a skilled psychotherapist, but the prognosis is naturally much less certain than in the younger age group.

In the light of the foregoing observations it can only be concluded that all or most exhibitionists are emotionally disturbed and in need of whatever treatment can be provided. Nevertheless, only some are referred from the Courts for psychiatric advice and others are punished out of hand. Yet Courts do have, under the Criminal Justice Act in Britain as well as in some North American jurisdictions, the power to put offenders of this sort on probation on condition that they accept medical treatment for periods of up to one year, provided that a suitable specialist shall have offered to be responsible for such treatment and thinks the patient may benefit from it. Since recidivism is common in this condition despite the use of legal punishments, it is to be hoped that medical investigation and, where possible, treatment will increasingly come to be preferred to retributive measures even though there is still a shortage of people capable of treating such offenders and even though the results of psychiatric treatment are uncertain and its value is unproven. Where psychiatric treatment is available the general practitioner should not fail to obtain it for his patient. In addition the practitioner will need aid in helping the patient's family to adjust to the scandal caused and it will be necessary to confirm that there is no underlying brain disease or psychosis of which the perversion is the first sign (cf. below).

The practitioner's biggest difficulties probably arise in endeavouring to interpret the situation to the patient and his family once treatment has been suggested. There is some evidence that a dominant father, or a severe reaction to the father, plays an important part in the genesis of exhibitionism. If there are associated family difficulties, with either the patient's parents or his wife, the practitioner will have to cope with the various reactions of these individuals, whether distressed, plaintive or hostile. As in the other situations of neurosis which we have discussed the important rule is to be sympathetic but to avoid involvement or the introduction of one's own emotional reactions into the situation.

ALCOHOLISM

Excessive drinking has been defined as follows by an expert sub-committee of the World Health Organization:*

> any form of drinking which in its extent goes beyond the traditional and customary 'dietary' use, or in the ordinary compliance with the social drinking customs of the whole community concerned, irrespective of the aetiological factors leading to such behaviour....

The more extreme forms of this excessive drinking are regarded as alcoholism by the subcommittee and alcoholics are defined as:

> those excessive drinkers whose dependence upon alcohol has attained such a degree that it shows a noticeable mental disturbance or an interference with their bodily and mental health, their interpersonal relations and their smooth social and economic functioning; or, who show the prodromal signs of such developments. They therefore require treatment.

More briefly one may say that by alcoholism we mean persistent drinking to excess such that the physical or mental health of the individual is impaired or his personal or public life disrupted.

Within this group of alcoholics two further categories are distinguished, viz: (1) 'Habitual symptomatic excessive drinkers', and (2) 'Addictive drinkers (alcohol addicts)'. In the first of these categories the sufferer, having developed the habit of drinking for emotional relief is unable to give up drinking day

*WHO techn. Rep. Series (1953), *48*, 15-16.

in and day out although he can, to some extent, moderate the quantities of alcohol which he takes, and the degree of his intoxication. In this phase he is 'unable to stop' drinking. Alcoholism of this sort is relatively common in wine-drinking countries and in some beer-drinking ones.

In the second category of alcoholics, that is, the addicts, the phenomena of the first category may or may not appear. There will always have been a habit of drinking for emotional relief but this may not have been a daily occurrence. The distinguishing feature of the second category is that once drinking starts the patient cannot regulate the quantities taken. It is often supposed that as soon as any small amount of alcohol enters the organism a demand for more is set up which is felt as a physical demand and which lasts until the drinker is too intoxicated or too sick to ingest more alcohol. Merry [48] has cast doubt upon this view by showing that the introduction of small quantities of alcohol in disguise to men who had ceased drinking did not result in a resumption of the habit. He thinks rather that the 'loss of control' precedes recourse to that first drink with which the patient relapses. Whatever the situation in regard to this matter once a bout has been started it will go on until the patient reaches the state just indicated. After recovery from such a bout, however, the physical demand does not lead to a repetition. For several days or weeks the patient may abstain until a renewal of the original psychological conflicts or a simple social situation leads the sufferer again to take a drink. Thus the patient may be able to stop drinking (unlike category 1), but once he takes a drink he suffers from 'loss of control'. The development of this repeated form of intoxication is commoner in spirit-drinking countries. Ultimately it too may become so common with the sufferer as to happen to him daily.

At the onset of the prodromal phase of addiction alcoholic amnesias become increasingly frequent, although they can occur with other types of drinking. Once addiction is established there is a steady trend to morning drinking, drinking alone and surreptitiously, the loss of friends and jobs and the neglect of family responsibilities. Ultimately, persistent drinking may cause chronic domestic friction, family arguments, separation or divorce, loss of employment or severe financial embarrassment and it may lead finally to suicide or attempted suicide.

As is well known there are yet other extreme effects upon the physical and mental state which should be mentioned. In some cases, particularly when there is some minor infection or when food intake has been neglected, the individual will develop delirium tremens. As mentioned later (Chapter 18) this is a confusional state. It is generally marked by considerable physical tremor, restlessness, attitudes of suspicion and terror, and vivid hallucinations. In other severe cases hallucinations may develop with less evidence of physical disturbance or peripheral neuritis may appear with less evidence of psychological change. Elsewhere in the body cirrhosis of the liver, cardiac myopathy, chronic gastritis and acne rosacea are well recognized as complications of persistent drinking, but it is now felt that other factors, especially vitamin deficiency may play a part in the development of these changes. By reason of their reduced intake of food, vitamin deficiency is something to which alcoholics are particularly liable. Sometimes as a sequel to the acute toxic deliria which it causes and sometimes without their supervention alcohol may also lead to permanent impairment of memory and cognitive function. The patient may thus develop a mild or moderate dementia; in some cases this impairment of memory will take the form of a Korsakow's syndrome which is described in Chapter 14.

In certain instances the disturbance resulting from alcohol has a markedly episodic quality. One such group consists of the very rare individuals who appear to undergo a 'mania a potu'—an episode of acute psychosis with subsequent genuine loss of memory for the incident. This is uncommon and may be due to an epileptic disturbance provoked either by the hydration associated with beer-drinking or by relatively small quantities of alcohol. More often sudden violent behaviour whilst drunk is caused by the disinhibiting effect of alcohol upon aggressive or antisocial personalities. Another rare condition associated with acute indulgence in alcohol is dipsomania. This is probably due to recurrent episodes of depressive illness in which the impulse to drink seems overwhelming although the individual may normally dread and avoid such behaviour.

Whilst these last are special cases they raise together with all the other types listed the fundamental question why men and occasionally women persist in heavy drinking to the detriment of their own health and prospects and those of their dependents and associates.

Aetiology

Social factors play a large part in the causation of alcoholism, but it is doubtful whether they can ever be regarded as its sole and sufficient cause. Otherwise when the balance of social advantage turned against drinking the practice would cease. This may happen in some people but never, by definition, in alcoholics who persist in drinking regardless of the physical or social harm which may ensue. Nevertheless it is true that those in occupations associated with the drink trade (barmen, publicans, and the like), those for whom drink is cheap in relation to their income (peasants in France, surtax payers in England) and those in occupations where drinking is socially favoured (heavy industrial workers and miners, expense account salesmen and service officers) are more exposed and vulnerable to the risk of becoming alcoholics. It is also the case that some social groups, for example, North American Indians and Inuit (Eskimo) who were not originally familiar with alcohol, have particular difficulty in achieving moderate patterns of consumption when it becomes available.

The particular social patterns of North American Indians have been adduced in explanation of their unusually high rates of alcoholism. For example, a culture which emphasizes reserve and restraint in personal contact may be most likely to lead to alcohol abuse once the disinhibiting agent becomes available; or a tendency to expect all food to be finished at a feast and all drink to be consumed once the bottle is opened has obvious hazards if the bottle is customarily large (for example, 40 ounces), and contains spirits. However the neighbouring Inuit (Eskimo) culture encourages extraverted behaviour, yet the Inuit suffers as much from excessive drinking as the Indian. Poverty cannot be blamed alone, since the pattern of alcoholism is also evident in some of the wealthy

Indian reserves. The effects of the White man's culture in depreciating the self-image of the Native, particularly when the original rich culture is despised, deserve some of the blame. Most likely the problem of extremely high rates of alcoholism in Native peoples is due to a complex of factors. The hereditary factor seems by far the least likely, especially when it is noted that Jews who have very low rates of alcoholism become subject to higher rates the further they move away from Orthodox Judaism and its traditional culture.

Once the habit of drinking has been established some temporary physical dependence upon alcohol may follow. However, it is not certain that there is any genetic predisposition to such dependence and hereditary and biochemical factors have not so far been shown to be important as primary causes of alcoholism. Therefore, if social factors alone do not account for the habit, it would seem likely, as we think, that the critical factor in its development is something in the personal characteristics of the individual and this view is supported by the common occurrence of neurotic and antisocial traits in the personal history of alcoholics, even before they ever took to drink. It is also supported by the truism that the habit of drinking is used both by people at large and by alcoholics in particular to relieve psychological stress and even in those groups where cultural patterns make alcoholism particularly common, it can still be recognized that individuals become more vulnerable when other circumstances in their lives are unsatisfactory. The psychological characteristics which predispose to excessive drinking are accordingly discussed next.

The cause of persistent drinking which is most readily obvious is persistent depression. This is sometimes endogenous, and once the patient is hospitalized and alcohol withdrawn the whole problem responds very readily to appropriate treatment. In the extreme and special case this appears recurrently in dipsomania (p. 325). In the common case depression appears in reaction to a series of disappointments, an unhappy married life, bereavement or other misfortune. The stable personality soon masters or relinquishes this method of keeping misery in check. The shy, insecure and sometimes paranoid individual tends to retain the habit. He does so perhaps for the well-known reason that alcohol tends to dull critical and perceptual faculties and improve self-confidence. He may also do so for the reasons advanced by psychoanalytic argument that taking alcohol provides oral gratifications for those who may specially need them together with the friendly company of members of the same sex for whom they may cherish repressed homosexual desires. These arguments are disputed but worthy of mention. They are derived as follows.

It was noted by Freud that paranoid psychotics appeared to have formed their delusions by projection and as a defence against latent homosexual wishes which they had repressed. Freud based his original argument upon the book, *Memoirs of My Nervous Illness*, by Judge Schreber, but clinical experience amply confirms the view that paranoid psychotics, if not actually latent homosexuals, at least often are preoccupied with homosexual ideas. Alcoholics also tend frequently to show paranoid ideas, to complain of impotence or to doubt their own virility and to cherish jealous delusions about the fidelity of their wives. From these associations it seems likely that alcoholics may have particular difficulty with repressed homosexual wishes and this view is said to be confirmed by the results in psychoanalysis with suitable patients. Whether or not this is true the company of other drinkers does provide the shy alcoholic with a form of social and emotional support which is particularly gratifying to him. A less recondite view of this problem arises from the observation that many alcoholics have a basically hysterical pattern in their personalities. Whether actively drinking or reformed, it is vitally important for them to maintain a façade which will be acceptable to themselves and to those whom they meet. This façade would appear to cover up feelings of insecurity, inadequacy and guilt which all too easily get out of hand. Alcoholics themselves regard their use of alcohol as a means of blurring over the defects in this image of themselves. However this may be, once the pattern is established the alcoholic, although normally conscientious and responsible, is liable to persist with his drinking in flagrant disregard of the bad consequences it may have for himself and his family.

A second sort of unstable personality which is predisposed to excessive drinking is that of the unstable inadequate or antisocial personality. This sort of vulnerable individual was described in a previous section. He, too, in the face of emotional stress, is liable to accept artificial comforts which later he finds hard to relinquish; he is the more predisposed to drink for consolation if he has any neurotic traits.

Besides those who drink for consolation or company there is one more group of drinkers which may be demarcated somewhat arbitrarily amongst the body of chronic alcoholics. These are people who drink, often alone, for the sake of the oblivion which alcohol brings. Some of these are abnormal personalities of either sort who drink episodically in response to isolated but frequent states of tense or depressed feeling. Others perhaps merely join in a practice which has been socially fostered. Vodka drinking in Russia seems by repute to be done in this way at times and student competitions as to who can drink most, most quickly, have something of the same 'do and die' quality. The most difficult cases are probably those which add this attitude to the other chronic alcoholic attitudes which we have already outlined.

Management

The patient should whenever possible be admitted to hospital and, if psychotic, may be detained compulsorily. Such admission is necessary to secure adequate nursing care in the case of those with delirium tremens, hallucinations, peripheral neuritis. It is also necessary in order to give all patients with an addiction the chance to cease their dependence upon alcohol which may best be provided by removal to a psychiatric hospital environment and away from the usual sources of temptation. Once in hospital no patient should receive any more alcohol but all cases where there are physical changes or confusional ones should receive treatment with high doses of vitamins by injection (see Appendix 1, p. 396). The acutely disturbed ones will require treatment with suitable sedatives or tranquillizers of which diazepam and intramuscular chlorpromazine are probably the most satisfactory. Together with these measures treatment for intercurrent bronchopneumonia or other physical complications may be required.

The patient is thus detoxicated by appropriate vitamin treatment, tranquillization and sedation and possibly the use of small doses of insulin (which may have a calming effect and of course help to put on weight). Following this, patients often declare how little they feel any need for alcohol. This is probably the truth for a significant number of cases and suggests that if the patient has come to have any biochemical or pharmacological dependence on alcohol, this can rarely exert a prolonged influence or be a substantial factor either in the aetiology or in the perpetuation of the condition. This may be contrasted with addiction to opium alkaloids where profound physical disturbances follow the withdrawal of the drug. In alcoholism the subsequent liability to relapse probably depends most on psychological factors. It follows that having accustomed the patient to be contented in hospital without alcohol the next step must be to plan his return to the general community in such a fashion that he can surmount or circumvent the sorts of difficulties which previously disposed him to drink. This is by far the most difficult part of the doctor's task and the procedure may require to be 'tailor-made' for each patient.

The sort of action that is generally taken is to support and encourage the patient, to interview the spouse and try and ease any causes of domestic friction, to provide alternative social outlets for the man who has been used to drink every night at his pub or club and sometimes to help in finding alternative employment. Where it exists one of the best helps possible for the alcoholic is to join Alcoholics Anonymous which often serves as a most vigorous and effective psychotherapeutic group, particularly for the newly abstinent. This often, too, provides an emergency service of members who will rally to the support of any of their fellows who call for help at times of special temptation such as loneliness. Alike for the clinic and the doctor it is important to maintain the follow-up since this especially encourages the patient against a relapse.

Besides psychological techniques physical methods of aversion therapy are also used. The theory underlying these treatments is essentially that if the patients can be made to feel sufficiently uncomfortable whilst having alcohol, they may be forming reflex feelings of disgust or distaste for alcohol. Accordingly some patients are given their favourite drink with injections of apomorphine which makes them vomit repeatedly.

An alternative treatment is disulfiram, a substance which in the presence of alcohol forms aldehydes in the body and brings about a toxic reaction. Disulfiram has the further advantage that so long as the patient continues to take it he is certain to have a toxic reaction with alcohol. These treatments require cooperative, even eager, patients, and may be dangerous. They are not suitable for those with heart or liver disease. They are, however, of some use as a prop where patient and spouse are both determined on a cure. They are, therefore, best used as supportive measures; the primary treatment of alcoholism is to attend to the personal needs and social stresses which have caused the individual to succumb.

In general we do not use aversion techniques ourselves, considering that they have little to offer compared with the risks and compared with the equally good or bad results of supportive and psychotherapuetic management. We also think that if the patient is to be treated with drugs it is probably better to use non-addictive medication which may ease some of his difficulties (for example, phenothiazines, antidepressants) rather than run the risk of toxic reactions in the patient who likes to experiment or is heedless of warnings.

The discussion of causes of alcoholism touched on many conditions and circumstances which would promote the illness. By the same token it must be recognized that some patients are much easier to treat than others. Prognosis varies considerably both with those who have alcoholism because of depression and with those who have alcoholism because of personality problems. On the whole, however, patients with an obvious cause for depression have the better prognosis and amongst those with personality problems there will be found some in whom the prognosis is quite good and others in whom it is relatively poor.

DRUG DEPENDENCE

As with alcohol so with drugs; patients rarely complain spontaneously of their undue dependence upon the favoured substance. More often others bring them to medical attention or else the doctor himself comes to feel that the patient is asking for too many tablets. Substances which give rise to this sort of problem are barbiturates and similar sedatives, codeine, some D-propoxyphene, pentazocine, cough medicines and amphetamine derivatives. Chronic dependence on benzodiazepines is also a definite problem.

Morphine, the opium alkaloids, pethidine and comparable synthetic analgesics used to affect only very small numbers, mainly members of the medical and nursing profession. However, in the last two decades there has been a rapid growth in the use of such drugs by young people, as well as a widespread use of cannabis and resort to lysergic acid diethylamide (LSD) which has given rise to much public concern and comment.

Once drug addiction is established its consequences are rather like those of alcohol. There is increasing interference with personal efficiency, occasional or more frequent intoxication during the course of the daily round, general impairment of physical health (especially with opium derivatives) and even the risk of a toxic psychosis (with amphetamines and LSD in particular) and peripheral neuritis. In two important respects, however, such addiction, with the possible exception of cannabis, differs from that to alcohol. First, pharmacological tolerance of increasing doses, and demands for ever-larger quantities of the drug, readily develop. Second, true physical withdrawal symptoms will occur, which is not necessarily the case with alcohol, and, therefore, when treatment of the addiction is begun, the stopping of the drug has to be done gradually. With barbiturates in particular there is a risk of convulsions or delirium if they are stopped abruptly.

Drug addictions again resemble alcoholism, however, in that they generally occur, with the possible exception of opium addictions, in people with a strong neurotic predisposition or unstable personality. Once established, they further resemble alcoholism in that they lead to deceitful and sometime ruthless behaviour on the part of the patient to secure further supplies. Only in the mildest instances, therefore, can they be treated outside hospital. When treatment is attempted there should be the same attention to underlying personal and social problems as with alcoholism and similar rehabilitative measures will be attempted. Withdrawal of the drug, however, will be gradual and may be eased by the use of antidepressant substances (like imipramine or the mono-amine-oxidase inhibitors) and/or phenothiazine tranquillizers (like chlorpromazine) none of which causes addiction. It should be emphasized of course that antidepressants and particularly mono-amine-oxidase inhibitors should not be given soon after the use of amphetamines.

Of all these drugs the use of cannabis is probably now the most widespread, particularly amongst the young and especially in those who are ill at ease in the civilization in which they find themselves. Many students have occasional experiments with this drug with no obvious ill effects except the legal penalties to which they are exposed if they are caught. Although there has been a report of brain damage following the excessive use of cannabis[13] this finding has yet to be confirmed. However, there is a consensus amongst clinical psychiatrists that cannabis intake appears to result in a number of psychotic illnesses in a susceptible group of patients. It is rarely possible to be sure that cannabis alone was responsible for the psychosis but, certainly, in our personal practice we have seen a number of patients in whom symptoms of anxiety, depression and depersonalization appear to have been precipitated by the use of cannabis. Reports by Kolansky and Moore[38] of psychotic illnesses due to cannabis are convincing. Symptoms may persist for some time after only a few occasions of smoking cannabis. Further, the chronic 'pot head' or apathetic chronic cannabis addict is said to be well known amongst those who take the substance.

The illegality of the practice may be one of the attractions of the habit, but any case for legalizing the utilization of cannabis at the present time appears to us to be flimsy. It may be that the drug is no more dangerous than alcohol or cigarettes, but if we could prevent those being used in society it would save much morbidity. It is impracticable to prevent the abuse of alcohol and cigarettes completely. It is still to be hoped that it may be practicable to abate the use of cannabis if not abolish it by maintaining legal restrictions upon it. It seems that cannabis is not addictive to the same extent as the opiates, but there is a further danger to young people in the possibility that those who sell cannabis may also try to sell other drugs such as heroin which is infinitely more dangerous. Yet coupled with LSD—as it often is by some users—there seems to us to be no real doubt about the toxic potential of cannabis.

In general practice the most common problem is probably to decide whether a patient who wants barbiturates or diazepam or a similar drug is truly dependent or merely seeking appropriate relief for symptoms of anxiety, tension, depression or insomnia. The same applies to a lesser extent with the use of the benzodiazepines. It has to be recognized that such substances in moderate dose can give valuable long-term relief to patients who might otherwise be severely disabled by such crippling conditions as intense phobic anxiety which we have known to confine patients indefinitely to their house. Yet after a while the doctor, and often the patient as well, may come to feel that the latter is addicted to drugs because he continues to depend on them and because the improvement they give is only temporary. It may be that this conclusion is as unreasonable as to suppose that a diabetic is addicted to insulin because he cannot forgo it without a recurrence of his symptoms. Yet we also suspect that the risk of the anxious patient wanting much bigger doses of benzodiazepines or hypnotics is somewhat greater than that of the diabetic requiring vastly greater quantities of insulin. Thus to withhold barbiturates, or the like, from many patients may be harsh, to give them to others is almost certainly wrong. To this dilemma we know of no perfect solution. We accordingly use antidepressants more readily than benzodiazepines for night sedation and for anxiety. Some patients who seem likely only to use occasional small doses of benzodiazepines are given them and patients already on such drugs who do not appear to be raising the dose, have their prescriptions maintained. We are prepared to give limited doses of benzodiazepines indefinitely to the more intractable cases of anxiety provided that the patient does not appear to be raising the dose.

NICOTINE ADDICTION

In the light of current evidence the majority of the medical profession have no doubt that the use of cigarettes is dangerous to health. What was formerly an agreeable pastime and method of easing tension must, therefore, now be regarded as a dangerous habit. It is certainly one which has always possessed the prime characteristic of an addiction since it is accompanied by an increasing physical tolerance to nicotine and in some cases may be the cause of minor withdrawal symptoms. Moreover, although the habit has been so common in the general population that it would have been hard to dispute its 'normality', it has always seemed that the majority of those who smoked heavily were unduly tense or frankly neurotic people. It therefore seems a proper subject for psychiatric attention. In giving it this attention we can offer no panacea. Fortunately we think there must be many people who, given suitable social support and encouragement, will be able to give up the habit by means of a positive effort of will and by the use of substitute oral gratifications to help them over the withdrawal phase.

In addition it is to be hoped that preventive measures and the withdrawal of advertising will play a large role in the reduction of the habit. In fact television advertising of cigarettes has been prevented in Britain and warnings also now appear on cigarette packets and on hoardings. After taking these considerations into account we would note that if cigarette smoking is a dangerous addiction it would be logical to treat people who smoke, say, more than twenty cigarettes a day like drug addicts or alcoholics and explore the neurotic basis of their habit. We would then admit them to a hospital to provide them with psychotherapy and social support which would enable them to be cured of it. This is, perhaps, a logical conclusion rather than a practical one and it may never be encompassed except for a few hypochondriacs who seek out novelties in treatment. What has happened is that some smoking cure clinics have been established which may succeed in giving help and emotional support in the withdrawal period, and also health education officers campaign against the habit in schools.

GAMBLING

Few readers, if any, can claim no experience of gambling, so it is important to define pathological gambling. Gambling can cause economic harm, social harm to the subject's family and reputation and psychological harm when the subject becomes preoccupied with it to the exclusion of all else. Gambling becomes pathological when the subject refuses to acknowledge the harm he is suffering or when he is unwilling or unable to limit the harm done.

Moran[60] proposes five syndromes of pathological gambling. *Symptomatic* gambling is consequent on a psychiatric illness which is the primary disorder. This is usually a depressive illness and must be distinguished from the reactive depressions which follow on a bout of unsuccessful gambling. Effective antidepressant treatment will often lead to the control of the gambling symptoms after a period of some weeks and therapy should be prolonged for six months.

Psychopathic gambling occurs in patients with personality disorders, usually of the antisocial type, and is associated with other signs of defective social adjustment. *Neurotic* gambling occurs as a response to an emotional disturbance such as an unhappy marriage or as a means of causing distress to the patient's family. This frequently improves when help is offered for the emotional troubles.

Impulsive gambling may be compared to some types of alcoholism. Once started there is 'loss of control' so that the gambling continues until the money runs out. This type of gambler struggles with the craving which he knows may ruin him. *Subcultural* gambling arises in situations of heavy gambling.

There are links between gambling and other deviant behaviour. The term 'loss of control' is borrowed from the literature on alcoholism, and there is evidence of an association between gambling and excessive drinking. The taking of risks which is essential to gambling is also present in some attempted suicides. After an overdose it is often a matter of chance whether the patient is discovered early enough to allow resuscitation or too late to save his life. There is some evidence that gamblers are more prone to attempt suicide. It might be thought that a disturbance of impulse control is common to gambling, alcoholism and attempted suicide.

There are several approaches to helping the gambler. In the first place it is important to treat effectively any underlying depressive illness and to deal with family conflict whether it is the cause or the result of the gambling. In the absence of these complications and when there is a sincere motivation for treatment (which excludes the majority of cases of personality disorder) behaviour therapy can be of value. In the most commonly used method an electric shock is administered to the patient as he is about to make the first move in starting to gamble. In one reported case the patient received the shock as he turned to the sporting pages of the newspaper. Success has been reported in 50 per cent of cases treated.

In recent years there has been a self-help group of gamblers called Gamblers Anonymous. Not all gamblers are prepared to make use of it, but it offers valuable support for those who do.

Social policy cannot be ignored. There is no doubt that the amount of gambling increased greatly after the liberalizing effect of the 1960 Betting and Gaming Act in Britain and there are clinical reports which show that for some patients the development of pathological gambling was to some extend dependent on the provision of facilities.

UNEMPLOYMENT

One of the characteristics of contemporary society is that gainful employment is now enjoined on all its members. Contempt is felt for those who, not needing to work, enjoy a life of leisure (witness the pejorative term *socialite*). Others who in not working are supported by the labours of their family or by supplementary benefits are liable to be treated as sick, condemned as lazy or prosecuted for failing to maintain their family. Yet this has not always been so. In more aristocratic times the definition of gentleman excluded gainful employment and many older people can still remember the shock of realizing that young ladies of gentle breeding were expected to go out to work during the first world war. It is still true, as Groddeck reminds us, that work was the curse laid upon man on his expulsion from Paradise. Nevertheless, failure to observe a general social obligation, whether it be for idleness or for occupation, is a sign of the social deviant. While some deviants rejoice in a peculiar independence of mind, it is generally true that an inferior social adjustment is often the sign of emotional or mental sickness.

This introduction was not intended as a philosophical digression but to point to the obvious fact that assessment of refusal to work (and this can take many forms) must have reference to the milieu in which the patient lives. In every large town in Britain there are areas in which a man with a large family is not expected to work: family allowances and supplementary benefit represent as good an income as that provided by a labouring job. In some parts of Canada, workmen have sought employment only for long enough to acquire entitlements to Unemployment Insurance Benefits. In much the same way in some districts not to be in trouble with the police is regarded as deviant behaviour. This refusal to work can take many forms. A constant succession of minor illnesses requiring a sick note, or rapid changing of job to job with long rest pauses in between are two of the more common. One characteristic of this behaviour is that it is perfectly adjusted to administrative regulations: the period of absence never lasts longer than thirteen weeks, at the end of which insurance benefits cease in the United Kingdom. It will be seen therefore that at least in some of these cases the pathology is not in the individual but in the local culture to which he conforms in evading work. Correct treatment of these cases lies in social action (perhaps rehousing into a different area where more conventional standards obtain) rather than in medical or psychological treatment.

Apart from such exceptions anxious consultations are sought because a certain member of the household cannot or will not go to work. The fact that a consultation is sought shows that the problem is not that of a work-shy sub-culture. Such cases can be divided into three groups:

1. *Staying in bed.* The typical history is of an adolescent boy or young man with a slowly deteriorating work record beginning after school leaving. By the time consultation is sought the boy has usually been unemployed for some time and spends a large part of his time in bed. Often refusal to get up may have been the cause of losing his job. When interviewed a striking feature is the absence of any convincing reason for this behaviour, even as regards neurotic symptoms. Almost all of these patients are suffering from simple schizophrenia. Once this diagnosis is in mind, the relatives can sometimes be prompted to recall episodes of bizarre behaviour; inexplicable cruelty or violence, fleeting paranoid trends or odd hypochondriacal notions. Little is made out on examination except the patient's lack of interest and lack of rapport.

2. *Periodic unemployment.* Many patients with a psychiatric illness succumb to the temptation to stay off work. Indeed in the case of a depressive illness this may be necessary owing to the very real impairment of concentration which so often happens in this illness. With neurotic illness, however, it is seldom necessary to stay at home and indeed it is usually harmful. Left to themselves most neurotic patients eventually return to work, but in one investigation it was noted that on average it took about three years for this to happen. This period can be considerably shortened by sensible and realistic advice at the outset of the illness. It has been noted that the tendency to stay off work is related more to the inadequacy of the personality rather than the severity of the symptoms. This perhaps gives the reason why patients who do not return to work fare so badly in psychotherapy, the common factor being an inadequate personality.

The work history of a patient with a chronic neurosis will show therefore relatively long periods of employment punctuated by episodes in which the symptoms got the upper hand and he stayed off work. With a more exacting and better-paid job it can be assumed that the personality has correspondingly greater resources and therefore the patient is more reluctant to resort to sickness absence and will respond more easily to treatment. Jobs of lower status frequently imply lack of personality assets as well as failing to provide adequate financial incentive to stay off the sick list. The prognosis is accordingly poorer. Even if intensive psychiatric treatment is not indicated or available supportive therapy will bring about a welcome improvement in the work record although symptoms may not be relieved.

Recurrent depression can sometimes hide under a welter of neurotic symptomatology and be the cause of periodic unemployment. This should be suspected if the family fail to describe a typical neurotic personality in between the attacks. Although depression may not be obvious, careful enquiry may reveal other depressive symptoms such as early waking, weight loss or the typical diurnal variation of being worse in the morning. Some of these patients respond well to antidepressant drugs which have to be made available at the start of each attack. By this means, recurrent unemployment can be avoided.

3. *Chronic unemployment.* It has already been noted that unemployment is related more to the assets of the personality than to the severity of the illness. It may be expected, therefore, that in a society of full employment, chronic unemployment is associated above all with abnormal personalities. To this group must be added chronic schizophrenia and subnormality (mental retardation), but at least in the former diagnosis it is the deterioration in personality which is the effective deterrent to would-be employers.

Chronic unemployment is a cardinal sign of the inadequate or asthenic personality disorder, but antisocial and paranoid personalities also have poor work records. Some of these men are bitter and full of grievances against the ill treatment which they believe they have received from society while others are quarrelsome and aggressive. It is clear that in such cases their tendency to pick quarrels and complain has played a large part in preventing their employment.

This group of inadequate and disturbed personalities makes a fascinating study for all who are interested in the problems of social adjustment. Their prognosis in treatment, however, is uniformly poor, and they constitute a disproportionate burden in time and money on the social services.

In a minority of young people unemployment forms part of their way of life. Delinquent boys are often unattracted by the rewards of hard work, and, for very different reasons, this also applies to young people who live in communes and belong to the hippie culture. Hippies are almost the opposite of delinquents and apart from drug-taking, they rarely break the law. They are quiet withdrawn young men and women who are affronted by a civilization which endorses conspicuous consumption. Their somewhat fragile existence retreats not only from the physical violence which is to be found in cities but also from the more subtle violence to their personalities which they have experienced when exposed to the pressures to conform to the values and morals of the families and social class. They attempt to achieve a style of living in which relationships are totally undemanding and they are often influenced by Buddhist thought. After a few years many become strong enough to face the challenge of a competitive society.

THE DROP-OUT

It could be argued that those who drop-out from general society are acting sensibly. Many, in their own view, claim to be giving up the 'rat-race' for the sake of inner peace. Reality accords less well with this view. Many drop-outs do not persist in that role, and on relinquishing it talk not of failure in achieving a worthy ideal but of recognition of a mistaken aim or idea. Others have had psychiatric treatment or evident emotional troubles. Moreover, as difficulty in finding employment for college graduates has become apparent, the current generation of students seems to have become more conventional, more openly concerned with the goals of graduation, employment and stable married life and less attracted to extreme or anarchic positions. Drop-outs increasingly appear to be young people with problems of adjustment.

Schizophrenia accounts (at all ages) for a number of dropouts. Drug dependence and personality disorders account for more. In general, the drop-out tends to be an individual with emotional conflicts, unable to adjust to the pressures of family, studies or work. The problem most often appears in children from families with disturbed relationships. But the conflict may arise from other sources, and in the recent past the influence of peer groups in encouraging drop-outs could also be postulated. In general, if 'dropping out' is not due to a psychosis, or to understandable depression at academic or job failure, the patient can be expected to show a selection from the gamut of personality disorders. In that case management is by techniques of psychotherapy and relationship with the sympathetic physician, if the patient is interested.

NEGLECT

A final social deviation which deserves brief comment is neglect. This is both an early sign of psychological illness and a common one. It may begin with the care of the person and his/her appearance, but often extends to household duties, social responsibilities and work obligations. Its connection with emotional disturbance was recognized by Shakespeare in the following lines about how to know a man in love: 'a beard neglected ... your hose ... ungartered, your bonnet unbanded, your sleeve unbuttoned, your shoe untied and every thing about you demonstrating a careless desolation ... (*As You Like It*, Act III, Sc. 2).

It may also obviously be a reaction of despair when nothing seems worth bothering with. In part for this reason, self-neglect has been cultivated in some groups (for example, hermits, nazirites, hippies and bohemian artists) to indicate indifference to one set of values, for example, bourgeois respectability, or to emphasize another—such as an intense artistic or spiritual life or concentration on holy matters without concern for the body. In many of these instances the emotional balance of the individual may well be suspect and neglect may be a prominent indicator of his social and psychological deviation. Also, the reasons given for self-neglect may well be rationalizations. Problem families often appear to live in a society of their own where current middle-class standards of cleanliness have no force. The insanitary conditions of these dwellings may offend the Health Visitor but do not provide *prima facie* evidence of the need to remove the inmates to the nearest mental hospital!

Recent work has shown[75] that there are complex determinants to the style of living found in problem families. Unexpectedly it was found that poverty itself is not an important factor, nor was there convincing evidence of a ghetto subculture which is found in the shanty towns of other countries. The most important factor was the lack of emotional stability in the father. This led to unemployment, marital conflict and psychological disorders in the children. The mothers became overwhelmed with their problems and lapsed into despair. The level of their emotional life regressed to that of children so that they became even less capable of rational adaptive responses. At this stage, to add to their difficulties, they were shunned by their neighbours and deprived of the help and support which they needed so desperately.

These interesting groups, however, come less often to medical attention than those in whom neglect is inadvertent or unplanned. With those who do appear in the surgery, whether voluntarily or at the instigation of others, neglect may be a symptom either of neurotic or psychotic illness. In some it stems from the will to reject the values of parents or other close kindred. One of us treated a student who habitually had untidy hair, greasy clothes marked with oil stains and motor-car dirt and filthy black fingernails. He agreed that he liked to be scruffy because he detested the attitudes of his parents who had always regimented him, insisting on tidiness and hoping that he would wear a white collar rather than be an artisan. In others, relative indifference to appearances (not amounting to neglect) may reflect preoccupation with other cares.

With psychotics self-neglect often serves as an indication of the severity of the illness. It is particularly common in the old who live alone and may be dementing but it will also at times appear in other organic confusional states, in chronic or acute schizophrenia and in endogenous depression. In all cases besides being able to use neglect as a mark of the severity of the illness the doctor may note how it fluctuates with improvement, such as the return of hope in the depressed.

Neglect of other responsibilities may be examined in a similar way. In the neurotic patient, even if unconsciously motivated, it may give great offence to his associates and justify psychotherapy for the personality disturbance.

In cases of brain disease it is often one of the early signs of illness being obviously related to the insidious failure of memory which marks senile dementia and other organic disturbance. It may occur too in schizophrenia or depression and, whatever its cause, it will often catch the doctor's attention and lead him to make further enquiries.

17

Compensation Cases

Many problems in consultation take place because the patient wants something other than advice or medicines from the doctor. The family want a difficult—usually elderly—member to be accommodated elsewhere, perhaps in hospital or in a local authority home. The breadwinner wants a sick note, the injured wife a witness who can be called upon for her subsequent divorce proceedings. The power of the doctor's note or his record is thus considerable, but it rests in a varying light according to circumstances and the patient's motives. Illness may be seen by him as very serious if it will help to secure a letter in favour of rehousing by the local authority, trivial if it has to be assessed for an insurance policy. Considerations of this sort are particularly relevant in compensation cases.

Many patients are entitled to claim Industrial Injuries Benefit or Workmen's Compensation if they are off work as a result of illness caused at their place of work. Some have a claim for damages as a result of accidents—especially motor vehicle accidents—which are attributed to the negligence of other people. In these circumstances the family doctor is often called upon to provide continuing sick notes or to support the claim of his patient. Even if he is not involved directly in providing legal evidence he may be under pressure to arrange protracted treatment. Sometimes this pressure is due more to litigation than to the patient's distress. For example, one man with post-traumatic headaches alleged to us that he attended his doctor's surgery, at some inconvenience, because of encouragement by his solicitor not to minimize the extent of his need for help. If he is uncertain of his ability to handle a problem, specialist help should be sought.

Doctors too are aware that a few patients may be malingering. The number who do so is probably very small. The number who give the doctor the unpleasant feeling that he is 'being used' is much larger, although it will of course vary from doctor to doctor in relation to the practitioner's sensitivity to the possibility that he is being manipulated. If this sensitivity is high the practitioner may become irritated and may be unhelpful to people who genuinely need his assistance. If it is too low he may go to the opposite extreme and espouse the case of his patient as a supporter rather than as a neutral observer. If he can adopt the latter role he may, fairly accurately, discriminate three main types of genuine post-traumatic psychological disorder. These are: firstly, psychological symptoms resulting from a very frightening experience; secondly, psychological symptoms complicating a physical disability; and, thirdly, psychological symptoms following head injury, in which some of the symptoms may be due to organic damage and others to psychological complications.

British and United States law, but not that of all continental countries, for example, France, accepts that psychological symptoms may follow from a very frightening accident and be compensatable, even though the individual was not physically injured. A mother who sees her child killed, a building worker who sees his companion suffer a fatal fall may each develop an anxiety or depressive reaction for which some damages will be awarded. A coal miner who was crushed by a fall of stone and suffered a ruptured pancreas developed claustrophobic symptoms for which damages were paid in addition to those for his injuries. The dispute in these cases is over the extent to which the individual might consciously overemphasize his symptoms in order to receive more money.

This last attitude has been alleged particularly in regard to those who have suffered minor head injury. Where head injury occurs with prolonged loss of consciousness or a depressed fracture or the appearance of neurological evidence of damage, it is normally accepted that headaches, forgetfulness, difficulty in concentration and depressive illness, including a typical endogenous depressive pattern, are attributable to the injury, as are focal signs like dysphasia. For many years, however, it has been disputed whether a so-called postconcussional syndrome was, or was not, a genuine sequel to head injury with brief or no loss of consciousness. It was argued that this condition was one in which conscious exaggeration played a large part and even that the symptoms were really due to the attempt to obtain money.[56]

The postconcussional syndrome in question generally starts two to three weeks after the injury and is accompanied by headaches, giddiness, difficulty in concentration and some degree of depression. Other symptoms at times include insomnia, fatigue, irritability, anxiety, loss of libido and hyperacusis. It is not appropriate here to argue the case in detail as to whether this is or is not basically an organic synsyndrome. The matter is still controversial but many current views[73] tend to the conclusion that the syndrome is basically organic in origin, and it has been shown that, although a majority of patients recover largely or wholly, there are some who do not get better even when their legal claim is settled.[53]

It should not be supposed that all the effects of head injury or other accidents are physical, however. Hospital admission, discomfort, reduced earning disability, altered domestic relationships, all combine to provoke psychological symptoms once injury has occurred. Rehabilitation can be slow and is not always successful particularly for those more elderly men who, because of increasing mental or physical frailty, were only just managing their work before the accident.

Legal proceedings themselves are also a stress, as is often recognized. For anyone involved they may require examination by doctors who are not necessarily sympathetic and cross-examination by barristers who can be distinctly unsympathetic. To appear in court is often a stress even for expert witnesses. It is likely to be much more of a stress, and the prospect of it can be terrifying, for those who have no special experience of speaking their thoughts in public and who are aware that the aim of the other side may be to discredit them as much as possible. Partly because it is recognized that legal proceedings are stressful to many people and partly because of a belief that the claim is being consciously exaggerated it is often said by doctors and others appearing for the defence in such cases that the symptoms will vanish promptly once the case is settled. As we have indicated this is not true, at least in a proportion of cases. However, it is true that many patients will feel easier once they know where they stand and no longer have the threat of court proceedings hanging over them.

The management of these patients requires a recognition of the problems outlined and sympathetic encouragement and support in regard to rehabilitation. The general practitioner is in a particularly good position in one respect compared with the specialist. He knows well, and should have good records of, the past history and behaviour of the patient in illness. This is sometimes the foundation of an accurate opinion and it is in any case a very good basis for an effective relationship in treatment and rehabilitation.

It is important for the practitioner to recognize which symptoms will improve quickly and which not. One of those which the patient can be assured is basically physical, but which will likewise diminish, is the distressing giddiness which frequently follows head injuries even of minor degree. With this symptom as with the others the practitioner must be prepared for spontaneous fluctuations which seem to occur without any necessary psychological or physical precipitant. On the whole these fluctuations do diminish with time and there is a general tendency towards improvement. Depressive features in the illness are particularly common between six weeks and six months after the head injury. Both at those times and later, antidepressant medication, carefully adjusted, can be of great use and aid the family doctor in supporting the patient. Lastly, it need hardly be said that throughout all this the doctor who maintains his tolerance and understanding of the patient and his dilemmas will find management of the case easiest and be the most helpful to the injured person.

Part Four

Psychiatric Emergencies

18

The Acutely Disturbed Patient

In emergency situations there is often a desperate call for something to be done quickly. Even if the call is not a desperate one there is always a pressing sense of urgency. This is reinforced in the case of psychiatric problems by the feeling—often, although not invariably, mistaken—that other people besides the patient are at risk too, and that everyone involved in the situation may rapidly be engulfed in a dire catastrophe. Often enough these feelings reflect the unconscious fears of the participant, including the doctor, rather than an objective assessment of the external situation. Nevertheless, they may be of considerable psychological importance.

The appeal character of attempted suicide will be considered later; however, the relatives of the attempted suicide, and the doctor who undertook to safeguard the patient's life, are only being realistic if they react not only in the light of the risk to life but also in the light of the guilt and remorse they would feel if the attempt caused death. For reasons like this there are two aspects to all emergencies and particularly psychiatric ones. The first is the need to bring efficient help in a material crisis—as a surgeon might conduct an operation. The second is the need to allay anxiety when the apparent emergency is a false one—to be able to create calm when the emergency is due to the tumult of people's reactions and not to the physical characteristics of the crisis. This, too, a surgeon might do in recognizing that an anxious young woman does not need to have her appendix removed. In psychiatry it is particularly relevant in the handling of panic attacks and domestic outbursts. As with surgery, the situation can only be managed if the practitioner has confidence in his ability to make the necessary technical distinctions between different kinds of illness.

Neurotic panic and hysterical excitement

The disturbance that can be caused by such conditions may be no less than that due to psychosis or delirium, indeed it is usually greater for the simple reason that these attacks are socially orientated. They are in effect an attempt on the part of the patient to communicate to his family his extreme distress. This usually succeeds so that by the time the doctor is called the relatives are more frightened than the patient. The entry of the doctor, with the offer of help implicit in his presence, has, therefore, almost always a calming effect which is diagnostic for this type of excitement. Any excitement which is cut short by the entry of an outsider (doctor, neighbour or policeman) is likely to be neurotic in nature. Even if the patient is not previously known to the doctor, a short history on the usual lines will speedily confirm the diagnosis: long-standing emotional instability on the part of the patient and an adequate precipitating cause such as a family quarrel.

A patient suffering from *extreme anxiety* can be a piteous spectacle; the trembling, the frightened air, the tears, all elicit spontaneous sympathy. At the same time the apologetic, dependent attitude will conciliate the irritation most of us may feel at being called out urgently to deal with a case of fright rather than with one of coronary thrombosis. But such a case, once the diagnosis has been made, presents greater difficulties than one of coronary thrombosis. Its treatment is apparently much less precise. A sedative may be given, say diazepam 10 mg. In doing this there is a sense of compulsion that one often has to treat effects even if unable always to determine their causes.

There is, too, a sense of unease, a feeling for the doctor as well as for the patient, that the situation is getting out of hand. However, it may not appear possible to handle the situation by psychological means. If the patient herself knows that the last thing she wants to do is to stick kitchen knives into her children or herself, as she fears, reassurance may seem useless and there would appear to be little scope for psychological manoeuvre. In fact the practitioner may take heart from the fact previously mentioned that the mere entry of an independent professional person (whether doctor or social worker) will serve as a *deus ex machina* and help provide a resolution of the crisis. At such a time the firm, kindly and correct reassurance that the patient is not going mad will in fact be very effective, the use of a moderate sedative will then be justified and the way to bringing the problem under control for the moment will have been found. Ultimately, such a case will then probably require routine psychological investigation and treatment if this is not already in progress. A more difficult tactical problem, however, often presents in a very similar way to the above. Hysterical patients may also present with symptoms of anxiety demanding urgent attention and here there is a situation which is superficially very similar to the foregoing, but fundamentally very different.

Whereas the hallmark of the patient with anxiety alone is his or her eagerness to give the minimum of trouble to others this is not so with the hysterical patient. We need hardly repeat at this stage that the hysteric uses symptoms unconsciously for gain. It follows that just as hysteria may mimic physical disease so it may mimic other types of psychological illness. Only very rarely does hysteria mimic psychotic conditions. Quite often now it mimics those types of psychological complaints to which we are willing to extend our sympathy. An example may illustrate this point.

One of us, in his first psychiatric appointment, was asked to see a patient at the door of the hospital—which was a completely open psychiatric unit in a general hospital group. The patient had been sent for in order to enter hospital for treatment. She arrived in her husband's car and then refused to leave it. Her bosom heaved; she was too frightened, she said, to enter this fearful place. She was offered a sedative by the doctor to help her overcome her anxiety and her relatives then lovingly persuaded her to enter the frightful place for the sake of her health. The house officer was afterwards teased gently by his consultant. He had offered medication to a patient to get her to enter hospital. Such a patient should have been offered the chance of seeing the unit and then making her choice whether to stay or go home. Instead the patient had imposed an improper obligation on the doctor—namely that he should treat an unreasonable complaint as if it were a rational one. This is the problem which may be presented to the practitioner very forcibly at times by hysterical patients. It can only be solved by a refusal to be hasty, by pausing to assess the meaning of the symptom and by careful consideration of the demand, overt or implied, which is being made upon the doctor and the patient's relatives. Urgent, demanding, noisy or even violent behaviour coming from a patient who is not psychotic should, therefore, be reviewed critically by the practitioner, particularly if it seems that it may be due to family conflicts. Uncomplicated anxiety may then be treated provisionally on the lines indicated. Hysterical behaviour, which may be defined as behaviour which tends to manipulate other people and has value in solving the patient's emotional difficulties, will require a different approach. The stress there will be first on the temporary nature of the symptoms and then on sedation as a minor and secondary measure. But any interpretation should be made cautiously so as not to provoke indignant denials and profound resentment.

Occasionally it may be necessary to accept the patient's threat of self-injury or violence as justifying restraint and admission to hospital. This may only be done if the threat of self-injury or attempted suicide or harm to others carries a minimum of conviction. Admission to hospital in such circumstances would have to be under compulsion, and it is wrong to use compulsion to solve a domestic problem. There are basically two alternatives open to the family and the patient in such a situation if the doctor's advice and presence is not enough to ease it. The family can be told that they may seek the help of the police if they fear damage either to themselves or to property. Alternatively they may leave the patient where he is, provided that the doctor is satisfied that this is a reasonably safe procedure. What is not right is for the doctor to deprive someone of his liberty because he has been engaged, or is engaging in, a violent domestic quarrel.

Little perhaps need be added about the treatment of those domestic quarrels which erupt in violence or threaten to do so. The practitioner will avoid taking sides, he will try to secure calm by persuasion and he will seek to define the situation as one for the contesting parties to resolve further themselves or as one in which at least the medical role is strictly limited. Above all he should avoid punitive attitudes such as calling for the police or threatening to do so.

Excitement in mania and schizophrenia

The excitement produced in these conditions has many similarities and contrasts markedly with neurotic excitement in that it is largely unaffected by the social environment. The doctor's entry into the situation, for example, may well pass unnoticed by the patient; if addressed by the patient, the content of the talk will be unchanged.

Mania is a rare form of manic-depressive illness. It does not mean merely 'disturbed' but rather disturbed in a special way. The less severe forms of this illness are known as hypomania. In mania or hypomania, as expected, many of the patient's reactions are the exact opposite of what may be seen in endogenous depression. His mood is euphoric (elated), his activity is excessive and he talks too much. Instead of seeing nothing good in the future he sees nothing bad in it; this is without justification and his judgement is correspondingly impaired. Characteristically in the more extreme forms he will bedeck himself foolishly and sing inappropriately. Throughout he shows such an overweening confidence in his good fortune that he may come in his exalted mood to cherish frank delusions of a grandiose type. He may think that he is Jesus Christ or that he has inherited a fortune. Nevertheless, his gaiety may be infectious and the observer will chuckle with the patient rather than at him. In his ceaseless activity two further points are of interest; in action many things are taken up and none concluded because of the continual restlessness; in speech the same happens and there is a torrent of words and ideas flowing logically but incessantly from one idea to the next, and known as flight of ideas. The connections between the ideas may all be followed but are often trivial and they may be presented with a fatuous satisfaction which is quite unwarranted. (For a graphic example of the most mild form and one which is acceptable socially the reader may care to consult Jane Austen's *Emma*,[2] where Miss Bates presents a very mild form of chronic hypomania.)

In two ways mania and hypomania become an emergency. First, if the patient is frustrated in his activities or if his delusions are forcibly denied by others, he may become paranoid. He may react with complaints and anger against those held responsible for causing him difficulties or opposing him. Second, in the milder states of hypomania, he may throw up his job for trivial reasons and invest in hare-brained schemes, or he may 'paint the town red' or roam the country spending his money freely and thoughtlessly. We can think of one temperate spinster secretary who gave up her economical lodgings and lived easily in comfortable hotels, travelling freely for many miles by taxi and lavishing her few hundred pounds of savings in these ways and on bottles of champagne which she hardly touched. Another woman, younger and normally virtuous, easily picked up a man in London and spent a dissolute weekend there with him.

States of excitement in schizophrenia may be very similar to mania; an experienced observer may detect a relative lack of warmth in the schizophrenic patient, as well as disturbances in the logic of the train of thought. It is probably wiser to assume the presence of a schizophrenic illness if the excitement occurs in a young adult, and certainly if there are any symptoms (delirium) of schizophrenia such as feelings of passivity (see Chapter 7). Schizophrenic excitements present if possible an even greater urgency than mania, owing to their unpredictable tendency to bizarre actions. When paranoid ideas are present, homicide has been known to occur, and other patients have attempted extraordinary forms of suicide such as setting fire to themselves.

Bearing in mind the difficulties of the differential diagnosis between excited schizophrenia and mania, it is perhaps fortunate that the immediate management and treatment of both conditions is similar. One difference lies in the prognosis that the manic patient will make a complete recovery, although liable to further attacks of either mania or depression; in a schizophrenic patient, the prognosis will be much less certain (see Chapter 7). Another difference lies in management with lithium carbonate. Although this treatment has its hazards it is very effective in the control of manic attacks and has a place in the prophylaxis of subsequent attacks of the mania and depression. This is discussed further in the Appendix on drug treatment.

Clouding of consciousness (delirium)

The next group of excited and disturbed patients to be considered is those with clouding of consciousness. Although clouding may occur in acute schizophrenia, it is more likely to be due to an acute functional interruption of central nervous system (CNS) activity. One extreme consequence of alcoholism and avitaminosis, delirium tremens, is named in part for the confused mental state which occurs. Similarly, a major infective illness, typhoid, gets its name from the Greek for a cloud because of the profound blurring of consciousness which is manifest at the height of the disease. These illnesses are typical examples of the acute organic confusional state. It is a good practice to describe them by the alternative title, delirium. They illustrate the fundamental characteristics of such conditions; that is, they are associated with organic disease of such a type, whether diffuse or local, that it can affect brain function and they are marked by a loss of awareness of the surroundings. The distinction between delirium and dementia often troubles clinicians. Strictly speaking a delirium or confusional state should be diagnosed not merely when consciousness is blurred but when it is observed to fluctuate. Lack of orientation, or a failure to identify the surroundings, is a feature common both to delirium and to dementia, as well sometimes as other conditions. In dementia these failures of knowledge or awareness are likely to be static, in confusional states they can be demonstrated to vary.

Any general disease which produces a systemic disturbance and any disease process affecting the brain, especially when there is a degenerative process present as well, may result in a dementia. Typhoid and delirium tremens have just been mentioned. The whole range of infective diseases may similarly be incriminated. In Great Britain pneumonia and chronic bronchitis are amongst the more likely infective causes; most often they will be associated in such cases with some degree of cor pulmonale, anoxia and carbon-dioxide intoxication. Similar results may follow from uraemia, dehydration and other electrolyte disturbances, for example, after surgical operations, and from diffuse metabolic disorders such as liver failure, pernicious anaemia and myxoedema. Likewise, any type of vitamin deficiency, but especially lack of vitamin B, will cause mental confusion. Centrally acting drugs given regularly in excessive dose will also cause such a syndrome; cortisone is notorious for this effect and amphetamines too may produce a delirium in addicts. Amongst general causes non-medical poisons such as lead, chemical sprays and any toxin ingested accidentally may have the same effect. Lastly, in disease of the brain itself or its coverings, meningitis, encephalitis, infections of the brain parenchyma, trauma including subdural haematoma, brain tumour and epilepsy may all cause delirium.

In the presence of many of these conditions there will be ample evidence of the physical disturbance. In other cases it will be the characteristics of the psychological disturbance which lead the practitioner to look again for physical disease even though he will in any case never fail to review the physical condition of psychotic patients. It has been said that clouding of consciousness is characteristic of these conditions. It is liable to fluctuate but may be recognized with little difficulty by the reduced awareness the patient has for his surroundings. Gross errors are common in the recognition of current dates and times, the description of the place and even the identification of people. Recent memory is particularly inaccurate and attention is distracted. At the same time the patient neglects the care of his person, talks in a rambling fashion and may become agitated, hallucinated or deluded. A prominent symptom may be panic or terror, and sometimes this is the most important presenting complaint whether it is directed to a particular object, like the little animals of delirium tremens, or whether it occurs as a generalized state of fright without a specific object.

Whilst these latter phenomena are common to all types of psychosis it should be noted that the memory disorder and the failure in orientation for time, place and particularly for people, is especially typical of the organic state. If it seems to occur in other conditions it usually happens because of the preoccupation of the patient with his own thoughts or because the mechanism of the illness interferes with the examination rather than with the patient's registration of events. Thus schizophrenics in periods of remission may reveal accurate memory for times when they were inaccessible to questions. In organic confusional states this does not happen. Recollection for the period of illness is never better subsequently than at the time of the illness and such memory as there is will be found to be hazy, the past events then having a dream-like quality. Moreover, if the disturbance of memory found on testing is due to a functional psychosis, there will usually be other evidence which permits such a condition to be diagnosed. There is sometimes a problem in distinguishing the organic psychosis from the functional one when the patient is not merely inaccessible but also actively resists attention and is agitated and restless. In such cases the matter of differential diagnosis may have to be postponed until the patient's agitation has been brought under control.

In those cases where the confusional process is due to a degenerative disease, such as Alzheimer's disease or multi-infarct dementia, there occurs irreversible damage to the brain, and these diagnoses therefore should not be used until the practitioner is satisfied that nothing more can be done to restore the patient's intellectual function to its former level. In old people it frequently happens that a chronic mild failure in cognitive (intellectual) function is made temporarily much worse by an intercurrent infection or other systemic disease. In these cases a partial and often a considerable improvement in the delirium may be hoped for. The same is true where the disease process affects the brain locally for whatever cause. In other cases of delirium the prognosis is that of the underlying disorder except where it has been so severe (as sometimes happens for instance in chronic bronchitis and emphysema) as to cause irreversible damage to cerebral neurones. The treatment of these conditions is partly that of agitation generally, which will be given later, and partly that of the basic physical illness. In addition benefit may be obtained from the administration during the acute phase of high parenteral doses of vitamins. There is some evidence that these need to be given in pharmacological rather than physiological doses to secure the best effect so that much more must be given than would be required for replacement therapy. Such treatment, however, has no value once the acute phase of the illness has been brought under control. Apathy, by its nature, is less quickly noticed. However, many patients with delirium are apathetic and the diagnosis in most cases is often missed. Opportunities to elucidate this important symptom may be looked for by the general medical intern, especially in post-operative cases and in those who have quite severe general systemic illness.

Epilepsy

It should be mentioned briefly that some disturbance of memory and orientation with irrational and perhaps threatening behaviour may result from *epilepsy*. This is almost invariably epilepsy associated with brain damage whether chronic or recent, and is generally due to epilepsy arising from lesions of the frontal or temporal lobes; most often it is the temporal lobes which are involved. Lesions in these sites may give rise to automatic behaviour with partial impairment of consciousness and must be considered as the possible explanation for short spells of disturbed behaviour accompanied by loss of memory for associated events. Characteristic of these attacks may be their acute onset and equally sudden termination, and they may last for up to two weeks. In Chapter 8 it was pointed out that the symptoms may be indistinguishable from those of schizophrenia; it remains to be pointed out that a confused and clouded state is more common (often with very marked retardation). Purposeless and repetitive behaviour (such as buttoning and unbuttoning a jacket) is also common. Violent and unrestrained behaviour (the epileptic furor) is well documented but extremely rare.

Agitated depression

Aspects of depression are considered in Chapters 4 and 7. Besides the risk of suicide there is a further emergency which may arise with depressive agitation. It has already been noted that there is a retarded form of depression which is generally opposite in type to manic illness and in which the patient is slow and even stuporous. More frequently, however, the severely depressed patient will show agitation—a combination most often of anxiety and special foreboding. So great may the patient's restlessness, panic and indifference to ordinary considerations become that he or she will completely wear down members of the family, for whom the situation becomes intolerable. Thirdly, there is a risk to the patient from self-neglect. In one unfortunate case which came to our notice an agitated housewife stopped eating or preparing food. She had previously had a partial gastrectomy and was referred to a physician as a suspected case of hypertension. The physician diagnosed an agitated depressive illness and advised referral of the patient to a psychiatrist. There was a brief delay and by the time she reached psychiatric consultation the whole clinical picture had changed; she was euphoric and free from depression, disorientated and forgetful. The syndrome was one of the states of delirium which we have just described. In this case it was due to vitamin deficiency and was accompanied by signs of peripheral neuropathy. Whilst the peripheral neuropathy improved and was not troublesome, the impairment of memory and intelligence was largely permanent and severely disabling. For the several reasons thus offered it is nearly always desirable for these patients to enter hospital. Failing this the general practitioner requires the fullest support of the specialist.

Stupor

Stupor is an uncommon but fascinating condition in which the patient, although fully conscious, is completely unable to initiate voluntary action. The patient will lie in bed, sometimes in a bizarre posture for weeks or occasionally months unless treatment is given. There are degrees of stupor, and some patients will unpredictably respond to conversation. Joyston-Bechal[33] has shown that it may arise in the course of schizophrenia, depression, neurotic states[5] and in organic cerebral disease.

Schizophrenic stupor is a variant of the catatonic syndrome (Chapter 7) and constitutes an emergency not only because of the danger of inanition but also because it may unpredictably erupt into a state of excitement which can only be cared for in a psychiatric unit. The differentiation between hysterical and schizophrenic stupor is not easy to describe: the observer is somehow aware that the patient is conscious that he is under observation whereas the schizophrenic is completely indifferent and detached in his autism.

TREATING THE DISTURBED PATIENT

The first essential, of course, is to know what disturbance one is treating. As we have just indicated there are essentially two types of furor to which the doctor may be called. One, which is an emergency calling for action, arises with any of the types of psychotic illness mentioned. The second, which is an emergency that calls paradoxically for inaction, arises with abnormal or neurotic personalities. In this second type of situation, which is more common than the first, we hope it will have appeared from the foregoing discussion that the doctor is often most effective when he plays a passive role. Occasionally, he will use a shrewd word, a sedative or provisions for compulsory admission if the local law permits, but for the most part he does best in such circumstances by avoiding error and commitment rather than by positive action. In the first type of emergency which we have mentioned he plays a more usual medical role, as follows.

The doctor, if he has not already done so, should attempt a physical examination. In the case of schizophrenic excitement, manic elation and the panic or restlessness of confused states the patient's behaviour disturbance may then be readily controlled with appropriate persuasion to accept the intramuscular injection of a phenothiazine drug (of which chlorpromazine 50 mg, repeated as necessary, is a convenient and safe form). It is surprising how frequently patients with paranoid delusions will accept that it is reasonable to have a physical examination and afterwards when told that their condition requires an injection accept it. This physical examination also serves a more fundamental purpose since it will assist in the differential diagnosis of delirium from schizophrenic or manic excitement or from agitated depression. Emergency drug treatment is also called for in the latter illness and it may be given with heavy oral doses of benzodiazepines especially diazepam, or with the phenothiazines such as perphenazine or trifluoperazine. If a delirium is diagnosed the treatment for the underlying condition, or else its investigation by the usual techniques will also be required. If the practitioner cannot secure this at home for the patient it is an overwhelming indication for admission to hospital whether a general one or a psychiatric one and whether the patient objects or not. In fact in all these acute psychotic conditions hospital admission is called for because of the further opportunities for treatment which it offers to the patient and for the protection which it affords to both him and his family.

Compulsory admission

Where the patient has not offended against the law so that he has neither come to the notice of the courts nor is liable to be charged by the police his admission to hospital must almost always be secured with the consent of his relatives if not his own. Of course, if the relatives are not available for consultation, action must be taken notwithstanding their absence. But in Britain their wishes can only be set aside by

very special procedures which need not concern us here* and
the next of kin of any patient compulsorily detained in
hospital have the right under Section 47 of the Act to order
the discharge of the patient unless a restriction is in force
which has been imposed by a court of law.

Unless the patient raises positive objection his admission to
any type of hospital should be undertaken informally. That
is, he will enter either a general hospital or a psychiatric hospital without signing any other document than the routine
consent to anaesthetic and operation which both require. He
may still be admitted to either type of hospital informally
in Britain and in most other jurisdictions even if unable to
give a valid signature to such a document provided that he
does not express opposition to the admission. If he does
express opposition then he should be admitted either under
Section 25 or Section 29 of the Mental Health Act.

The Mental Health Act provides for the compulsory admission of patients to any hospital in the British National Health
Service and to other approved hospitals and nursing homes
so long as the managers of the hospital are prepared to accept
such patients. Under Section 25 of the Act patients are
'detained for observation' on the recommendation of two doctors (one of whom must be approved as specially experienced in psychiatry and the other of whom should where
possible be previously acquainted with the patient). There is,
therefore, no difficulty in admitting to hospital any patient
for whom a bed is available and in whose case the general
practitioner and the consultant psychiatrist are agreed that
compulsory admission is required. For such admission under
either Section 25, 26 or 29 of the Mental Health Act, the
appropriate method, having made sure that there is a bed
available, is to contact the Mental Welfare Officer, complete
the necessary forms which he will provide and advise the
relatives that this procedure will not be carried out unless
they permit it.

The Mental Health Act (1960), Scotland, makes similar

---

* Application to a County Court on the grounds of their unreasonable-
ness is involved.

provisions to the foregoing except that a Sheriff (magistrate) as well as two doctors must approve compulsory admissions.

In North America arrangements vary for compulsory admission according to the rules made in each American state or Canadian province. In Canada patients may be admitted either informally or compulsorily both to psychiatric hospitals and psychiatric units in general hospitals. Usually this is arranged on a medical request, certificate or recommendation and the period of detention may be extended by the hospital specialist. Review boards and appeal processes are normally available. A practitioner in Canada will need to ascertain the exact details of the law in whichever province he practises. The same applies in the United States of America where state rules vary. Not all state psychiatric hospitals in the United States can accept informal admissions however. Nevertheless, all states except Alabama provide for voluntary admission on the written request of the patient. This last procedure was abandoned in Britain in 1960. Compulsory admission in the USA may be either by medical certificate or after a judicial hearing. The only safe advice for the physician wishing to be informed about requirements in the USA as in Canada is to discover for himself the exact legal rules which are in force in his locality.

19

Suicide and
Attempted Suicide

The preceding chapter contained a description of conditions
which presented emergency problems. We now wish to discuss a condition which produces such a state of alarm that it
always calls for an immediate response by the medical practitioner. It is true that some of the implications of attempted
suicide, especially from a psychiatric point of view, may be
considered at leisure by the practitioner once the medical and
surgical aspects of the problem have been dealt with. However, it is often a matter of urgent concern to decide whether
the patient will repeat his attempt, whether he needs to be
admitted to hospital or whether there are any other steps
which should be taken to prevent its repetition.

Attempted suicide is a topic upon which knowledge has
been advanced in recent years by clinical psychiatric research
so that we have attained a better understanding of the
motives and effects of suicidal actions. We, therefore, present
here a résumé of modern views on attempted suicide and in
the light of these some conclusions about its management are
offered.

There are certain contrasts between suicide and attempted
suicide. Suicide is more common in men, attempted suicide
in women. Suicide is more frequent in older than in younger

people; but the reverse holds for attempted suicide which is more frequent in younger persons. There are great variations in reported suicide rates from different countries. In the USA the reported suicide rate is some 12 per 100 000. In Canada the rate is 11 per 100 000 and the British rate lower still and apparently falling. Spain, Italy, Ireland and the Netherlands report low rates of suicide (under 10 per 100 000) whilst Austria and many other European countries (not only Scandinavian ones) and Japan report rates of more than 25 per 100 000. Such figures are often not reliable. Religious and social attitudes influence whether or not a death is classified as suicide, and under-reporting is thus common.

In England and Wales about 3000 people die by suicide every year. Recently the numbers have fallen a little, whether because of improved psychiatric and other services or because of better medical facilities in resuscitating patients suffering from overdoses, or because of the change from coal gas to North Sea gas remains uncertain. At a conservative estimate at least 50 000 to 60 000 people in Britain hazard their lives annually in some episodic action, for example, taking an overdose of drugs which deliberately courts the risk of death. The ratio is similar in North America. Most general practitioners will be familiar with this ratio. From their own experience they may know that attempted suicide is one of the commonest causes of admission to general medical wards. Within a year or two of starting practice they will nearly all have seen several attempted suicides amongst their own patients, whilst actual suicides will have been much less frequent. The numbers of patients who attempt suicide have risen regularly and sharply in the last ten to twenty years. The reasons for this are not wholly known. Some allowance has to be made for a failure of recording in previous years. Nevertheless, a substantial real rise has taken place. The most popular explanation suggests that it relates to the increasing isolation of individuals in our society. As extended family structures become more amorphous and only the small group of parents and one or two children becomes common so the supportive links between individuals become less numerous, and any rupture in the remaining bonds of affection between people leaves the individual more alone and more likely to have recourse to a suicidal attempt. A general relaxation of social attitudes and rules also contributes to this situation.

Amongst these attempts the degree of seriousness of the risk will be noted to have varied quite considerably between different cases and there may have been some tendency on the practitioner's part to regard his patients as either people who really meant to kill themselves and bungled it or else as people who never really wished to die and did what they did to attract attention or as a bluff to blackmail others. As it happens, such a natural view is an oversimplification of a complex phenomenon. It is a bad error to think of attempted suicide as either 'failed suicide' or merely a trivial act to call attention to the patient. In fact the degree of risk involved in a suicidal attempt or a suicide is often not related to the seriousness of the intent. Some who give evidence of a firm wish to die take only minor and trivial steps in that direction. Others who would appear to have resolved merely on making a gesture do so with a thoroughness or vigour which readily puts their lives in great danger. Of those who do die it is frequently typical that they take more care for their suicidal action to remain concealed from others for an effective period, whilst those who do not die commonly take some steps towards contact with others not long after their suicidal action. That these steps do not always save the individual from death may be seen in the case of the film star Marilyn Monroe who died while attempting to make a telephone call.

Nevertheless, in those who survive the chance of discovery by others will have been greater than in those who die. It is one thing for a woman living alone to lock the door and take a hundred antidepressant tablets; it is another for a wife whose husband is returning from work to take half a dozen tablets, lie down on a sofa and leave an empty container for tablets beside her. However, the practitioner who meets with a case of attempted suicide will have to bear in mind that a large minority of such individuals will repeat the attempt in the future and a small but significant number of them will ultimately kill themselves whether or not they have seemed to intend doing so. Suicides and attempted suicides apparently represent two different yet overlapping populations. How then is the attempted suicide to be viewed?

Perhaps the first consideration must be to recognize that in every attempted suicide there are some motives which incline the patient to death and others to life. The patient is nearly always ambivalent about the outcome and his ambiguous deeds represent the result of his conflicting feelings. Indeed it has been said that if one had to design a pictorial symbol for attempted suicide one would present this act as Janus-faced, with one aspect directed towards destruction and death and the other towards human contact and life.

It is true that many attempted suicides will deny that they intended to take their life, but this must not mislead the doctor into underestimating the seriousness of the situation. Often if the question is rephrased: 'When you took the tablets, did you care whether you lived or died?' the patient will admit that he did not care to live. Apart from what the patient says, his actions speak for themselves. Although the patients may be unaware of their self-destructive urge and even ascribe it to 'an accident', it is as well to remember that healthy people are careful not to make mistakes when handling potentially lethal instruments such as sleeping tablets or a gas oven.

On the other hand, the actions of the suicide also provide much evidence for the existence of socially oriented motives. Occasionally, these may be almost entirely absent, as in the patients who withdraw from social contacts, but in the majority suicidal acts are acts of communication as well as of self-destruction. Patients often show great concern with the events which may follow their death and this is reflected in the suicide notes which they frequently leave. Even without this overt communication, the relatives are usually in little doubt as to the meaning of the act. Most frequently it is a simple appeal for help, 'I can't cope any longer', but often it is a reproach or a threat. One patient set fire to the house as well as taking an overdose. As with the self-destructive impulse, the patient may not be clearly aware of the message which his suicidal act conveys so clearly to his family, but their reactions leave little doubt as to its meaning. It must be repeated that in the majority of suicidal acts both self-destructive and socially orientated motives are present and if, in one instance, the appeal or threat aspect appears predominant it must be remembered that the reverse may be true (with fatal consequences) if the suicide act is repeated. This is more likely to happen when the first suicide act has failed to change the patient's social milieu.

The final consideration then is to ask whether the suicidal attempt has altered the situation. In many patients it has been noted that the so-called failure of a suicidal attempt will be accepted without demur at least for a time and in many patients also the depression disappears immediately after the attempt. To some extent this change is probably due to what has been called the 'ordeal character' of the attempt. Patients sometimes explain their attitude as one of 'kill or cure' and imply that their survival means Fate did not intend them to die. To an equal or greater extent the change may depend upon the altered attitude of those surrounding the patient. In other words the appeal, whether conscious or unconscious, often succeeds in changing social relationships.

In the light of these considerations the experienced practitioner will, therefore, enquire into three major facets of every suicidal attempt. He will look for the antecedent events and especially the precipitating incident which is almost always to be found in personal relationships, he will note the severity of the attempt and the direction in which the patient moves after the potentially fatal action—whether towards or away from other people, and lastly he will observe very carefully whether the threat or act of suicide has changed the circumstances of the individual as it frequently does. These considerations all apply no matter what the particular diagnosis or form of psychological illness which may be present in the patient. They, therefore, provide an extended illustration of the rule offered earlier that what characterizes neurosis is a disturbance of personal relationships. Even in psychotic conditions the suicide attempt may be closely linked to the attitudes of other people, for example, in treating the patient as ill, freeing him from an imagined or delusional criticism and so forth.

However, it is also necessary to take account of diagnosis when the subsequent management of the patient is being considered. Although attempted suicide may occur with any diagnostic category it is not known what the commonest diagnosis is in such cases in general practice. In hospital practice the predominant group consists of reactive or neurotic depressions and then nearly as commonly endogenous ones. Substantial numbers also occur with schizophrenics and with antisocial personalities. It seems likely that the same distribution may be true for general practice but with even greater proportions of neurotic and reactive depressions.

Management

Some attempted suicides manage themselves in that having taken an overdose of tablets or some other similar step they and their relatives see the crisis through without calling for medical aid. Only afterwards, in the course of psychiatric history-taking on another occasion, may the previous attempt be disclosed. In others the general practitioner takes immediate steps to secure emergency medical treatment and the problem is subsequently handled by the hospital.

In Britain it is recommended that every attempted suicide should be seen by a psychiatrist and this will now be arranged in most hospitals following admission for treatment. In many it is the practice for a psychiatrist to see even those who attend at Casualty for such attempts and this practice should be adopted everywhere. There is some recent evidence that trained junior medical staff (registrars/residents) can select patients for appropriate management as well as specialist psychiatrists. But this evidence is not strong enough to justify a change in current practice in Britain or to hold back on the provision of adequate psychiatric services elsewhere. At the very least the junior medical staff and a skilled social worker should be able to call readily on the help of a consultant psychiatrist.

Failing hospital attendance or admission, the practitioner must decide whether or not to seek psychiatric help and if so how. We need not discuss the mechanism of this procedure except to say that in the event of admission to a psychiatric unit being recommended urgently this can be arranged informally but, if not, the use of compulsory powers may be necessary. Such compulsory powers are justified in Britain if the patient refuses to enter hospital and if the doctor considers he is suffering from a mental disorder which requires or is capable of benefiting from treatment. In effect almost anyone who still seems to be suicidal, regrets that he has survived or threatens suicide convincingly can be detained by these provisions. They are nearly always appropriate in cases diagnosed as psychotic and in some others as well. Obviously, however, the decision to use compulsory powers will most likely be made after discussing the case with the staff of the receiving hospital who may be expected to give some advice in the matter if required. The position varies in North American jurisdictions. Ontario, for example, in the face of strong medical opposition has made compulsory admission dependent upon the likelihood of harm to the patient or others; these are features which figure in the British criteria for compulsory admission but are not obligatory in the United Kingdom where susceptibility to treatment may be the sole criterion provided that the patient is regarded as mentally ill.

If the practitioner continues to treat the patient at home, the essential thing is that he should satisfy himself that the situation which called forth the attempt has altered sufficiently for the attempter not merely to say he no longer wishes to commit suicide but also to be content with the changes that ensued. The practitioner would be ill advised to make such a decision unaided in the case of manic-depressive illnesses and with schizophrenics, but he will be obliged to make it on his own in some cases of domestic argument and neurotic reactions. In that event his best criterion for immediate decision is 'How has the suicidal attempt altered the social situation?', but he should still endeavour to obtain psychiatric confirmation of his decision by consultation at a later date.

The long-term prognosis after recovery from a suicide attempt is uncertain, but patients who do attempt suicide are a vulnerable group and have an increased rate for future attempts as well as probably an increased death rate by suicide. There have been reports that 30 per cent of attempts were repeated within one year at certain clinics. Amongst patients who have attempted suicide more will ultimately die by suicide than from the normal population, but the precise ratio is unknown. The figure is probably between 1 and 10 per cent depending on the sample of patients. Between one half and two-thirds of patients who commit suicide have significant physical illness (not always known to them). Similar proportions of suicides communicate the possibility of their action to others. Alcoholics, the unemployed or retired and people living alone are at particular risk of a further fatal outcome. So also are older patients and those who have made a serious attempt. However, even patients who have made trivial attempts may remain at risk, particularly if the initiating circumstances remain unchanged.

Appendix 1
Drug Treatment

There are a few simple principles which can effectively guide the practitioner in selecting drugs for his patients with psychological illness. The first, of course, is that many psychological complaints respond to sympathy, interest and the psychotherapeutic approach so that drugs may have less real benefit than is thought. The response to a placebo occurs to a great extent because of this—perhaps more than because the patient thinks he is getting a magic, or wonderful scientific, potion. A second and related consideration is that some illnesses will in any case remit spontaneously and a drug which tides the patient over the acute difficulty may not be a radical therapy. However, it can still be a very valuable, even life-saving, aid.

The third consideration is the most important that we need to stress here. It is that there are many good drugs with similar actions (for example, the phenothiazines) and amongst these it is more important for the doctor to be thoroughly familiar with the use of one or two than to think that good results may be got by ringing the changes through half a dozen related compounds. Such familiarity is important because few of these drugs have a set dose. Their efficacy tends to vary in different patients even when account is taken of body build. This may be because of marked individual differences in intestinal absorption or because some severe conditions, for example, mania, require relatively larger doses than others or because of individual differences in sensitivity to such side effects as hypotension. Particularly with the phenothiazines and antidepressants, therefore, the optimum dose may have to be found by a process of empirical trial. In some situations, for example, mania, it is more important to give a dose which will readily abate the worst effects of the disturbance even if this means making the patient too drowsy. In others, such as paranoid schizophrenia and senile psychoses, the dose may require to be built up gradually because otherwise the patient, who may doubt any need for tablets, may reject them as their side effects are obviously troublesome even though harmless. Naturally, higher doses can be employed under hospital conditions and these often serve to establish a level which can be maintained subsequently in general practice. A further point which must be stressed, even though well recognized, is that the drugs prescribed for a potentially suicidal patient should be kept by a responsible relative.

Only official drug names are used in this discussion but a list of proprietary names is provided at the end of this appendix. Readers in Canada and the United States may note with some regret that certain useful drugs approved in Britain are not available in either or both of these countries.

Treatment in particular clinical situations can now be considered.

Hypnotics

Hypnotics are generally well known. They all have disadvantages. Flurazepam 15 to 30 mg at night has been shown to interfere with subsequent daytime concentration. Nitrazepam 5 to 10 mg can be expected to have the same effect. Antidepressants used as hypnotics often need to be given 2 to 3 hours before retiring and their sedative effect may be prolonged into the morning. Nitrazepam or flurazepam are still acceptable however. The hypnotic of choice is nitrazepam 5 to 10 mg at night. Barbiturates ought no longer to be used and preparations containing methaqualone ought probably to be avoided also since it appears to have some addictive potential. Chloral hydrate or dichloralphenazone is an acceptable hypnotic but tends to interfere with the action of anti-depressant and other medication and for that reason should be avoided unless it is being used alone. The same applies to glutethimide. Most patients who need more than one or two 5 mg tablets of nitrazepam probably have an additional disturbance apart from mild insomnia. In such cases rather than use barbiturates or other unsatisfactory hypnotics it is best to supplement the nitrazepam with substantial doses of sedative antidepressants or, if the patient is not depressed but agitated, with equally full doses of the sedative phenothiazines. It is in any case quite a good practice to give all or nearly all the antidepressant medication which patients require at night since in that way the sedative effects become available for a useful purpose instead of serving merely as a complication of treatment if the drug is given during the day. The patient who needs 50 mg or 100 mg daily of amitriptyline may best be given it in a single dose at night rather than in divided doses through the twenty-four hours. Very similar principles apply to the use of phenothiazines at night, since the tranquillizing action which they may have is likely to be partly long term and not directly related to sedation.

In patients whose hypnotics are being reduced, one or two sleepless nights may occur but reduction should be continued unless there is a clear sequence of several nights of insomnia without drugs and the patient shows the effects of sleeplessness.

Depression, especially of the endogenous variety, is the main indication for hypnotics, but they will also be necessary in conditions of excitement, for example, hypomania and mania, excited schizophrenia and some confusional states.

Sedation

For anxious or depressed patients mild sedation can often be achieved with chlordiazepoxide 5 to 10 mg t.d.s. or with diazepam 2 to 5 mg t.d.s. Double or even treble doses can be of use for a short time unless they make the patient drowsy. These drugs have the excellent advantage that there is almost no suicidal risk with them. Their main side effect is drowsiness, and even that is often not marked. They are not known to be harmful in pregnancy. The main toxic effects are induced sensitivity with skin rashes and agranulocytosis, but the latter is extremely rare. Habit formation can occur with the benzodiazepine group of drugs of which chordiazepoxide, diazepam, oxazepam, medazepam and nitrazepam are common forms in use.

One substance which may have useful sedative effects and which belongs to none of the previously mentioned groups is oxypertine. In some patients 10 mg of this is a suitable alternative to 10 mg of chlordiazepoxide. Curiously, larger doses of this drug have long been known to be effective in schizophrenia. As with the benzodiazepine group its lethal dose appears to be almost unattainable in man. Experience is less with it than with the benzodiazepines as a sedative, but raising the dose does not appear to increase the effectiveness of the drug against anxiety and this is an indication that it may have less addictive potential than the other group.

The butyrophenones of which haloperidol is the most popular closely resemble the phenothiazines in their effects and use.

Tranquillizers

The phenothiazine group of tranquillizers were the first true tranquillizers to be introduced. It was soon confirmed that chlorpromazine could calm psychotic agitation without producing drowsiness. Some of this group (especially fluphenazine, trifluoperazine and perphenazine) can be useful in small doses in certain types of neurosis and mild depression, but the outstanding value of the drugs still lies in their ability to abate excitement or the florid psychological disturbances which accompany psychotic illness. They are, therefore, appropriate in mania and hypomania, in overactive confused patients and in schizophrenic patients who are overactive, restless, deluded or hallucinated or showing other signs of active psychosis. They tend to abolish or at least reduce the effects of many of these disturbances and are useful in short- or long-term inpatient and outpatient control of these illnesses. In long-term illnesses, particularly, the optimum dose may have to be found by repeated adjustment. This is considered further below.

Neuroleptic Drugs

The following are the main oral neuroleptics and butyrophenones available in Britain:

Preparations	Strength	
Drugs with dimethylaminopropyl side-chains		
Chlorpromazine hydrochloride	10	mg
	25	mg
	50	mg
	100	mg
Methotrimeprazine	5	mg
	25	mg
	100	mg
Promazine hydrochloride	25	mg
	50	mg
	100	mg
Drugs with piperazine side-chains		
Fluphenazine dihydrochloride	2·5	mg
	1	mg
Perphenazine	2	mg
	4	mg
	8	mg
Prochlorperazine dimaleate	5	mg
	25	mg
Thiopropazate hydrochloride	5	mg
	10	mg
Trifluoperazine dihydrochloride	1	mg
	5	mg
	10	mg
Thioridazine hydrochloride	10	mg
	25	mg
	50	mg
	100	mg
Butyrophenones		
Haloperidol	1·5	mg
	5	mg

Based on *Prescribers' Journal*, Vol. 2, August 1962.

As emphasized above the practitioner should be familiar with two or three of these and not worry about others. All of them have a tendency to produce some drowsiness, a dry mouth, postural hypotension and a parkinsonian syndrome in excessive dose. There is a risk with all of them of agranulocytosis and of obstructive (cholestatic) jaundice. These risks are low but the development of a pyrexia is an urgent indication for checking the leucocytes or suspending the drug. If the leucocytes are to be checked this should be done promptly. We have known a fall in the leucocyte count be corrected within forty-eight hours on withdrawing the drug. The phenothiazines have been widely used in pregnancy but there is no evidence with them of fetal malformation in excess of random expectation. Troublesome side effects can be photosensitivity and acute dystonic reactions. The latter are particularly liable with trifluoperazine, thioproperazine and perphenazine. Convulsions can occasionally be provoked in susceptible subjects; nevertheless epileptics can still be given these drugs.

We ourselves tend most to use chlorpromazine, perphenazine, trifluoperazine, promazine and thioridazine. They are all good all-round members of the group. Examples of doses are shown in the following table:

	Routine	*Higher Level**
Chlorpromazine	25 to 75 mg thrice daily	100 to 200 mg thrice daily
Perphenazine	4 to 8 mg thrice daily	16 mg twice daily
	5 mg daily	or thrice daily
Promazine	25 to 75 mg thrice daily	100 to 200 mg thrice daily
Thioridazine	25 to 50 mg thrice daily	100 to 200 mg thrice daily
Fluphenazine	1 mg daily	2·5 mg thrice daily
	or thrice daily	
Trifluoperazine	1 mg thrice daily	5 mg or 10 mg thrice daily

* The higher level doses should be used with caution and the upper limits only approached gradually.

Anti-parkinsonian drugs, for example, benzhexol, are sometimes given routinely with the higher doses; intravenous benztropine 1 to 2 mg is an effective antidote for the acute dystonic reaction. Thioridazine tends to have less risk of photosensitivity but a greater one of drowsiness.

The effect of all these substances, and especially trifluoperazine, tends to be cumulative. Adjustment of dose may require a week's delay therefore with trifluoperazine and even two or three days' delay with those like chlorpromazine whose action appears relatively rapidly. It may also take such periods of time or longer to get some impression of the usefulness of the drug. As much as a month may be necessary. Some patients are prone to stop their drugs with bad effects, such as a recurrence of delusions, which may only appear after an interval of three or four weeks.

The phenothiazines are used at times for neurosis. The evidence that they are of any value is doubtful but fluphenazine and thioridazine are sometimes thought to be useful. Because of their antiemetic and antihistamine actions phenothiazines can be preferred to barbiturates in tense or agitated patients where symptoms of those types are prominent.

It is perhaps worth mentioning that some phenothiazines are very useful in the treatment of chronic pain when this is due to nerve lesions or to neoplasms. Chlorpromazine, pericyazine and methotrimeprazine are particularly helpful in this respect. It is appropriate to supplement such medication with other drugs which are in more ordinary use as analgesics, for example, paracetamol (acetaminophen), dextropropoxyphene and pentazocine.

Some phenothiazines, especially perphenazine and trifluoperazine, have an undoubted exciting effect, producing restlessness (akathisia) in a proportion of cases. It is much less certain whether these drugs have a euphoriant effect though this has been claimed. Whenever phenothiazines are used, a careful watch should be kept for the possibility of depression appearing. Chlorpromazine and pericyazine seem particularly prone to cause this effect. It has also been shown quite clearly with fluphenazine given to patients with schizophrenia by long-acting intramuscular injection. In schizophrenic patients the possibility of changing the phenothiazines should be considered if they become depressed or, if necessary, of using ECT (EST) to alleviate the condition. This is more a technical psychiatric problem than one to be found often in general practice, but it may confront the practitioner from time to time. If the practitioner is using phenothiazines for sedation or for the relief of pain it is wise to give small doses at least of a tricyclic antidepressant with them to counteract the potentially depressing effect of the phenothiazines. This is not advisable in schizophrenia because of the risk of provoking hallucinations, excitement and confusion with antidepressants.

Another important side effect of the long-term use of phenothiazines is the provocation of dyskinesias especially in the facial, buccal and lingual musculature. These extrapyramidal dyskinesias are both promoted and relieved by phenothiazine drugs, particularly in elderly people. The result is that if one comes across patients who have been having phenothiazines for some time and starts reducing the dose these movements may appear more than was evident previously, yet they are probably originally attributable to the drug. The long-term use of phenothiazines is essential for many patients and yet it should always be kept to a minimum because of the risk of this particularly unpleasant complication amongst others. It is noteworthy that although a minimum continued dose may produce the symptom, it is more likely with higher doses. Estimates of the frequency of this complication with long-term use range as high as 20 to 30 per cent. If patients having neuroleptic drugs are observed carefully and regularly and if the drugs are stopped at the first sign of a facial dyskinesia, the latter usually remits. If allowed to develop steadily, the complication is much less likely ever to disappear.

Long-acting injections for schizophrenia

In the treatment of schizophrenia it has been shown in recent years that patients who fail to take their drugs can nevertheless be maintained in the community by the organization of suitable clinics and routine appointment systems concerned with the provision of long-acting depot injections of a phenothiazine. The one most used has been fluphenazine, first introduced as fluphenazine modecate and now in use as fluphenazine decanoate. Alternative preparations are flupenthixol decanoate which we also discuss below in connection with antidepressants, and fluspirilene.

Substantial numbers of patients who were otherwise seemingly hopeless chronic hospital cases maintain themselves now in the community as a result of this preparation. Injections are required every one to six weeks depending on the preparation, and the disadvantages are the same as those attaching to the other phenothiazines.

Antidepressant substances

The antidepressant substances fall into five main groups:
1. Stimulants, such as amphetamines
2. Tricyclic drugs, for example, amitriptyline
3. Mono-amine-oxidase inhibitors
4. Flupenthixol, a thiaxanthene compound
5. L-Tryptophan.

Stimulants

Except for proved cases of narcolepsy amphetamines should no longer be used because of the danger of addiction. This probably applies to all effective stimulants, including methyl phenidate.

Tricyclic antidepressants

We group together here imipramine, desipramine, amitriptyline, trimipramine, nortriptyline, protriptyline, clomipramine, dibenzepin, dothiepin, doxepin, maprotiline, iprindole and butriptyline. This list is not exhaustive but includes all the very active drugs at present available from this group. All these are closely related and they are derived from modifications of the phenothiazine nucleus. Certain other drugs with a tetracyclic structure, viz. maprotiline, mianserin and nomifensine have also recently become available.

The tricyclic drugs are all effective antidepressants. Minor side effects from them tend to be the result of peripheral cholinergic and anticholinergic actions. The relative advantages of one over the other vary somewhat but the leading ones currently are probably trimipramine and amitriptyline amongst the sedative ones and dothiepin and dibenzepin amongst the less sedative ones. They tend to have a calming as well as a euphoriant effect. The most common side effects are a dry mouth, constipation, postural hypotension and drowsiness. Toxic effects are rare and include blood dyscrasias and jaundice. ECG changes, especially flattening of T-waves, occur with some of these drugs and there is evidence that amitriptyline may occasionally provoke sudden death in patients with pre-existing heart disease. The provocation of glaucoma is an occasional risk. The retention of urine both in younger and in older people, especially men, occurs more often.

The three new tetracyclic drugs seem to have less anticholinergic effects and therefore less side effects. This is particularly true of mianserin and may also be the case with butriptyline (a tricyclic) and nomifensine. Cardiotoxic actions may well be less with some of these drugs, especially mianserin. Almost all tri- and tetra-cyclic antidepressants can provoke an epileptic fit in susceptible individuals. Nomifensine is a singular exception in that respect.

It is important to find the dose suited to the individual patient. The dose for dothiepin may be 25 to 50 mg t.i.d. or 150 mg given just on one occasion daily at night. One of the commonest reasons for the failure of tricyclic antidepressant drugs in practice is that not enough care is taken over the adjustment of the dose. We normally advise patients with whom a few days can be taken for this purpose that they must commence with only one or two tablets or capsules a day and gradually increase the dose by one tablet or capsule each day until they reach a level which is slightly too sedative for them. Once that level has been reached they are advised either to maintain it or to drop back by a small amount to a previous tolerable dose level and then to keep on this established quantity of the medication. Once this has been done a period of three to four weeks is necessary to judge if improvement is taking place. Advice may be needed in regard to postural hypotension, for example, care in rising, especially after sleep or a bath. Constipation may be relieved sometimes by Tab Carbachol BP 2 mg daily. Distigmine bromide, a potent but expensive preparation, may also relieve constipation when given as a 5 mg tablet. Care must be exercised with the dose of these substances and although also effective for the relief of retention, for which purpose they may also be given by injection, they ought not to be used unless bladder neck obstruction has been ruled out.

There are risks in giving certain tricyclic and mono-amine-oxidase inhibitors together, but some combined administration is feasible as we discuss below. There are also risks in treating with tricyclic drugs patients who are having hypotensive medication, and these risks are discussed later.

Mono-amine-oxidase inhibitors (MAOI)

The mono-amine-oxidase inhibitors and the tricyclic antidepressants are of substantial value in endogenous depression and have a place too in reactive depression. Mono-amine-oxidase inhibitor drugs as the name indicates inhibit the enzyme mono-amine-oxidase which plays some part in the metabolism of substances like 5-hydroxy-tryptamine, adrenaline and noradrenaline. These substances are concentrated in the hypothalamic and limbic regions of the brain. It is not clear how the MAOI produce their effect on depression but it is not related directly to their ability to inhibit mono-amine-oxidase *in vitro*. Of those in current use we prefer phenelzine dihydrogen sulphate in doses of 15 mg thrice daily or four times daily, or isocarboxazid 10 mg twice or thrice daily. Tranylcypromine which is a rapidly effective member of the group is not advised because of a tendency to cause hypertensive crises.

All members of this group are similar in their side effects to those of the tricyclic substances (dry mouth, hypotension, and the like) but occasionally they have a stimulant effect. Damage to the liver and blood dyscrasias are very rare except with iproniazid which is relatively hepatotoxic.

The more serious risks of the MAOI arise with certain foods and drugs. Hypertensive crises may be provoked if foods are taken which contain excess or relatively large quantities of tyramine. This particularly applies to cheese and Marmite and similar yeast extracts and other protein concentrates which are rich in amines.

Another most serious risk which occurs with the MAOI, but not with imipramine and related compounds is that adrenaline and noradrenaline can have paradoxical effects in patients on these drugs who have also been given meperidine or morphine. Two or three weeks may have to elapse after giving mono-amine-oxidase inhibitor substances before meperidine and adrenaline can be given and this is a considerable hazard for patient and anaesthetist if acute surgery is contemplated and particularly if the patient's treatment is unknown to the anaesthetist.

Because of the numerous risks and awkward characteristics of MAOI, all patients to whom they are being given should be issued with a card. An example of a suitable card is shown below.

This patient is receiving an MAOI (Mono-Amine-Oxidase Inhibitor). All drugs affecting the CNS should be given at reduced dose.

Drug . . . .

Dosage. . . . .

---

1. Take only the correct dose, as instructed.
2. Do not eat cheese of any type, cooked or uncooked. Avoid Bovril, Oxo, Marmite, yeast extracts, broad beans, lentils, spinach, pineapple, grapefruit, bananas, shell fish, crabs, lobster, tinned fish, game, meat extract, liver, yoghurt, chocolate and fermented foods.
3. Alcohol, for example, beer, cider, stout, wines, spirits and the like, should not be taken. Diluted soft drinks such as orange squash are permitted, but not pure citrus juices.
4. Should you develop a severe headache, report it to your doctor immediately.
5. Do not use cold cures or other proprietary remedies sold by chemists without your doctor's consent.
6. Always carry this card with you while you are being treated with the MAOI tablets. If you go to another doctor, into hospital or to the dentist, show this card.

Because the risks mentioned are either more common with the MAOI group, or unique to it, we use these substances only as second or third choice after tricyclic drugs have been tried. They can also be used in certain ways with a limited number of tricyclics. This is discussed again later. However a tribute to the efficacy of these drugs (and the tricyclics also) is that they can sometimes provoke hypomania. They should only be given to depressed patients with schizophrenia on specialist recommendation because they may also provoke excited schizophrenia. Like the tricyclics they can safely be given in conjunction with phenothiazines.

Flupenthixol and other antidepressants

Flupenthixol is an unusual substance pharmacologically although not in its structure. Chemically it is a thiaxanthene and, therefore, quite closely related both to the phenothiazine and the tricyclic groups of drugs. It was introduced originally in Scandinavia for the treatment of schizophrenia and is now available in Britain for that purpose in the form of flupenthixol decanoate. The usual maintenance dose for schizophrenia is some 20 mg of flupenthixol as the decanoate intramuscularly every two or three weeks. When used by mouth doses of up to 9 mg daily of flupenthixol have been employed, the main side effect being Parkinsonism. In small doses of 1 to 2 mg a day it is a powerful antidepressant which, if it is going to work, shows its effect very quickly. In those doses it is usually free of any significant side effects, except for increased appetite and weight gain and sometimes Parkinsonism.

It has no contraindications, moreover, in regard to food or other drugs. Sometimes, its effect diminishes after some weeks or months and when this happens it does not help to raise the dose. This probably indicates that the slight stimulant action which is sometimes noticed with it is not a reason to fear addiction. It can be well given simultaneously with tricyclic drugs, say flupenthixol 0·5 mg in the morning and afternoon and at tea time being given with a night time dose of a tricyclic preparation. Because of its quickness of action, freedom from side effects and lack of contraindications we think it will quickly prove useful in general practice.

L-tryptophan

The use of L-tryptophan has been suggested because it is the precursor of 5-hydroxytryptamine and there is some evidence to suggest that low levels of brain 5-hydroxytrypta-

mine are related to depression. It is normally given in a dose
of 1.0 g t.d.s. either as four tablets of Optimax equal to
1.0 g L-tryptophan or as a chocolate-coated powder. It is
cumbersome to take and some patients find it provokes
nausea, but many also develop a more satisfactory sleep
pattern when taking it. There is controlled evidence that it
has an antidepressant action, and, if tolerated orally, it has
no awkward side effects. Because of the large size of the
tablets and perhaps relative lack of efficacy it is best used
as a supplement to the tricyclic or MAOI groups or else
for patients who cannot tolerate other types of antidepressants. For theoretical reasons discussed shortly (page 393)
it might be expected that amongst the tricyclic drugs clomipramine would be the best to combine with L-tryptophan
and there is some controlled evidence to this effect. If an
MAOI is used with L-tryptophan in normal doses of each, a
combination of slurred speech, ataxia, nystagmus, apathy and
even confusion may result. This usually happens after 3 to 4
weeks when the patient appears to have responded to the
medication. It is important to watch for this complication
which is easily treated by moderate reductions in the dose of
one or both drugs. It should be noted also that L-tryptophan
is relatively expensive (about 1 dollar per gram dispensed in
Canada) and not all North American drug plans will pay for
it.

Hypotensive and antidepressant medication

Special problems arise when depression occurs in patients
receiving antihypertensive medication. For several years now
it has been known that drugs such as methyl-dopa and reserpine directly affect brain amines and can precipitate depression in certain patients. Fortunately, patients receiving these
drugs usually have milder forms of hypertension and in this
situation, if hypotensive drugs are specifically indicated, the
drug can usually be stopped in agreement with the physician,
and a diuretic or one of the less depressant drugs, for
example, adrenergic blocking agents such as debrisoquine, or
β-blockers like propranolol can be given in small doses instead. Frequently, just stopping the drug is all the therapy

that is required for the depression, but in the more severe depressions or ones which do not improve after stopping the drugs it may be necessary to give tricyclic antidepressants or to consider ECT (EST). In patients receiving reserpine, depression becomes much more likely if doses greater than 0.4 mg per day are given, and it is in any case not advisable to use this substance. Depression can, of course, occur in patients on methyldopa and reserpine and be unrelated to the drugs, but the more 'endogenous' qualities the depression has the more likely it is to be drug induced. A patient who has had a depressive episode on methyldopa should not have the drug again.

Adrenergic blocking agents such as guanethidine, bethanidine and debrisoquine have very little or no effect on brain amines, and so when patients receiving these drugs become depressed the drug is not usually the cause and one should look more into the patient's personality and life situation for clues as to the aetiology of the depression. If it is felt that the depression requires antidepressants it is important not to use tricyclics in addition to the adrenergic blocking agents because when the two groups of drugs are taken together, control of the blood pressure is lost. Patients maintained on adrenergic blocking agents are generally more severely hypertensive and so it is important to maintain reasonable control over the blood pressure throughout.

The interaction of adrenergic blocking agents and tricyclics was demonstrated very clearly in 1967 by Mitchell, Arias and Oates.[57] They stabilized patients on either guanethidine or bethanidine and then started them on the tricyclic drug desipramine and found a mean rise of 26 to 29 mm pressure in patients on guanethidine and 42 mm in patients on bethanidine compared with the pre-tricyclic period.

The pharmacological basis for this is found to be in the respective actions of the two groups of drugs. The adrenergic blocking agent is concentrated within the adrenergic neurone and prevents the release of noradrenalin. It is taken up initially into the neurone by the same mechanism responsible for the uptake of noradrenaline, but this action is blocked by the tricyclic group of drugs. Thus, with the uptake of the hypotensive drug blocked, and more noradrenaline available at the receptor site, the blood pressure rises.

In treating depressed patients on adrenergic blocking agents we aim to achieve maximum alleviation of the depression with minimum loss of blood pressure control. If the patient is severely depressed, ECT (EST) is the treatment of choice and, in the hands of a skilled anaesthetist, should carry very little increased risk. The less severe depressions can be managed best by gradually stopping the blocking agent and at the same time adding a diuretic, for example, Navidrex-K and a β-blocking agent, especially propranolol, to maintain some degree of blood pressure control. It is, of course, important to monitor the blood pressure at frequent intervals during this period. When the adrenergic agent has been stopped and a few days have elapsed to allow for its effects to wear off, the tricyclic drug may be introduced to the diuretic, or diuretic-propranolol combination. The tricyclic also has a hypotensive effect and when the patient is receiving adequate doses of the antidepressant it may sometimes be possible to stop either the diuretic or propranolol or both.

When reinstating adrenergic blocking agents, the reverse procedure should be carried out, but allowing seven to ten days for the effects of the tricyclics to wear off to avoid a paradoxical rise in blood pressure.

For patients who have had depressions, debrisoquine or bethanidine are usually the best drugs for the further management of their blood pressure, because they do not directly affect brain amines. Some of the difficulties of treating depressed hypertensive patients with antidepressants may be avoided by prescribing mianserin if bethanidine is being given since there is evidence that the action of the former does not block the latter.

Clonidine is coming into vogue in the treatment of some forms of hypertension (as well as migraine), but has not yet had a wide enough use for us to be certain about any definite psychological side effects. However, a report of a trial of the drug done in 1970 by McDougall et al.[47] reported three out of twenty-eight patients becoming depressed while taking it. These patients had all had previous depressive episodes, but it suggests that the doctor should be on the lookout for depressive swings in patients on clonidine and, for the time being at least, avoid it in patients with previous histories of depression.

Pargylene which is an MAOI with marked hypotensive as well as thymoleptic effects is now little used in hypertension owing to the dangers of the MAOI group of drugs. Its only feasible use is for the chronically neurotically depressed mild-to-moderate hypertensive who proves intolerant to the more usual antihypertensive drugs.

A policy for antidepressant drugs

Antidepressant drugs should not be given routinely for cases of neurosis or transitory brief reactive depression. They are the treatment of choice, however, in mild and moderate endogenous depression, and it is very appropriate to give them also in persistent reactive depression. If urgent relief of the depression is necessary, ECT (EST) will have to be given. Antidepressants can, however, readily be given in addition to ECT (EST). When we initiate treatment with an antidepressant drug we expect that about 70 to 80 per cent of suitable patients seen in consultation will be better at the end of one month. The response rate in general practice should be higher.

In one general practice series of patients with depression 50 per cent of patients recovered in two weeks without active drug treatment. Sixty-five per cent recovered with flupenthixol. Thus many patients need no drug even though the drug in the trial quoted was shown to have a very significant effect. In Canada and the United States flupenthixol is not available as an antidepressant. In Britain, flupenthixol or a tricyclic should be the drug of first choice. The writer's preference when in Britain was to use flupenthixol first. If flupenthixol fails or if the initial drug is in fact a tricyclic, the question arises which tricyclic should now be used. The first line of action is to review the patient's history in case a particular antidepressant previously appeared to be successful. If this is the case it should be resumed. If it failed, it should be discarded and an alternative may be selected according to the following tentative argument.

It is believed from pharmacological evidence that two main

types of biogenic amines are significantly depleted or reduced in their effectiveness in depression. One is serotonin (5-hydroxytryptamine or L-tryptophan). The other is the catecholeamines (norepinephrine and epinephrine). The tricyclic antidepressants are thought to prevent breakdown of transmitter amines after their discharge into the synaptic cleft (the space between the terminal of one nerve and the adjoining cell). Most of the tricyclic drugs affect both types of amines. It seems however that clomipramine affects 5-hydroxytryptamine to a greater extent than other tricyclic antidepressants, whereas maprotiline, mianserin and nomifensine affect catecholeamines to a differentially greater extent. It has been postulated that some depressions are related to 5-hydroxytryptamine deficiency, others to catecholeamine deficiency. Clinically, there is no satisfactory way at present to decide this point. However, if a patient has failed to improve after one month's adequate treatment with one of these drugs it is logical to try one with a different action. Similarly, if significant recovery has not taken place with one of the more widely active tricyclic antidepressants then clomipramine and a noradrenergic blocking drug may be tried in turn for about three to four weeks each if necessary. All tricyclic antidepressants have a good improvement rate of about 70 per cent after one month so that there is no clear way to decide which should have preference initially. The writer normally commences with amitriptyline or trimipramine and then if these have failed, tries the benefits of clomipramine. Some patients tolerate this latter drug very well. Some complain of added malaise or other unpleasant side effects in which case clomipramine is stopped and maprotiline is next used.

If none of these measures so far described is satisfactory, and if the patient can still afford not to have ECT (EST), L-tryptophan can be tried. Most often it can be given with clomipramine as already mentioned. If all these measures are not enough MAOIs can then be employed. The patient in this situation will have been ill for some months and specialist help is likely to be overdue. If the family doctor should wish to use MAOIs or if his patient is receiving them on specialist advice, he should know the following. First, some adverse reactions have occurred when MAOIs and tricyclic antidepressants have been given together. In the writer's view, and in that of most British psychiatrists, the risk of such reactions has been considerably overstated in North America. But they do exist. Four rules allow safe prescription of combined antidepressants. First, always avoid using any except the following tricyclic antidepressants with MAO inhibitors: amitriptyline, trimipramine, doxepin, dothiepin or maprotiline. It is known that these have been safely combined. Second, always introduce the tricyclic antidepressant first, usually at night. There is evidence that most reactions appear to have followed the reverse order of introduction of MAOI and TCAD. Third, use about one-half to two-thirds of the usual dose of each of the drugs being combined (the ordinary side effects like hypotension are additive). Fourth, introduce only one tablet a day of the MAOI for two days and then increase the dose to that which is intended. A gap of about ten days has proved necessary in the writer's experience to allow transition to the use of MAOIs from those tricyclic antidepressants which can cause adverse interactions (especially clomipramine or imipramine). However a longer interval can be used for the sake of caution whilst the patient takes, say, amitriptyline or dothiepin. Few, if any, adverse reactions due to the combination of MAOI and tricyclic antidepressants are known with these precautions.

In all cases of depression for which an antidepressant is prescribed liberal sedation may also be needed. It is often not enough to prescribe the antidepressant. Benzodiazepines or oxypertine are useful in this respect. A new sedative, chlormethiazole, which is also useful sometimes as a hypnotic may be used as a supplement for very agitated patients. Careful checking and adjustment of the proportions of all these drugs will often produce most rewarding results. It is axiomatic, however, that careful enquiry into the suicide risk is essential and that psychotherapeutic management of the patient and his family are no less important than the administration of drugs.

Lithium carbonate

It has been known for some time that lithium carbonate is

an effective treatment for mania. In this role it is peculiar in that it can restore apparent normality of thought processes. By contrast the usual tranquillizers such as chlorpromazine leave a patient somewhat restless or disordered in his thought but damped down by sedative and tranquillizing medication. The difficulty with lithium for the treatment of mania is that the dose used for therapeutic purposes (about 1·6 mmol per litre) tends also to be near to the doses which can be fatal.

Lithium has, however, become much more popular since reasonably sound evidence began to become available that it actually had a prophylactic action against recurrent mania or against recurrent attacks of endogenous depression. The decision in regard to the use of lithium for such illnesses is properly a specialist one, but the general practitioner will find himself engaged in supervising patients who are taking lithium carbonate. Before giving lithium routine checks on the cardiovascular, renal, hepatic and thyroid function are undertaken. Lithium carbonate is available in ordinary preparations as a 250 mg tablet in Britain and 300 mg in the United States and Canada. Sustained release preparations do not appear to have any great advantage but side effects are less if the dosage is given at 12-hourly or 8-hourly intervals. It is usual for the psychiatrist to take the responsibility for adjusting the dose of lithium and checking that it is within the prophylactic range viz. 0·8 to 1·6 mmol per litre measured as nearly as possible 12 hours after the last dose was taken. (The level fluctuates by about 30 per cent over that time interval.) Minor side effects of lithium include tremor, abdominal distention and constipation. More troublesome side effects include vomiting. In general vomiting for any reason is an indication to suspend the use of lithium temporarily until serum levels can be checked and the current position established accurately.

Patients taking lithium suffer no real restrictions but should attempt to keep the approximate quantity of salt in their diet constant. Excess salt will reduce the lithium level in the blood and a reduced intake of salt with be liable to result in an increased serum lithium level. Side effects which may appear in the longer term include a mild non-toxic goitre. This is provoked apparently by a blocking of the effect of thyrotropic hormone in the production of thyroxine. It can be satisfactorily treated by the administration of L-thyroxine in small doses. Once a stable dosage is established, psychiatrists usually undertake 3-monthly serum lithium and T4 estimations. The T4 generally falls somewhat in the first six months but this can be accepted if it is not below normal and signs of hypothyroidism such as impaired energy or limited powers of concentration have not reappeared. Another side effect which may be troublesome is the development of diabetes insipidus.

The decision to place a patient on lithium will not be taken lightly. Pregnancies have been satisfactorily concluded without harm to the fetus in patients who have been taking maintenance lithium carbonate. Nevertheless, both in pregnancy and for the long term, which the administration of lithium requires, it is hard, indeed impossible, to predict what side effects may appear over decades. However, there are a number of patients whose lives have been transformed by the use of this substance and there are many in whom there are reasonable indications for its regular use for periods of two to five years.

Vitamins

Ordinary doses of oral preparations of compound vitamin tablets are sometimes useful for patients who have neglected their diet. In confusional states and alcoholism, however, higher non-physiological doses may be valuable. In such instances the usual procedure is to give a proprietary preparation, which is available in both high dose and maintenance dose ampoules. The high dose ampoules may be given once daily for two or three days and the low dose once daily for about a week. Patients needing such injections should probably be in hospital.

OFFICIAL AND OTHER NAMES OF SOME NEUROLEPTICS, ANTIDEPRESSANTS, MAOIs and COMBINATIONS

Official names	Proprietary names		
	Britain	*Canada*	*United States*
Neuroleptics			
Chlorpromazine	Largactil	Largactil	Thorazine Chlor-PZ Cromedazine Promachel
Metho-trimeprazine	Veractil	Nozinan	Nozinan
Promazine	Sparine	Sparine	Sparine
Fluphenazine	Moditen	Moditen	Prolixin Permitil
Fluphenazine decanoate (depot injection)	Modecate	Modecate	Prolixin
Perphenazine	Fentazin	Trilafon	Trilafon
Prochlorperazine	Stemetil	Stemetil	Compazine
Thiopropazate	Dartalan	Dartal	Dartal
Trifluoperazine	Stelazine	Stelazine	Stelazine
Pericyazine	Neulactil	Neuleptil	Not licensed
Thioridazine	Melleril	Mellaril	Mellaril
Mesoridazine	—	Serentil	Serentil
Piperacetazine	—	Quide	Quide
Haloperidol	Serenace	Haldol	Haldol
Thiothixene	Navane	Navane	Navane
Chlorprothixene	Taractan	Tarasan	Taractan
Loxapine	Not licensed	Loxapac	Loxitane
Hydroxyzine	Atarax	Atarax	Vistaril
Clopenthixol decanoate (depot injection)	Clopixol	Not licensed	Not licensed

Note: Official names of drugs are mostly the same in the British Isles and North America. There are occasional differences, the most notable perhaps being paracetamol (Britain) for acetaminophen (Canada and the USA). Only selected drugs are listed here, the basis for selection being to take those names which the student or physician may meet most often. The absence of any entry for a drug in one or other country indicates that the author is uncertain either that a drug is licensed in the country concerned or that it has a proprietary equivalent at the time of compilation of the table.

Official names	Proprietary names		
	Britain	*Canada*	*United States*
Neuroleptics, cont'd.			
Fluspirilene (depot injection)	Redeptin	IMAP	Not licensed
Pimozide	Orap	Orap	
Flupenthixol decanoate	Depixol	Not licensed	Not licensed
Flupenthixol	Fluanxol	Not licensed	Not licensed
Antidepressants			
Amitriptyline	Tryptizol	Elavil	Elavil
	Lentizol	Deprex	Endep
	Saroten	Novotryptin	
	Laroxyl	Levate	
Butriptyline	Evadyne	Not licensed	Not licensed
Clomipramine	Anafranil	Anafranil	Not licensed
Desipramine	Pertofran	Norpramin (cf. Imipramine) Pertofrane	Norpramin Pertofrane
Dibenzepin	Noveril	Not licensed	Not licensed
Dothiepin	Prothiaden	Not licensed	Not licensed
Doxepin	Sinequan	Sinequan	Sinequan Adapin Curatin
Flupenthixol	Fluanxol Depixol	Not licensed	Not licensed
Imipramine	Berkomine	Tofranil	Tofranil
	Ethipram	Impranil	Janimine
	Dimipressin	Impril	Imavate
	Tofranil	Novopramine	Presamine
	Praminil	Praminil	SK-Pramine
	Norpramine (cf. Desipramine		
Iprindole	Prondol	Not licensed	Not licensed
L-tryptophan	Optimax	Tryptan*	Not licensed
Maptrotiline	Ludiomil	Ludiomil	Not licensed
Mianserin	Norval Tolvin	Not licensed	Not licensed
Nomifensine	Merital	Not licensed	Not licensed
Nortriptyline	Allegron Aventyl	Aventyl	Aventyl

* Only licensed as a dietary supplement.

Official names	Proprietary names		
	Britain	*Canada*	*United States*
Antidepressants, cont'd.			
Opipramol	Insidon	Not licensed	Ensidon Insidon
Protriptyline	Concordin	Triptil	Vivactil
Trimipramine	Surmontil	Surmontil	Surmontil
Viloxazine	Vivalan	Not licensed	Not licensed
Mono-Amine-Oxidase Inhibitors			
Iproniazid	Marsilid	Marsilid	Marsilid
Isocarboxazid	Marplan	Marplan	Marplan
Phenelzine	Nardil	Nardil	Nardil
Tranylcypromine	Parnate	Parnate	Parnate
Combinations			
Amitriptyline 12.5 mg Chlordiazepoxide 5.0 mg	Limbitrol 5		
Amitriptyline 25 mg Chlordiazepoxide 10 mg	Limbitrol 10		
Amitriptyline 10 mg Perphenazine 2 mg	Triptafen Minor	Etrafon 2-10	Triavil 2-10 Etrafon 2-10
Amitriptyline 10 mg Perphenazine 4 mg	Not licensed	Etrafon A	Triavil 4-10 Etrafon A
Amitriptyline 15 mg Perphenazine 3 mg	Not licensed	Triavil	
Amitriptyline 25 mg Perphenazine 2 mg	Triptafen DA	Elavil Plus Etrafon D	Triavil 2-25 Etrafon 2-25
Amitriptyline 25 mg Perphenazine 4 mg	Triptafen Forte	Etrafon F	Triavil 4-25 Etrafon Forte
Nortriptyline 10 mg Fluphenazine 0.5 mg	Motival	Not licensed	

Official names	Proprietary names		
	Britain	*Canada*	*United States*
Combinations, cont'd. Tranylcypromine 10 mg Trifluoperazine 1 mg	Parstelin	Parstelin	Parstelin

Appendix 2

Partial Synopsis of Adult Psychiatric Conditions

The purpose of this synopsis is to provide the reader with a broad guide to the main psychiatric symptoms, which will serve as a framework for the conditions discussed in the text, where the emphasis is on the differentiation of symptoms. However, many readers who have appreciated that approach have also wished for a concrete structure of the traditional type to facilitate systematic learning. It is possible for the reader to achieve the latter aim with the help of the Index, but it is hoped that this additional synopsis will serve the same purpose.

The synopsis is deliberately incomplete since certain conditions, for example, subnormality and child psychiatry, are presented in a structured fashion within the text. It is therefore meant to be used as a supplementary aid, particularly for those disorders which are dealt with in more than one place. However, some cross-reference to the text is still recommended.

The synopsis is based in part on the 9th Revision of the International Classification of Diseases (ICD-9, 1977) and in part on the draft guidelines of the Diagnostic and Statistical

Manual–III (DSM–III) of the American Psychiatric Association (1978). It is by no means in accordance with all the recommendations of those sources and represents the author's individual decisions, mostly in accordance with current and standard views. Where a non-standard view is being offered in terms of British or North American practice, this is so far as possible indicated. The information given is necessarily condensed and approximate.

One special point worth noting is that the most important general factor affecting prognosis is the length of time for which the illness has been present. As a rule the longer a patient has had a psychiatric illness, the less likely is recovery to occur, except in some cases of depression. The more acute, and sometimes the more dramatic, the onset, the better the prognosis.

Delirium (confusional states)

Delirium may occur at any age including children, but occurs with increasing frequency in older age groups. The main *symptoms or signs* are fluctuating attention or awareness, failures of registration or orientation; visual and other hallucinations may occur, and apathy and/or agitation, and/or restlessness. Slowing of EEG rhythms is usual. Complications include self-neglect, accidental exposure to danger, etc. *Causes* are systemic or cerebral illness affecting brain function, e.g. pneumonia with anoxia, infections (classically typhoid = 'clouding'), diabetes, head injury, meningitis, encephalitis, drugs or alcohol in excess or their withdrawal. *Differential diagnosis* is mostly from dementia, rarely from hysteria or simulation; also from drug-induced hallucinations, 'normal' or physiological hallucinatory states (e.g. hypnagogic and hypnopompic hallucinations), schizophrenia and other psychotic illness. Paranoid illnesses require special distinction.

It is *important* to exclude treatable illnesses, e.g. thyroid disease, meningitis, etc. *Prognosis* is for recovery with successful treatment of curable primary causes but a residuum of dementia may persist, especially after severe head injury, anoxia in older persons, prolonged CO poisoning, etc. *Treatment* is of the primary cause if possible. Ensure a proper electrolyte balance, nutrition (parenteral vitamins may help), oxygenation if appropriate, correction of any metabolic deficits, etc. Maintain optimum conditions of sensory input, e.g. good lighting, and give repeated simple explanations to patient about his environment. Encourage presence of familiar persons. Use neuroleptic tranquillizers as first choice for agitated patients.

Dementia

Dementia occurs at any age, increasingly in older age groups; it affects 4 to 5 per cent of the population over 65, either moderately or severely. Multi-infarct dementia is commoner in men, Alzheimer's dementia is commoner in women. Before the age of 60 or 65 dementia is called pre-senile, usually if no external cause is evident. It is marked by global impairment of intellectual function, especially cognitive skills, memory and judgement. First *signs* are often failure of judgement in social situations or failure of impulse control or subtle personality changes. Later evident deterioration of personality appears. Memory impairment is usually prominent. Disorientation is common in moderately severe dementia. Emotional lability, particularly sudden tears, is a feature of dementia due to multiple cerebral infarcts, or severe multiple sclerosis. Delusions of persecution or hallucinations may occur. Focal loss of function, e.g. aphasia or a dysmnesic state, is sometimes called partial dementia. Self-neglect is a common complication. Hazards arise from forgetfulness, e.g. inattentive use of matches. Superimposed delirium is common. *Causes* include local or general cerebral disease, e.g. tumour, head injury, syphilis, normal pressure hydrocephalus, multi-infarct disease. Systemic disorder is the second main type of cause, e.g. intoxication chronically affecting brain function, anoxia, alcoholism, some cases of myxoedema. The commonest cause of dementia is Alzheimer's disease. Treatable causes amount to 15 to 30 per cent of cases.

Differential diagnosis is from delirium (confusional states). The key to dementia is persistent loss of function. In delirium, impairments fluctuate. Distinction from depression is important. *Treatment* depends on cause. Complete or partial recovery is possible in certain cases, e.g. myxoedema, head injury, normal pressure hydrocephalus, depression mimicking dementia. Survival over 2 years is rare in hospitalized Alzheimer's or multi-infarct dementia. Any concomitant delirium requires urgent treatment. Primary conditions need treatment. Maintain simple, constant and familiar environment as much as possible to allow patient to make maximum use of residual skills and knowledge. In advanced cases neuroleptic drugs may be used for agitation.

Organic hallucinosis*. Organic hallucinosis is marked by persistent or repeated hallucinations, usually visual, with organic cause and without loss of alertness or impaired wakefulness. It does not meet the criteria for delirium, dementia or organic delusional syndrome. The commonest *causes* are alcohol and abuse of hallucinogens.

Organic delusional syndrome*. In the organic delusional syndrome, the occurrence of delusions is attributed to a defined organic factor in a state of full wakefulness and in absence of signs sufficient for diagnoses of delirium, dementia or organic hallucinosis. *Causes* include amphetamines, cannabis, hallucinogens, brain lesions, e.g. with temporal lobe epilepsy.

Organic affective syndrome*. The organic affective syndrome is characterized by mood changes of depression or elation resembling those seen in affective illnesses, and attributable to definite and substantial organic causes (e.g. reserpine, ACTH treatment or steroids, Cushing's syndrome, viral illnesses, direct brain trauma). It should not meet the criteria for dementia, delirium, organic hallucinosis or organic delusional syndrome.

Organic personality syndrome*. In the organic personality syndrome, a marked change in personality occurs due to some clearly defined organic factor. This syndrome does not meet the criteria for any other organic brain syndrome. The 'frontal lobe syndrome' with apathy, contentment, lack of concern, social or sexual indiscretions, or inappropriate

---

* It is particularly important to be on the alert for these conditions. A high 'index of suspicion' is the best guide to diagnosis.

behaviour is one variant. The nature and localization of the pathological process determines the clinical pattern.

The schizophrenias

Onset of schizophrenia is rare in childhood, occasional in early adolescence, and most frequent from age 18 to 30 years. The paranoid type occurs more often in the late twenties and after. Slightly more males are affected than females. The incidence is 0.4 to 0.8 per cent of individuals over their lifetime.

There are five main types according to symptomatology. *Simple schizophrenia* is marked by loose associations of thoughts and flat affect. *Hebephrenic schizophrenia* resembles simple schizophrenia with, in addition, marked emotional incongruity and fleeting hallucinations. *Catatonic schizophrenia* is marked by immobility or rigidity, posturing, mannerisms, mutism and, rarely nowadays, waxy flexibility. Catatonia may alternate with excitement. *Paranoid schizophrenia* shows relative predominance of delusions or hallucinations which may be persecutory or grandiose. *Residual schizophrenia* (chronic defect state) resembles simple schizophrenia in a patient who previously has had a more florid/active episode, usually with more evidence than in simple schizophrenia of odd ideas, delusions or hallucinations persisting in attenuated form.

The onset may be insidious or abrupt, always with disorganization by comparison with a previous level of functioning. Multiple psychological processes are disturbed including some of the following: language, thought content, perception, emotion, sense of self ('ego boundaries'), volition, relationship to external world and motor behaviour. Characteristic delusions include being controlled, thoughts being broadcast, thought insertion or withdrawal, other bizarre delusions, somatic delusions and hallucinations. Auditory hallucinations are characteristic, often in the form of commentary on the patient by a distant voice or voices. Complications include self-neglect, accidental hazards, loss of employment, diverse changes in social relationships, conflict with legal agencies, a significant risk of suicide, etc.

Causes: Studies of twins and of children of schizophrenic

mothers adopted away confirm the presence of hereditary (genetic) factors. Children or siblings of schizophrenic patients have a 10 to 15 per cent chance of developing schizophrenia. Amphetamines and some drug-induced psychoses (especially from hallucinogens like LSD) closely resemble schizophrenic illnesses. There is no definite evidence of cause but effective drugs block dopaminergic synapses, suggesting that dopamine may be instrumental.

There is an increased incidence of schizophrenic-like psychoses in patients with temporal lobe epilepsy/brain damage, especially those with lesions near the third ventricle, which indicates the possibility of organic causes. Acceptable evidence exists also of brief schizophrenia-like illnesses resulting from acute stress, and of prolonged paranoid schizophrenia-like illnesses occurring after concentration camp experiences.

Differential diagnosis is from schizophreniform psychosis (an acute illness marked by prominent paranoid hallucinatory or depressive features but without disintegration of personality); some exclude all illnesses of less than six months' duration from diagnosis of schizophrenia; from hypomania and mania by absence in them of alienation (passivity) phenomena and predominance of mood change, from delusional or hallucinatory states due to organic disease; from confusional states and from dementia; from reactive acute stress-induced psychoses in which patient may be irrational, deluded or hallucinated, without characteristic schizophrenic features; from hysterical psychoses (rare) which resemble reactive psychoses; from amphetamine, cannabis, LSD and other drug- or alcohol-induced psychoses; from affective and neurotic illnesses and from personality disorders.

Prognosis. In acute illnesses, about 50 per cent recover without relapse; 35 per cent are improved; 10 to 15 per cent remain chronic with little improvement. *Treatment* is with neuroleptic drugs (phenothiazines and butyrophenones, see Appendix on drug treatment, p. 380). It is also important to manage the patient's environment. Some patients do better away from relatives. Relapses often occur after stopping medication or after life-stresses.

Paranoid disorders

Paranoid disorders are persistent encapsulated persecutory delusions or delusions of jealousy, not explainable by either schizophrenic, schizophreniform, affective or reactive psychoses or organic mental disorders. Onset is rare after 30 years of age. The boundaries between paranoid schizophrenia and paranoid personality are difficult to define; paranoid disorders often occur in socially isolated, seclusive, eccentric individuals whose intellect is usually well preserved. Immigration, deafness and other social stresses predispose to paranoid disorders. *Differential diagnosis* is from schizophrenia and those conditions from which schizophrenia has to be distinguished. Highly systematized delusions without hallucinations are sometimes called paranoia. With hallucinations they are difficult to distinguish from schizophrenia. Confusional states often have paranoid features that show disturbances of consciousness.

Affective disorders

Mania and hypomania. Mania and hypomania are less common than schizophrenia or depression. Attacks recur at variable intervals, often alternating with depression. The first attack is usually in the thirties; more females than males are affected. Spontaneous remission is usual. Signs are insomnia, elation, over-activity, rapid speech, flight of ideas and grandiose delusions (rarely hallucinations). Patients are commonly full of schemes and frustration may lead to aggressive responses. There is a hereditary pattern with 20 per cent risk to children. The disorder may be provoked by stress, disappointment or bereavement, and lasts for weeks rather than months. There is about 50 per cent risk of mania or depression in first 12 months after an attack, diminishing thereafter. *Differential diagnosis* is from schizophrenia, confusional states, dementia with excitement, other psychoses especially drug- and treatment-induced, e.g. organic affective psychosis after ACTH or steroid treatment for multiple sclerosis. *Treatment* should be carried out in hospital to prevent substantial social and other misfortunes resulting from patient's behaviour, e.g. aggression by men, promiscuity by normally restrained women. Many psychiatrists consider compulsory detention unequivocally humane but not all jurisdictions necessarily agree. This is an outstanding example of lack of insight by civil libertarians into human needs. After recovery, patients almost invariably regret their behaviour and are grateful for protection. They are best managed by quiet, confident persuasion on medical model. Chlorpromazine and lithium are acute treatments. ECT is sometimes live-saving. Lithium is a very effective prophylactic treatment.

Bipolar depression. Bipolar depression may occur at any age; it is usually first diagnosed in the thirties. Depression occurs in patients who have had mania. Common signs are low spirits, guilt, ideas of unworthiness, and sometimes delusions. Bipolar depression may be distinguished from paranoid illnesses by the presence of guilt, and evidence that the patient feels that he *deserves* any misfortunes which he experiences or anticipates. Biological signs of depression occur including loss of interest and enthusiasm, loss of weight, impaired concentration, terminal insomnia, and morning exacerbations. It is provoked by bereavement, departure or other loss of loved person or loss of some role (loss of the loved object). It is to be distinguished from paranoid illnesses, dementia, endogenous depression, secondary depression (American terminology), and neurotic reactive depression. Spontaneous recovery is usual, but the depression may last from one week to many years. Its duration is shortened by antidepressants, and if necessary ECT (EST) will bring relief. Management rarely requires treatment of the original psychological cause.

Endogenous depression. Endogenous depression is the term used in Britain, Australia and to some extent in North America for depression with characteristics of the depression in bipolar affective illness, whether or not associated with mania. It often occurs in obsessional personalities.

Unipolar depression. Unipolar depression roughly corresponds to endogenous depression or bipolar depression in the absence of any history of mania or hypomania. Patients should not have a history of any prior psychiatric disorder unless it was similar to the present one. Secondary depression is a depressive disorder in patients who have a prior history of anxiety, alcoholism or other psychological disturbance (North American alternative diagnosis to primary unipolar depression).

Reactive (neurotic) depression. Reactive (neurotic) depression lacks 'endogenous' features, especially delusions, guilt and self-blame, and usually shows initial insomnia and evening worsening of depressed mood. It is more related to precipitating environmental causes than endogenous depression, but this distinction is not absolute. Patients tend to be less stable and less obsessional than in endogenous depression.

Neurotic depression. Neurotic depression is broadly equivalent to reactive depression in Britain. It tends to imply a depression arising from understandable emotional or neurotic conflicts. In the USA the term is used to imply less severity than *psychotic depression* which is a controversial term sometimes used to indicate that certification of the patient is appropriate because of suicidal risk or break from reality. Psychotic depression is also used to indicate a depression similar to, but more severe than, neurotic depression, or to indicate the presence of delusions or hallucinations. In view of the obvious variation in usage, psychotic depression is one term with which we could well dispense.

The types of depressive illness need to be distinguished from one another but there is still no universally agreed system. A practical arrangement is to recognize:

1. The bipolar type of depressive illness
2. Depressive illness, single or recurrent, with an endogenous *pattern*
3. Exogenous depressive pattern
4. Mixtures of (2) and (3)
5. Depressive personality (see later)

Students in the USA particularly should be able to distinguish bipolar, primary unipolar and secondary depressive illnesses (see also pp. 88–9) for discussion of this topic). Alternatively, they can use the APA DSM–III draft guidelines arrangement of bipolar affective disorders; depressed; and major depressive episode, the last with the qualification of the main contributory factors. Depressive disorders need to be distinguished from the following: depressive personality, cyclothymic personality, dementia, organic affective illness, schizophrenia with depression, alcohol with depression, neurotic illnesses such as obsessional or anxiety disorders with depression, and lastly somatic psychological symptoms with depression. For discussion of treatment, see pp. 123-7.

Anxiety disorders

Anxiety appears in many psychiatric illnesses. A different underlying diagnosis, e.g. schizophrenia or endogenous depression, may be required. Neurotic anxiety disorders are only independently diagnosed in the absence of such other conditions. The personality of the patient may also be more important than the diagnosis. Overt anxiety symptoms affect all ages but are common in females and present most commonly between the ages of 16 and 30. Two to four per cent of the general population have had a disorder described as an 'anxiety state' or a 'phobia' (specific fear). They are characterized by fear which the *patient* (not the physician) considers to be unreasonable.

Phobic anxiety. Phobic anxiety is marked by unreasonable fear in specific situations, e.g. the dark, closed rooms, crowds, open spaces, or of specific objects, e.g. spiders. It is often found with more generalized anxiety or depression, conversion symptoms, obsessional illnesses, schizophrenia and yet other psychiatric conditions. *Causes* include predisposed personality, childhood experiences promoting insecurity, and current stresses. *Differential diagnosis* is from those conditions with which it is associated, also from thyrotoxicosis and very rarely from phaeochromocytoma. The *prognosis* is variable, said to be one-third remission in 2 years, one-third improved and one-third unchanged. Behaviour therapy and psychotherapy have both been shown to improve on the natural prognosis. The prior duration of symptoms is relevant. *Treatment* includes behaviour therapy, and reassurance, medication, management of environment, and all degrees or types of individual psychotherapy, group therapy and cognitive therapy. The choice of treatment depends on the individual case but environmental changes, behaviour therapy and psychotherapy are preferred. Benzodiazepines and anti-depressants may help but are over-used. If drugs are employed, antidepressants should be preferred to benzodiazepines, because of the addictive characteristics of benzodiazepines.

Generalized anxiety. Generalized anxiety occurs at all ages and is more common in females than males. It is often associated with phobias, somatic anxiety (see below) and depression. It is marked by a pervasive feeling of impending doom. *Causes* are as for phobic anxiety. *Treatment* is similar but with more emphasis on psychotherapy and medication.

Somatic anxiety. Somatic anxiety includes tension head-aches, palpitations, tremor and other physical symptoms due to disturbed autonomic physiology. Occurrence, causes and treatment are as for generalized anxiety. Relaxation treat-ment is helpful in some cases.

Obsessional neuroses

Obsessional neuroses are relatively rare. Onset occurs at any age, and there is often a history of many brief episodes in childhood. The disorder is marked by intrusive thoughts which the patient cannot resist and feels obliged to enter-tain. *Differential diagnosis* is from other neuroses and from delusional states. In delusional states, patient *believes* in reasonableness of his ideas. *Prognosis.* About one-third recover or improve within 3 years, perhaps two-thirds in 5 years. *Treatment* with clomipramine or phenelzine may be effective in some cases, also highly specialized behaviour therapy.

Conversion symptoms (hysteria)

In conversion symptoms, a loss of bodily function (motor/sensory) corresponds to the patient's ideas, not to an organic disorder, e.g. paresis of limb not according to innervation. Classical *symptoms* include paralyses, ataxias, aphonias, blindness, deafness, (hemi)anaesthesias. Classical symp-toms are rare in sophisticated populations except in (1) pa-tients with neurological disease, (2) compensation cases and (3) military psychiatry. Many symptoms mimic anxiety, e.g.

a headache may have an hysterical basis but this is hard to prove. Conversion was explained by Freud as resulting from repressed emotional conflict based on sexual difficulties. The first part of this formulation is generally accepted, the second part not, but sexual disturbances/conflicts are common in patients with conversion symptoms. The more modern analytical view states that the conflict can arise in many areas other than sexual, such as conflict over dependency needs, aggression, etc. Resolution of the fundamental conflict constitutes the primary gain. Secondary advantages accruing from the symptom constitute the secondary gain.

Dissociative symptoms (hysteria)

Dissociative symptoms include conversion symptoms and also psychological impairments such as hysterical memory disorder. There is some evidence of predisposition (hysterical/dependent personality in 40 per cent of cases). Childhood experience is probably relevant but its features are ill-defined. The disorder is usually precipitated by emotional conflict. Occasional cases are seen mainly to be the consequence of change in the patient in response to physical illness or brain damage. *Differential diagnosis* of hysterical symptoms is from physical disease and almost all other psychiatric syndromes (schizophrenia, depression, anxiety, organic psychoses). The *prognosis* depends on the length of history. About 70 per cent of new cases recover within 12 months. Relapses are liable to occur. Response to suggestion often occurs but not invariably. The *treatment* of choice is psychotherapeutic exploration, support, and changes in the patient's environment.

Factitious disorders. Factitious disorders are self-induced but not malingering, and include hospital addiction syndrome ('Munchausen's syndrome'), Ganser syndrome and deliberate disability. These disorders may be distinguished from malingering by relative lack of environmental gain.

Anorexia nervosa

Anorexia nervosa was formerly rare, now possibly increasing; about 90 per cent of patients are young females or in their twenties and thirties. It often occurs in girls who have been plump. 'Weight-phobia' (fear of weight gain) is the central phenomenon. The disorder is characterized by anorexia, weight loss and secondary amenorrhoea. Subjective overestimation of their bodies as fat is found even in very thin patients. Induced vomiting and laxative abuse may occur to reduce weight and can cause dangerous complications. A few patients have other major psychiatric illnesses. Estimates of mortality rate range from 1 to 20 per cent at 5 years. About half of the patients have histrionic/dependent personalities and about one-third have some obsessional characteristics. The weight-phobia appears to be a maladaptive response to earlier experiences, family and social pressures and puberty. *Differential diagnosis* is from endocrine disorders and other causes of amenorrhoea, and other psychiatric conditions. Prognosis is uncertain. The disorder is hard to treat. *Treatment* includes psychotherapy, behaviour therapy, persuasion to gain weight and psychotropic drugs, especially chlorpromazine and antidepressants. Management requires sympathetic but quite strict supervision for the patients who often cheat about their intake. Occasionally episodes of gorging (bulimia) occur.

Personality disorders

People differ in their habitual characteristics and ways of response. There is no final, competely satisfactory way to classify the different patterns of behaviour which seem most common. Recurrent maladaptive behaviour leads to the label of some type of personality *disorder*, e.g. sociopathic personality. Other personality *types* are recognized which may lead on to illness; obsessional personalities are liable to develop obsessional neurosis and more often depression. However, such types are not necessarily pathological. A 'personality disorder' should not be diagnosed as pathological unless it is causing problems for the patient and/or his environment. Some commonly used categories are outlined; in practice individuals often show mixed patterns.

Sociopathic personality disorder (also called psychopathic in the past). Incidence figures for sociopathic personality disorder depend upon the stringency of criteria; it is common in legal offenders. The disorder is defined in the Mental Health Act (England and Wales 1959, Scotland 1960) as marked by abnormally aggressive or seriously irresponsible conduct. Its essential feature is failure to learn from previous experience (despite adequate intellect), but this is a *relative*, not absolute, failure. Callous disregard of others is common. Typical past history see (pp. 310–13) includes impaired opportunities for emotional bonding in childhood, truancy, poor educational attainment, poor job record, law-breaking, impulsive suicidal or aggressive behaviour, poor social and marital adjustment. There is an increased percentage of non-specific EEG abnormalities in psychopathic patients. *Differential diagnosis* is from schizophrenia, other personality disorders and organic personality disorders. *Causes* are occasionally organic, e.g. post-encephalitic; there is a clear but not invariable relationship with deprivation of maternal care in younger children, especially those aged 18 months to 4 years. *Treatment* is often very difficult but may consist of management of situational problems, supportive relationship, and passage of time.

Inadequate personality disorder. Inadequate personality disorder often resembles sociopathic personality disorder but without its aggressive features. Childhood deprivation is usually less severe. The disorder is characterized by the patient's inadequacy in most aspects of his life, such as the social, physical, psychological, etc.

Passive aggressive personality disorder. Passive aggressive personality disorder is a controversial category, little used in Britain, popular in North America. It is marked by passive resistance in people who lack assertiveness and self-confidence. Such people are often dependent on others and resent those on whom they depend. Obstructive behaviour is manifested by stubbornness, intentional forgetfulness, etc.

Obsessional personality disorder. The obsessional personality is conscientious, meticulous or obstinate. The disorder is often a normal variant. It frequently provides a substrate for depression, occasionally for obsessional illness. The alternative term, *compulsive personality disorder* (DSM–III), emphasizes the restricted ability to express warm and tender emotions; preoccupation with rules, order, organization and detail; contrasting indecisiveness and attempts at dominance, often depressed or angry.

Anxious personality disorder. The anxious personality disorder can be a normal variant depending on severity; tendency to worry unduly; increased number of phobic symptoms, somatic signs of anxiety, depression, etc.

Depressive personality disorder (chronic depressive disorder). Depressive personality disorder is recommended to describe individuals who suffer sustained non-psychotic depressive mood or loss of interest or pleasure in most usual activities for a period of at least two years (DSM–III). Essentially it describes people in whom depression appears to arrive readily and persists perhaps on a basis of other personality disorder. DSM–III makes this a new category of affective illness rather than personality disorder. The former concept was of chronically pessimistic worrying individuals with occasional periods of improved mood and cheerfulness.

Cyclothymic personality type. The cyclothymic personality type is non-pathological but ICD-9 recognizes a pathological version. Relatively sustained periods of increased activity and cheerfulness alternate with periods of depression that seem to come on without external precipitants. Distinguish from emotional lability which is common in hysterical personalities.

Borderline personality disorder. Borderline personality disorder is a very controversial and confusing American term, best avoided. (*Borderline state*, also to be avoided, refers to psychosis in *borderline personality*.)

Hysterical (histrionic) personality disorder or type. Depending on severity, the hysterical personality is dramatic, immature, manipulative, dependent, emotionally shallow and labile, superficially warm and appealing, flirtatious but sexually inhibited with tendency to retreat into physical ill-health. The disorder is often not nearly as bad as the description makes it sound. Hysterical personality in mild degree can be an asset in salesmen, teachers, lecturers, doctors (although they never recognize it) and others in service occupations because of associated concern with looking after needs of others.

Dependent personality disorder or type. The dependent personality is quiet and lacking in self-confidence, gets others to assume responsibility for major areas of his/her life, and accepts subordination of his/her own needs in order to avoid relying on self. The type shades into hysterical personality.

Narcissistic personality disorder or type (DSM–III). Narcissistic personality is a new category, partly abstracted from aspects of older views of hysterical, borderline and anti-social personalities (q.v.). It takes account of psychodynamic observation of individuals who lack the capacity to relate to others and require constant evidence of others' respect for them. They have a strong sense of self-importance with usually unrealistic fantasies of success. They are cool and indifferent in interpersonal relationships but are anxious to receive attention and admiration. Some display exhibitionist features.

Paranoid personality disorder or type. The paranoid personality is marked by pervasive mistrust and diffuse suspiciousness of people in general. He/she is often hypersensitive and easily slighted, is rigid, and may be energetic, argumentative, stubborn, hostile, litiginous and intense, and occasionally dominant.

Introverted personality disorder (DSM–III). The introverted personality is reserved, withdrawn, solitary, seclusive, often vague, indecisive and detached, and self-absorbed, with little capacity for any sort of emotional display. The diagnosis is not made if characteristics of *schizotypal personality disorder* are apparent.

Schizotypal personality disorder (DSM–III) (new category). The essential features of a schizotypal personality are various oddities of thinking, perception, communication and behaviour. Social isolation and other features of introverted personality disorder are also present.

Schizoid personality disorder. The term *schizoid personality* which was formerly used to mean detached, introverted, cold and eccentric, should be avoided and *introverted personality disorder* or *schizotypal personality disorder* used instead.

Psychosexual disorders

Gender identity disorder. Gender identity disorder is a rare condition in which the individual feels that his/her anatomic sex is inappropriate and incongruent with his/her 'true' sexual make-up. In adults gender identity disorder is known as trans-sexualism.

Trans-sexualism. Trans-sexualism is very rare. It is marked by a wish to be rid of one's original genitals and to live as one of the opposite anatomic sex; these feelings are usually lifelong but for diagnostic purposes, should have been present for at least two years with absence of physical intersex, genetic abnormality or other psychiatric illness such as schizophrenia. Cross-dressing, employment in cross-sex roles and persistent requests for physical change are characteristics. Male/female ratio is approximately 4:1.

Homosexuality. The American Psychiatric Association (DSM–III) refuses to classify homosexuality as abnormal as it only regards as abnormal those deviations from standard sexual behaviour that involve gross impairment in the capacity for affectionate sexual activity between adult human partners. Other views hold that homosexuality is abnormal because it inevitably and always separates affectionate sexual activity from possibility of reproduction, a fundamental biological function.

Other sexual abnormalities. Other forms of sexual abnormality which are recognized in addition to those mentioned include fetishism, exhibitionism, voyeurism, pedophilia, zoophilia, sexual masochism, sexual sadism and necrophilia. In all these cases aberrant stimulus or situation is needed for orgasm to be reached.

For *psychosexual dysfunctions*, see pp. 265–78.

References

1. Daisy Ashford (1919). *The Young Visiters or Mr. Salteena's Plan*. Lighthouse Books, London: Chatto & Windus (1949).

2. Jane Austen (1816). *Emma*, ed. R. W. Chapman, Vol. 3, Chap. 2, 3rd ed. Oxford: Clarendon (1933).

3. T. X. Barber (1969). *Hypnosis—A Scientific Approach*. New York: Van Nostrand Reinhold.

4. J. C. Barker & A. A. Baker (1959). Deaths associated with electroplexy. *J. ment. Sci., 105*, 339-48.

5. H. K. Beecher (1956). Relationship of significance of wound to pain experienced. *J. Am. med. Ass., 161*, 1609-13.

6. A. T. Beck (1976). *Cognitive Therapy and the Emotional Disorders*. New York: International Universities Press.

7. K. Bergmann (1971). The neuroses of old age. In *Recent Developments in Psychogeriatrics*, ed. D. W. K. Kay and A. Walk. *Brit. J. Psychiat.*, Special Publications 6, 39–50.

8. E. Bott (1957). *Family and Social Network*. London: Tavistock.

9. J. Bowlby (1952). Maternal care and mental health. *Monograph Ser. W.H.O.*, 2.

   J. Bowlby (1962). Deprivation of maternal care. A reassessment of its effects. *Publ. Hlth Pap. W.H.O.*, 14.

10. J. Bowlby (1977). The making and breaking of affectional bonds: I. Aetiology and psychopathology in the light of attachment theory. *Br. J. Psychiat., 130*, 201–10.

11. G. W. Brown (1967). The family of the schizophrenic patient. In *Recent Developments in Schizophrenia*, ed. A. Coppen and A. Walk. Royal Medico-Psychological Association. London: Headley Bros.

12. G. W. Brown and J. L. T. Birley (1968). Crises and life changes and the onset of schizophrenia. *J. Hlth soc. Behav., 9*, 203-14.

13. A. M. G. Campbell, M. Evans, J. L. G. Thomson and M. J. Williams (1971). Cerebral atrophy in young Cannabis smokers. *Lancet, ii*, 1219-24.

14. P. Chodoff and H. Lyons (1958). Hysteria, the hysterical personality and 'hysterical' conversion. *Am. J. Psychiat.*, *114*, 743-50.

15. M. B. Clyne (1961). *Night Calls. A Study in General Practice.* London: Tavistock.

16. A. J. Cooper, A. A. A. Ismail, C. G. Smith and J. A. Loraine (1970). Androgenic function in 'psychogenic' and 'constitutional' types of impotence *Br. med. J.*, *iii*, 17-20.

17. K. Dalton (1964). *The Premenstrual Syndrome.* London: Heinemann.

18. H. V. Dicks (1967). *Marital Tensions.* London: Routledge and Kegan Paul.

19. M. R. Eastwood (1975). *The Relation Between Physical and Mental Illness.* Clarke Institute of Psychiatry Monogr. No. 4. Toronto: University of Toronto Press.

20. L. Eitinger (1961). *Concentration Camp Survivors in Norway and Israel.* London: Allen and Unwin.

21. J. L. Emery (1972). Welfare of families and children found unexpectedly dead ('Cot deaths'). *Br. med. J.*, *i*, 612-5.

22. H. J. Eysenck, ed. (1960). *Behaviour Therapy and the Neuroses.* Oxford: Pergamon.

23. M. Frankignoul and M. Dongier (1971). Personnalité du coronarien et psychodynamique. *Psychol. Médicale*, *3*, 495-522.

24. L. J. Friedman (1962). *Virgin Wives.* London: Tavistock.

25. F. Galton (1883). *Inquiries into Human Faculty.* London: Macmillan.

26. General Register Office (1968). *A Glossary of Mental Disorders.* Studies on Medical & Population Subjects No. 22. London: HMSO.

27. G. Gorer (1971). *Sex and Marriage in England Today.* London: Nelson.

28. J. L. Halliday (1937). Psychological factors in rheumatism: a preliminary study. *Br. med. J.*, *i*, 213-7.

29. D. K. Henderson (1939). *Psychopathic States.* New York: Norton.

30. B. N. Herzberg and A. Coppen (1970). Changes in psychological symptoms in women taking oral contraceptives. *Br. J. Psychiat.*, *116*, 161.

31. F. Henriques (1961). *Love in Action.* London: McGibbon and Kee.

32. B. Isaacs (1972). *Studies in Illness and Death in the Elderly in Glasgow.* Scottish Health Service Study No. 17. Edinburgh: Scottish Home and Health Department.

33. M. P. Joyston-Bechal (1966). The clinical features and outcome of stupor. *Br. J. Psychiat.*, *122*, 967-81.

34. D. W. K. Kay and D. Leigh (1954). The natural history, treatment and prognosis of anorexia nervosa, based on a study of 38 patients. *J. ment. Sci.*, *100*, 411-31.

35. G. A. Kelly (1963). *A Theory of Personality.* New York: Norton.

420   References

36. D. G. Klee, S. Ozelis, I. Greenberg and L. J. Gallant (1959). Pain and other somatic complaints in a psychiatric clinic. *M. St. med. J.,* 8, 188-91.

37. G. L. Klerman (1978). Affective disorders. In *The Harvard Guide to Modern Psychiatry*, ed. E. P. Nicholi, Jr. Cambridge, Mass.: Harvard Univ. Press, pp. 253-81.

38. H. Kolansky and W. T. Moore (1971). Effects of marijuana on adolescent and young adults. *J. Am. med. Ass.,* 216, 486.

H. Kolansky and W. T. Moore (1972). Toxic effects of chronic marijuana use. *J. Am. med. Ass.,* 221, 1.

39. I. Kolvin (1972). Emotional problems of childhood and adolescence: infantile autism or infantile psychosis. *Br. med. J.,* iii, 753-5.

40. E. Kraft, A. Schillinger, N. Finby and M. Halperin (1965). Routine skull radiography in a neuropsychiatric hospital. *Am. J. Roentg.,* 89, 1212-19.

41. T. Lidz and S. Fleck (1960). Human integration and the role of the family. In *The Etiology of Schizophrenia*, ed. D. D. Jackson. New York: Basic Books.

42. K. Lorenz (1966). *On Aggression.* London: Methuen.

43. A. H. Mann (1973). Cortical atrophy and air encephalography. *Psychol. Med.,* 3, 374.

44. C. D. Marsden and M. J. G. Harrison (1972). Outcome of investigation of patients with pre-senile dementia. *Br. med. J.,* ii, 249-52.

45. W. H. Masters and V. E. Johnson (1970). *Human Sexual Inadequacy.* Edinburgh: Churchill.

46. W. Mayer-Gross, E. Slater and M. Roth (1969). *Clinical Psychiatry*, 3rd ed. London: Baillière Tindall.

47. A. I. McDougall et al. (1970). Clondine in hypertension. *Br. med. J.,* iii, 440-2.

48. J. Merry (1966). The 'loss of control' myth. *Lancet, i,* 1257.

49. H. Merskey (1968). Psychological aspects of pain. *Postgrad. med. J.,* 44, 297-306.

50. H. Merskey (1971). An appraisal of hypnosis. *Postgrad. med. J.,* 47, 572-80.

51. H. Merskey and P. R. F. Clarke (1962). Determinism, responsibility and illness. *Lancet, ii,* 291-4.

52. H. Merskey and R. N. Hester (1972). The treatment of chronic pain with psychotropic drugs. *Postgrad. med. J.,* 48, 594-8.

53. H. Merskey and J. M. Woodforde (1972). Psychiatric sequelae of minor head injury. *Brain, 95,* 521-8.

54. V. Meyer and E. S. Chesser (1970). *Behaviour Therapy in Clinical Psychiatry.* Harmondsworth, Middlesex: Penguin Books.

55. N. E. Miller (1948). Studies of fear as an acquirable drive: 1. fear as motivation and fear-reduction as reinforcement in the learning of new responses. *J. exp. Psychol., 38,* 89.

56. H. G. Miller (1961). Accident neurosis. *Br. med. J., i,* 919-25; 992-8.

57. J. R. Mitchell, L. Arias and J. A. Oates (1967). Antagonism of

the antihypertensive action of guanethidine sulfate by desipramine hydrochloride. *J. Am. med. Ass.*, *202*, 973-6.

58. M. E. de Montaigne (1580). *Essais.* Book I. Chap. 14. Tr. E. J. Trechmann. Oxford: Oxford University Press (1927). (In some editions chap. 14 and chap. 40 are transposed.)

59. M. E. de Montaigne (1580). *Essais*, trans. E. J. Trechmann, Bk. 1, chapter 21. Oxford: Oxford University Press (1927).

60. E. Moran (1970). Varieties of pathological gambling. *Br. J. Psychiat.*, *116*, 593.

61. G. O. Morris and L. C. Wynne (1965). Schizophrenic offspring and parental styles of communication. *Psychiatry*, *28*, 19.

62. J. O. Ottosson (1962). Electro-convulsive therapy—electro-stimulating or convulsive therapy? *J. Neuropsychiat.*, *3*, 216-20.

63. C. M. Parkes (1972). *Bereavement.* London: Tavistock.

64. W. D. Rees and S. G. Lutkins (1967). Mortality of bereavement. *Br. med. J.*, *iv*, 13-16.

65. M. Roth (1952). A theory of ECT action and its bearing on the biological significance of epilepsy. *J. ment. Sci.*, *98*, 44-59.

66. I. Rubin (1966). *Sexual Life after Sixty*. London: Allen and Unwin.

67. A. J. Rush, A. T. Beck, M. Kovacs and S. Hollon (1977). Comparative efficacy of cognitive therapy and pharmacotherapy in the treatment of depressed outpatients. *Cognit. Therapy and Res.*, *1*, 17-37.

68. M. Schofield (1965). *The Sexual Behaviour of Young People.* Harlow: Longmans.

69. K. Schneider (1958). *Psychopathic Personalities*, trans. M. W. Hamilton. London: Cassell.

70. B. F. Shaw (1979). Personal Communication.

71. B. F. Shaw and A. T. Beck (1977). The treatment of depression with cognitive therapy. In *Handbook of Rational Emotive Therapy*, ed. A. Ellis and R. Grieger. Berlin: Springer, pp. 309-26.

72. E. B. Strauss (1950). Impotence. *Br. med. J.*, *i*, 697-9.

73. A. R. Taylor (1967). Post-concussional sequelae. *Br. med. J.*, *iii*, 67-71.

74. W. L. Tonge (1955). The neurasthenic psychopath. *Br. med. J.*, *i*, 1066.

75. W. L. Tonge, D. S. James and S. M. Hillam (1974). *Families Without Hope: A Controlled Study of 33 Problem Families.* London: British Journal of Psychiatry Special Publication.

76. C. E. Vaughn and J. P. Leff (1976). Influence of family and social factors on the course of psychiatric illness. *Br. J. Psychiat.*, *129*, 125-37.

77. World Health Organization (1973). *The International Pilot Study of Schizophrenia.* Geneva: WHO.

Index